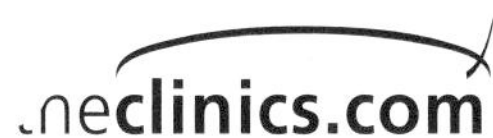

HEMATOLOGY/ ONCOLOGY CLINICS OF NORTH AMERICA

Antithrombotic Therapy: Current Practice and Future Trends

GUEST EDITOR
Rodger L. Bick, MD, PhD, FACP

February 2005 • Volume 19 • Number 1

SAUNDERS

An Imprint of Elsevier, Inc.
PHILADELPHIA LONDON TORONTO MONTREAL SYDNEY TOKYO

W.B. SAUNDERS COMPANY
A Division of Elsevier Inc.

The Curtis Center • Independence Square West • Philadelphia, Pennsylvania 19106

http://www.theclinics.com

HEMATOLOGY/ONCOLOGY CLINICS OF NORTH AMERICA
February 2005
Editor: Kerry Holland

Volume 19, Number 1
ISSN 0889-8588
ISBN 1-4160-2772-6

Hematology/Oncology Clinics of North America (ISSN 0889-8588) is published bi-monthly by W.B. Saunders Company. Corporate and editorial offices: The Curtis Center, Independence Square West, Philadelphia, PA 19106-3399. Accounting and circulation offices: 6277 Sea Harbor Drive, Orlando, FL 32887-4800. Periodicals postage paid at Orlando, FL 32862, and additional mailing offices. Subscription prices are $210.00 per year (US individuals), $315.00 per year (US institutions), $270.00 per year (foreign individuals), $380.00 per year (foreign institutions), $240.00 per year (Canadian individuals), and $380.00 per year (Canadian institutions). Foreign air speed delivery is included in all *Clinics* subscription prices. All prices are subject to change without notice. POSTMASTER: Send address changes to *Hematology/Oncology Clinics of North America,* W.B. Saunders Company, Periodicals Fulfillment, Orlando, FL 32887-4800. **Customer Service: 1-800-654-2452 (US). From outside the US, call 407-345-4000.** E-mail: hhspcs@harcourt.com

Hematology/Oncology Clinics of North America is covered in *Index Medicus, EMBASE/Excerpta Medica, and BIOSIS.*

Printed in the United States of America.

GUEST EDITOR

RODGER L. BICK, MD, PhD, FACP, Clinical Professor, Departments of Medicine and Pathology, University of Texas Southwestern Medical School; and Director, Dallas Thrombosis Hemostasis & Vascular Medicine Clinical Center, Dallas, Texas

CONTRIBUTORS

WILLIAM F. BAKER, Jr, MD, FACP, Associate Clinical Professor, Center for Health Sciences, University of California–Los Angeles, Los Angeles, California; Director, Thrombosis, Hemostasis, and Special Hematology Clinic, Kern Medical Center; and California Clinical Thrombosis Center, Kern Medical Center, Bakersfield, California

RODGER L. BICK, MD, PhD, FACP, Clinical Professor, Departments of Medicine and Pathology, University of Texas Southwestern Medical School; and Director, Dallas Thrombosis Hemostasis & Vascular Medicine Clinical Center, Dallas, Texas

LESLIE CHO, MD, Assistant Professor, Division of Cardiology, Loyola University Stritch School of Medicine, Loyola University Medical Center, Maywood, Illinois

ERWIN COYNE, PhD, Research Associate, Hines Veteran's Affairs Hospital, Hines, Illinois

BARBARA B. HALEY, MD, Professor, Department of Medicine, Harold C. Simmons Comprehensive Cancer Center, University of Texas Southwestern Medical School, Dallas, Texas

JAWED FAREED, PhD, Professor, Departments of Pathology & Pharmacology and Cardiovascular Surgery, Loyola University Chicago, Maywood, Illinois

EUGENE P. FRENKEL, MD, Professor, Departments of Medicine and Radiology, Harold C. Simmons Comprehensive Cancer Center, University of Texas Southwestern Medical School, Dallas, Texas

DEBORAH A. HOPPENSTEADT, PhD, Professor, Departments of Pathology & Pharmacology and Cardiovascular Surgery, Loyola University Chicago, Maywood, Illinois

RUSSELL D. HULL, MBBS, MSc, Department of Medicine, University of Calgary, Foothills Hospital, Calgary, Alberta, Canada

WALTER P. JESKE, PhD, Associate Professor, Thoracic and Cardiovascular Surgery, Loyola University Stritch School of Medicine, Cardiovascular Institute, Loyola University Medical Center, Maywood, Illinois

DAVID J. KUTER, MD, DPhil, Chief, Clinical Hematology, Hematology/Oncology Unit, Massachusetts General Hospital; and Associate Professor, Harvard Medical School, Boston, Massachusetts

WENDY LEONG, PharmD, MCPS, MBA, Burnaby Research, University of British Columbia, Vancouver, British Columbia, Canada

FRED S. LEYA, MD, Professor, Division of Cardiology, Loyola University Stritch School of Medicine, Loyola University Medical Center, Maywood, Illinois

HARRY L. MESSMORE, Jr, MD, Staff Physician, Hines Veteran's Affairs Hospital, Hines, Illinois; and Professor, Loyola University Stritch School of Medicine, Cancer Center, Loyola University Medical Center, Maywood, Illinois

SOHRAB MOBARHAN, MD, Professor, Department of Gastroenterology, Loyola University Stritch School of Medicine, Loyola University Medical Center, Maywood, Illinois

JOHN F. MORAN, MD, Professor, Division of Cardiology, Loyola University Stritch School of Medicine, Loyola University Medical Center, Maywood, Illinois

GRAHAM F. PINEO, MD, Department of Medicine, University of Calgary, Foothills Hospital, Calgary, Alberta, Canada

RACHEL P. ROSOVSKY, MD, Clinical Fellow, Hematology/Oncology Unit, Massachusetts General Hospital; and Instructor, Harvard Medical School, Boston, Massachusetts

YU-MIN SHEN, MD, Assistant Professor, Department of Medicine, Harold C. Simmons Comprehensive Cancer Center, University of Texas Southwestern Medical School, Dallas, Texas

JEANINE WALENGA, PhD, Professor, Departments of Pathology & Pharmacology and Cardiovascular Surgery, Loyola University Chicago, Maywood, Illinois

WILLIAM WEHRMACHER, MD, Adjunct Professor, Department of Physiology, Loyola University Stritch School of Medicine, Loyola University Medical Center, Maywood, Illinois

CONTENTS

FORTHCOMING ISSUES

April 2005

Multidisciplinary Approach to Lung Cancer
Gregory A. Masters, MD, *Guest Editor*

June 2005

Sarcomas
Robert G. Maki, MD, PhD, *Guest Editor*

August 2005

Primary Central Nervous System Lymphoma
Lisa M. DeAngelis, MD, and
Lauren E. Abrey, MD, *Guest Editors*

RECENT ISSUES

December 2004

Non-Malignant Disorders of the Blood in Infants and Children
George R. Buchanan, MD, *Guest Editor*

October 2004

Angiogenesis and Anti-Angiogenic Therapy
Lee M. Ellis, MD, and
Michael S. Gordon, MD, *Guest Editors*

August 2004

Chronic Lymphocytic Leukemia
Manlio Ferrarini, MD, and
Nicholas Chiorazzi, MD, *Guest Editors*

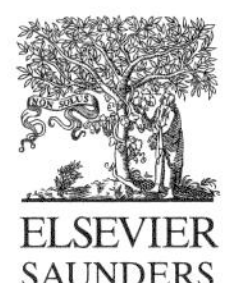

ELSEVIER
SAUNDERS

Hematol Oncol Clin N Am
19 (2005) ix

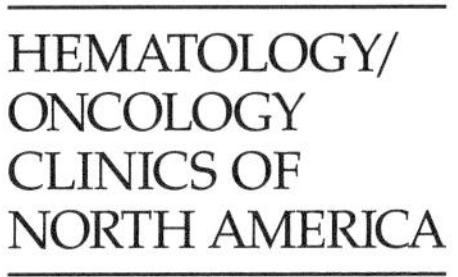

Dedication

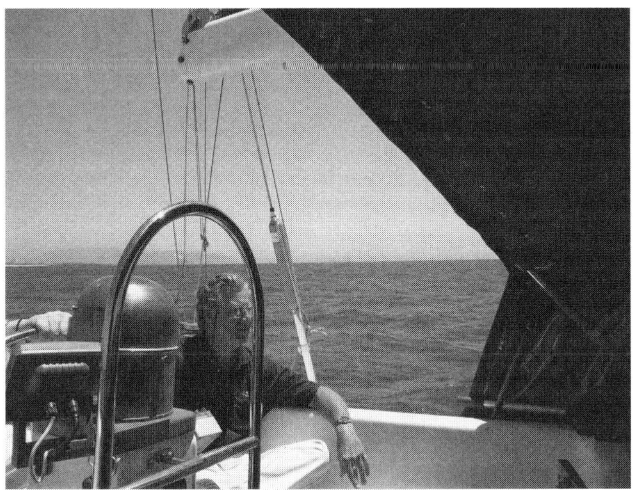

This issue is dedicated to Paul A. Bick, PhD, for his unwavering commitment to morals, ethics, and humanity.

Rodger L. Bick, MD, PhD

doi:10.1016/j.hoc.2004.09.001
hemonc.theclinics.com

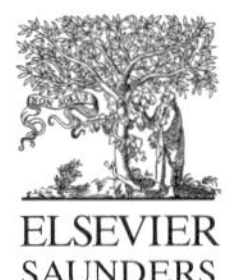

ELSEVIER
SAUNDERS

Hematol Oncol Clin N Am
19 (2005) xi–xvi

HEMATOLOGY/
ONCOLOGY
CLINICS OF
NORTH AMERICA

Preface

Antithrombotic Therapy: Current Practice and Future Trends

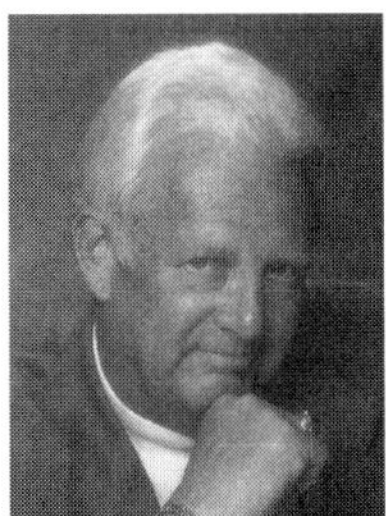

Rodger L. Bick, MD, PhD, FACP
Guest Editor

Thrombosis is clearly the most common cause of death in the United States. Approximately 2 million individuals die each year from an arterial or venous thrombosis or the consequences thereof [1]. Approximately 80% to 90% of all causes of thrombosis can now be defined with respect to cause. Of these, over 50% of all patients harbor a congenital or acquired blood coagulation protein or platelet defect that caused the thrombotic event. Because thrombosis is a major health problem, scientists, clinicians, and the pharmaceutical industry are constantly striving to develop better, more targeted, and more successful thrombotherapeutic and thromboprophylactic antithrombotic agents. It is obviously of major importance to define those individuals who harbor prothrombotic defects or risk factors, because this (1) allows appropriate antithrombotic therapy to decrease risks of recurrence, (2) helps determine of the length of time the patient must remain on therapy for secondary prevention, and (3) allows for testing of family members of those who harbor a blood coagulation protein or platelet defect that is hereditary (approximately 50% of all coagulation and platelet defects mentioned above). These and common clinical defects leading to thrombosis are discussed later and can be found in Table 1. Aside from mortality, significant additional morbidity occurs from both arterial or venous thrombotic events, including—but not limited to—paralysis (nonfatal thrombotic stroke),

0889-8588/05/$ – see front matter
doi:10.1016/j.hoc.2004.09.009

Table 1
Causes of thrombosis

Clinical conditions		
Arterial	Venous	Blood protein and platelet defects
Atherosclerosis	General surgery	Antiphospholipid syndrome
Cigarette smoking	Orthopedic surgery	APC resistance
Hypertension	Arthroscopy	Factor V Leiden
Diabetes mellitus	Trauma	Sticky platelet syndrome
LDL cholesterol	Malignancy	Prothrombin G 20210A
Hypertriglyceridemia	Immobility	Protein S defects
Positive family history	Sepsis	Protein C defects
Left ventricular failure	Congestive heart failure	Antithrombin defects
Oral contraceptives	Nephrotic syndrome	Heparin cofactor II defects
Estrogens	Obesity	Plasminogen defects
Lipoprotein (a)	Varicose veins	TPA defects
Polycythemia	Post-phlebitic syndrom	PAI-1 defects
Hyperviscosity syndrome	Oral contraceptives	Factor XII defects
Leukostasis syndrome	Estrogens	Dysfibrinogenemia
Inflammation/sepsis	Inflammation/sepsis	Homocystinemia
		MTHFR mutations
		Factor V Cambridge
		Factor V Hong Kong
		Factor V HR2 mutation
		Immune vasculitis

cardiac disability (repeated coronary events), loss of vision (retinal vascular thrombosis), fetal wastage syndrome (placental vascular thrombosis), stasis ulcers and other manifestations of postphlebitic syndrome (recurrent deep vein thrombosis), and so forth. It is anticipated that newer agents, as well as clearer indications for time-proven older antithrombotic agents, will enhance efficacy while decreasing or minimizing adverse reactions, particularly hemorrhage.

Deep vein thrombosis

The incidence of deep vein thrombosis in the United States is approximately 159 per 100,000 or around 398,000 per year [1,2]. A definable etiology can be found in 80% to 90% of these patients; this allows effective therapy to be delivered and allows for the other advantages of defining the blood coagulation protein or platelet defects, mentioned above, to be instituted. For example, approximately 28% of these patients will have antiphospholipid syndrome, and if treated with oral anticoagulants, approximately 65% will fail (rethrombose) [2]. Also, approximately 30% to 50% of these patients will have coagulation protein or platelet defects that are congenital; consequently, family members should be assessed and, obviously, antithrombotic therapy for the afflicted patient should be long-term, not 6 weeks to 3 months.

Pulmonary embolus

The overall incidence of pulmonary embolus (PE) in the United States is approximately 139 per 100,000 or about 347,000 cases per year (clinical data); the incidence of fatal PE is 94 per 100,000 or about 235,000 deaths (autopsy data) [1–3]. The same scenario as that for deep vein thrombosis prevails for PE. If the PE is not fatal, every attempt should be made to define the blood coagulation protein or platelet defect responsible.

Coronary artery thrombosis

One and a half million individuals in the United States will have an acute myocardial infarction per year; 50% of these will be fatal, while the other 50% will be a premature/precocious event [1,4]. Thus, there are approximately 750,000 deaths from coronary artery thrombosis per year. Of these coronary thrombotic events, 67% of patients harbor a coagulation blood protein or platelet defect leading to thrombosis. Fifty percent of these coagulation protein or platelet defects will be hereditary, thus emphasizing the importance of defining the presence and type of defect in survivors of acute myocardial infarction. Defining the defect will also allow one to optimize antithrombotic therapy for secondary prevention.

Cerebrovascular thrombosis

Cerebrovascular thrombosis occurs in over 1.5 million individuals yearly in the United States; of these, 66% suffer death or severe permanent paralysis. In those individuals who suffer from cerebrovascular thrombosis, including transient cerebral ischemic attacks, small stroke syndrome, and frank thrombotic stroke, at least 30% harbor a blood coagulation protein or platelet defect causing thrombosis. Like the disorders discussed above, the need for defining the presence or absence and type of defect is of obvious importance.

Although the incidence of retinal arterial or venous thrombosis is unclear and death does not occur, significant visual morbidity is a major problem. Like cerebrovascular thrombosis, approximately 30% of individuals sustaining retinal vascular thrombosis harbor a blood coagulation protein or platelet defect; reasons for defining these are as obvious as for the other disorders discussed.

Recurrent miscarriage syndrome

Many women suffer miscarriages. Although there are anatomic, hormonal, and genetic/chromosomal causes, defects in blood coagulation proteins or platelets leading to early placental vascular thrombosis and nonviability of the

Table 2
Incidence of thrombosis in the United States

Disease	Prevalence/incidence	Total cases per year	Definable reason
Deep vein thrombosis	159/100,000	398,000	≈90%
Pulmonary embolus	139/100,000	347,000	≈90%
Fatal pulmonary embolus	94/100,000	235,000	≈90%
Myocardial infarction	600/100,000	1,500,000	≈67%
Fatal myocardial infarction	300/100,000	750,000	≈67%
Cerebrovascular thrombosis	600/100,000	1,500,000	≈30%
Fatal cerebrovascular thrombosis	396/100,000	990,000	≈30%
Total serious thromboses	1498/100,000	3,742,000	≈50%
Total deaths from above thrombosis	790/100,000	1,990,000	≈50%
All cancer in 1996	544/100,000	1,359,150	
Cancer deaths in 1996	222/100,000	554,740	

fetus account for approximately 30% to 50% of all cases of FWS [5]. Clearly defining the coagulation defect almost always allows for antithrombotic therapy, which will lead to normal term pregnancy.

Comparative incidence rates for thrombotic deaths compared with cancer deaths in the United States are found in Table 2; note only the most common thrombotic problems leading to significant morbidity or mortality are included [6]. Table 1 summarizes the etiologic factors known to be responsible for many of these events; this table serves to illustrate the types of defects and prevalence that should be considered, thus allowing appropriate therapy to be instituted when such defects are found.

The etiologies of hypercoagulability and overt thrombosis are becoming more clear and often definitive with enhanced knowledge of hemostasis and the development and extended use of testing systems useful for evaluating patients with thrombotic and thromboembolic disorders. Using these test systems, in conjunction with careful clinical assessment of patients, approximately 80% to 90% of patients with thrombosis will have a defined etiology. Many of these will have an obvious clinical condition leading to thrombosis, and at least 50% to 80% will have an underlying hereditary or acquired blood protein/platelet defect causing thrombosis. Many clinical conditions are associated with an increased risk of arterial or venous thrombosis and thromboembolism; the more common of these are summarized in Table 1.

It must be remembered and emphasized that a diagnosis of thrombosis is similar to and as generic as a diagnosis of "anemia"; in all instances, one must ask: What is the etiology of the thrombosis? Like anemia, the specific and appropriate therapy is highly dependent upon defining the etiology. Thrombosis, be it arterial or venous, can no longer be viewed as a generic diagnosis; approaching thrombosis in this manner probably accounts for not only many treatment failures, but also for often confusing and conflicting results of clinical trials. Most clinicians and most trialists approaching thrombosis as a generic diagnosis fail to note that a very heterogeneous population is likely to be present and outcomes will depend upon designing therapy specific for a given etiology. As a simple example, it would not make sense to treat a patient who has thrombosis and harbors sticky platelet syndrome with heparin or coumadin when they actually need aspirin; nor would it make sense to treat a patient who has antiphospholipid syndrome and thrombosis with aspirin (no response) or warfarin (65% failure rate) when they respond most ideally to heparin.

Because of new drug developments, this issue of the *Hematology Oncology Clinics of North America* is dedicated to new antithrombotic drugs as well as new indications and potential new uses for albeit older but time-tested drugs. The first article offers new perspectives on heparin and low molecular weight heparin. The second article addresses the all-important issues of potential generic low molecular weight heparins and the potential advantages and greater potential for problems that may occur. In the third article, Drs. Pineo and Hull discuss new concepts and indications for warfarin drugs. In the fourth article, Dr. Messmore and associates discuss the rapidly growing field of new antiplatelet agents. The fifth article is a masterful review of the new direct thrombin inhibitors by Dr. Frenkel and associates. Br. Baker offers new perspectives and new indications for thrombolytic therapy. The final article is a topic of much concern to hematologists and oncologists—that of catheter-related thrombosis—written by Dr. David Kuter and associates, all well-recognized experts in this area.

Rodger L. Bick, MD, PhD, FACP
Departments of Medicine and Pathology
University of Texas Southwestern Medical Center
Dallas Thrombosis Hemostasis Clinical Center
10455 North Central Expressway
Suite 109, PMB 320
Dallas, TX 75231, USA
E-mail address: rbick@thrombosis.com

References

[1] Bick RL, Fareed J. Current status of thrombosis: a multidisciplinary medical issue and major American health problem—beyond the year 2000. Clin Appl Thromb Hemost 1997; 3(Suppl 1):1.

[2] Bergqvist D, Lundblad B. Incidence of venous thromboembolism in medical and surgical patients. In: Bergqvist D, Comerota A, Nicolaides A, et al, editors. Prevention of venous thromboembolism. London: Med-Orion Press; 1994. p. 3.

[3] Ramaswami G, Nicolaides AN. The natural history of deep vein thrombosis. In: Bergqvist D, Comerota A, Nicolaides A, et al, editors. Prevention of venous thromboembolism. London: Med-Orion Press; 1994. p. 3.

[4] American Heart Association. Heart and stroke—1997. Dallas (TX): American Heart Association; 1996.
[5] Bick RL. Recurrent miscarriage syndrome and infertility caused by blood coagulation protein or platelet defects. Hematol Oncol Clin North Am 2000;14:1117–31.
[6] American Cancer Society. Cancer. Facts and figures: 1996. American Cancer Society; 1996.

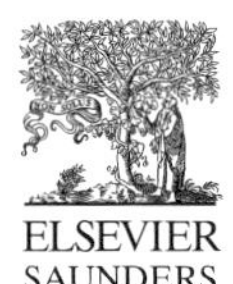
ELSEVIER
SAUNDERS

Hematol Oncol Clin N Am
19 (2005) 1–51

HEMATOLOGY/
ONCOLOGY
CLINICS OF
NORTH AMERICA

Unfractionated Heparin, Low Molecular Weight Heparins, and Pentasaccharide: Basic Mechanism of Actions, Pharmacology, and Clinical Use

Rodger L. Bick, MD, PhD, FACP[a,b,*],
Eugene P. Frenkel, MD[c], Jeanine Walenga, PhD[d],
Jawed Fareed, PhD[d], Deborah A. Hoppensteadt, PhD[d]

[a]*Departments of Medicine and Pathology, University of Texas Southwestern Medical School, 2201 Inwood Road, Dallas, TX 75235-8852, USA*
[b]*Dallas Thrombosis Hemostasis & Vascular Medicine Clinical Center, 10455 North Central Expressway, Suite 109, PMB 320, Dallas, TX 75231, USA*
[c]*Departments of Medicine and Radiology, University of Texas Southwestern Medical School, 2201 Inwood Road, Dallas, TX 75235-8852, USA*
[d]*Departments of Pathology & Pharmacology and Cardiovascular Surgery, Loyola University Chicago, 2160 South First Avenue, Maywood, IL 60153, USA*

During the past decade, a large number of new anticoagulant and antithrombotic drugs have been developed. As shown in Fig. 1, these agents represent a wide variety of substances that are derived using natural sources, biotechnology-based methods, and synthetic approaches [1]. Because of the structural and molecular characteristics, these agents exhibit physicochemical and functional diversities. Thus, each of these classes of drugs controls thrombogenesis by way of distinct mechanisms.

The main classes of these new drugs include peptides, peptidomimetics, heparinomimetics, and recombinant proteins. In addition, there are several antiplatelet drugs such as the platelet glycoprotein IIb/IIIa complex inhibitors

* Corresponding author. Dallas Thrombosis Hemostasis & Vascular Medicine Clinical Center, 10455 North Central Expressway, Suite 109, PMB 320, Dallas, TX 75231.

E-mail address: rbick@thrombosis.com (R.L. Bick).

doi:10.1016/j.hoc.2004.09.003 **hemonc.theclinics.com**

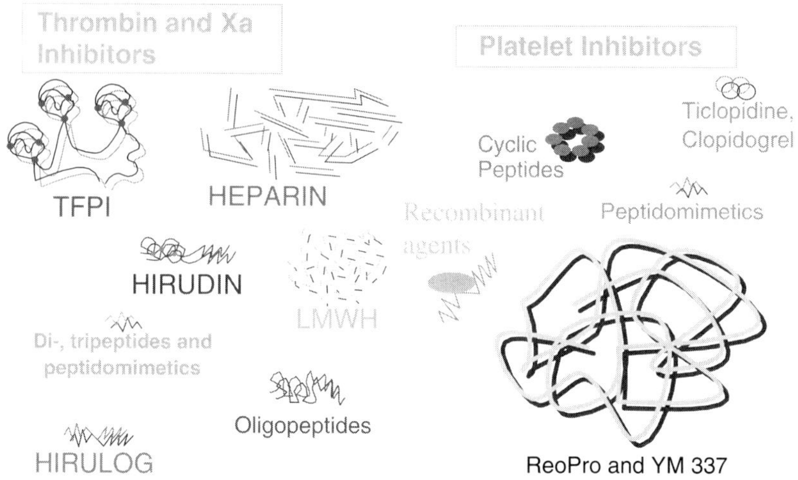

Fig. 1. A comparison of the newer anticoagulant and antithrombotic drugs. The newer drug classes include thrombin and Xa inhibitors that are prepared by biotechnology, isolation and purification from the natural sources, and using newer biotechnology-based methods. LMWH, low molecular weight heparin; TFPI, tissue factor pathway inhibitor.

and ADP receptor antagonists that have played a major role in the management of cardiovascular disorders. Despite these significant developments, heparin and heparin-derived drugs have continued to play a major role in the management of thrombotic and cardiovascular disorders.

Heparin, low molecular weight heparins (LMWHs), and related derivatives will continue to be used clinically for decades even though new related compounds, derivatives, and indications will continue to evolve, be modified, or otherwise undergo clinical change.

There remain several unanswered important issues related to the current practices of anticoagulant therapy because many of the newer drugs are monotherapeutic. The widely acclaimed notion that these new drugs will eventually replace conventional anticoagulants such as warfarin (Coumadin) and heparin/LMWHs requires objective validation. Drugs such as the pentasaccharide Arixtra and antithrombin agents (Hirudin, Angiomax) target only one site, whereas the conventional anticoagulants are polytherapeutic. It is therefore difficult to perceive that a monotherapeutic agent will produce all of the polytherapeutic effects of conventional drugs without the potential toxicity associated with their use.

Unfractionated heparin (UFH) is a strongly anionic polyelectrolyte, which at physiologic pHs, contains three acidic functional groups that are fully dissociated. Because of this, heparin has a large number of pharmacologic properties. Among these properties are its antilipemic and antihemolytic actions [1]. Heparin also is known to inhibit a variety of enzymes including myosin

ATPase, RNA-dependent DNA polymerase, elastase, and renin [1]. Heparin inhibits tumor growth and exhibits antibacterial and antiviral properties [1].

Heparin is administered by intravenous (IV) infusion or by subcutaneous (SC) injection. After entering the blood stream, heparin binds to a variety of plasma proteins, thereby lowering its bioavailability and producing a variable anticoagulant response. These proteins include histidine-rich glycoprotein, platelet factor 4, vitronectin, and von Willebrand factor. Heparin exhibits complex pharmacokinetics and is cleared by two mechanisms. The rapid, saturable phase of elimination is thought to be due to receptor-mediated internalization of heparin by endothelial cells and macrophages. A slower, nonsaturable renal mechanism also clears heparin from the plasma. The anticoagulant effect of heparin, therefore, is not linearly related to dose when in the therapeutic range. The biologic half-life of heparin increases from 30 minutes following an IV bolus dose of 25 U/kg to 150 minutes following a bolus dose of 400 U/kg.

Heparin is used in the therapy of several cardiovascular disorders including prevention and treatment of arterial and venous thromboembolism, treatment of unstable angina, acute myocardial infarction, cardiac and vascular surgery, coronary angioplasty, stent implantation, and as an adjunctive agent during thrombolysis. Heparin also is the anticoagulant of choice during pregnancy.

Studies have demonstrated that there is a reduction in mortality in patients receiving heparin for the treatment of pulmonary emboli. In addition, recurrent thrombosis is not common during the heparinization period but increases significantly when heparin is stopped and no other anticoagulant therapy is used. Heparin is effective in treating venous thrombosis. This effectiveness has been shown to be dependent on the anticoagulant effect achieved. Heparin also is effective prophylactically, reducing the risk of venous thrombosis and pulmonary embolism 60% to 70%. Heparin is effective short-term in preventing acute myocardial infarction and recurrent refractory angina in patients with unstable angina. This beneficial effect is lost on cessation of heparin therapy. In patients who have previous myocardial infarction, heparin administration has been shown to significantly reduce reinfarction and death compared with untreated controls. Heparin has been tested as an adjunct in thrombolytic therapy and appears to increase patency during the initial stages of recanalization by preventing rethrombosis. Heparin is the anticoagulant of choice in pregnancy because it does not cross the placental barrier and is not known to cause unwanted effects on the fetus.

UFH has remained the anticoagulant of choice for interventional and surgical indications despite the development of newer agents. Several newer LMWHs are now routinely used for specific indications in arterial and venous indications. It is important to note that each LMWH is a distinct drug and that the different LMWHs cannot be interchanged for specific indications until parallel clinical trials have been done to show equivalence. Each of these products has its own specific dosage for a given indication. LMWHs have gradually replaced heparin for prophylaxis and treatment of deep vein thrombosis, however, the role of these agents as surgical and interventional anticoagulants is not clearly established. Although LMWHs are widely used for various other indications, there still are several unresolved questions related to the development of these drugs:

1. Are different LMWHs distinct drugs?
2. Can we interchange various LMWHs for specific indications?
3. Will LMWHs replace UFH for anticoagulation indications?
4. Will antithrombin drugs and anti-Xa agents eventually replace LMWHs in anticoagulation indications?
5. What is the feasibility of oral LMWHs for specific indications?
6. What is the possibility of the introduction of generic versions of LMWHs? Are there any adequate guidelines to compare these drugs with the branded products?

Currently, several newer agents are being investigated as possible substitutes for heparin. These new agents include antithrombin, anti-Xa, anti–tissue factor, heparinoids, oral formulations of heparin, glycosaminoglycans mixtures, activated protein C, and biotechnology-derived serpins such as recombinant antithrombin III (ATIII) and heparin cofactor II. All of the agents currently are developed for indications in arterial and venous thrombosis. Each of these agents may be used for a specific and relatively narrow range of indications and may not have a broad clinical spectrum, as is observed with the heparins.

UFH and LMWHs are chemically and functionally heterogeneous in nature. Fig. 2 describes the depolymerization of heparin that results in a LMWH product (4–8 kd). The resulting LMWHs also exhibit differences in molecular and functional properties due to significant differences in the procedures used to prepare each LMWH. Initial attempts to standardize LMWHs based on their biologic and physiochemical properties have failed. Each LMWH has distinct properties that are largely dependent on the molecular composition. Each LMWH differs in its biochemical, physicochemical, clinical, and pharmacologic profile and, thus, these products are not equivalent. Each product is individually developed for a given indication, and the data from one product are not interchangeable with those of another product.

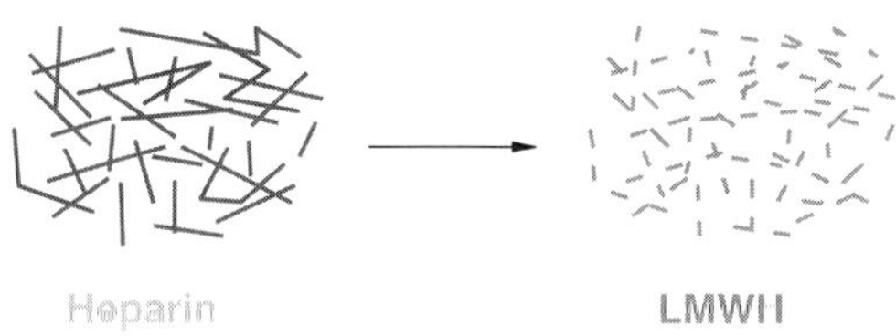

Fig. 2. A comparison of the molecular heterogeneity between UFH and LMWH. The mean molecular weight of UFH range is between 12,000 and 16,000 d, whereas the LMWHs exhibit the molecular weight of 4,000 to 7,000 d. Because of the enzymatic and chemical digestion, the LMWHs exhibit additional structural alterations that add to their uniqueness.

Table 1
Molecular and chemical characteristics of various low molecular weight heparins

LMWH	Characteristics
Nadroparin	Presence of 2,5-anhydro-D-mannose at reducing terminus
Enoxaparin	Presence of 4,5 unsaturated uronic acid at nonreducing terminus
Dalteparin	Presence of 2,5-anhydro-D-mannose at reducing terminus
Certoparin	Presence of 2,5-anhydro-D-mannose at reducing terminus
Tinzaparin	Presence of 4,5 unsaturated uronic acid at nonreducing terminus
Reviparin	Presence of 2,5-anhydro-D-mannose at reducing terminus
Ardeparin	Labile glycosidic bonds

The depolymerization of heparin to prepare LMWHs can be accomplished by chemical, enzymatic, physical, and radiochemical methods. The resulting LMWHs exhibit marked differences in their chemical and biologic activities. These differences may be due to the procedure-inflicted structural differences and molecular weight component distribution [2,3]. Different LMWHs show distinct chemical groups that make these agents distinguishable. As listed in Table 1, nadroparin, dalteparin, certoparin, and reviparin have a 2,5-anhydro-D-mannose at the reducing terminus, whereas enoxaparin and tinzaparin have a 4,5 unsaturated uronic acid at the nonreducing end. These differences contribute to the uniqueness of each product. Additional structural differences in each product also can be found.

Table 2 lists the currently available LMWHs, along with the trade name and the manufacturer. Most of these LMWHs are sodium salts of depolymerized porcine mucosal heparin, with the exception of nadroparin, which is a calcium salt. Each LMWH is designated by an International Nonproprietary Name and a trade name; however, additional commercial names may be given to different LMWHs by various companies in different countries.

The LMWHs usually are characterized by their anti-Xa and anti-IIa potencies. A comparison of the molecular weight, anti-Xa and anti-IIa potency, and the ratio of Xa/IIa of the different LMWHs is shown in Table 3. Dalteparin has the highest

Table 2
Commercially available low molecular weight heparins

International nonproprietary name	Trade name	Manufacturer
Ardeparin sodium	Normiflo	Wyeth-Ayest
	Indeparin	Gland
Certoparin sodium	Sandoparin	Novartis
Dalteparin sodium	Fragmin	Pfizer
		Kissei
Enoxaparin sodium	Clexane	Aventis
	Lovenox	
Nadroparin calcium	Fraxiparin	Sanofi-Winthrop
Panaparin sodium	Fluxum	Alfa Wassermann
Reviparin sodium	Clivarin	Abbot
Tinzaparin sodium	Innohep	Braun
	Logiparin	Novo/Leo/Pharmiom

Table 3
Characterization of low molecular weight heparins

LMWH	Median molecular weight (d)	Anti-Xa (IU/mg)	Anti-IIa (IU/mg)	Xa/IIa
Enoxaparin	4800	104	32	3.3
Dalteparin	5000	122	60	2.0
Nadroparin	4500	94	31	3.0
Tinzaparin	4500	90	50	1.8
Clivarine	3900	130	40	3.3

median molecular weight and the highest anti-IIa activity, whereas clivarine has the lowest molecular weight. The other LMWH values are in between the values for dalteparin and clivarine. Although the anti-Xa and anti-IIa actions of LMWHs usually are designated for pharmaceutical characterization, this also reflects on the functional diversity in each LMWH.

The *United States Pharmacopeia* (USP) assay usually is employed for the potency evaluation of UFH; however, at high concentrations (> 10 μg/mL), the LMWHs also show anticoagulant actions in the USP assay. The USP potency of several LMWH preparations compared with UFH is shown in Fig. 3. The USP activity is measured using a standard USP coagulant method. As can be seen, the USP activity of most LMWHs is lower than UFH; however, each of these LMWHs exhibits a distinct USP potency that is largely dependent on the components (oligosaccharides). The molecular and structural features also contribute to the in vivo pharmacodynamic effects. Because LMWHs are expected to be used in surgical and interventional indications, it is therefore recommended that these drugs be characterized in terms of their USP U/mg.

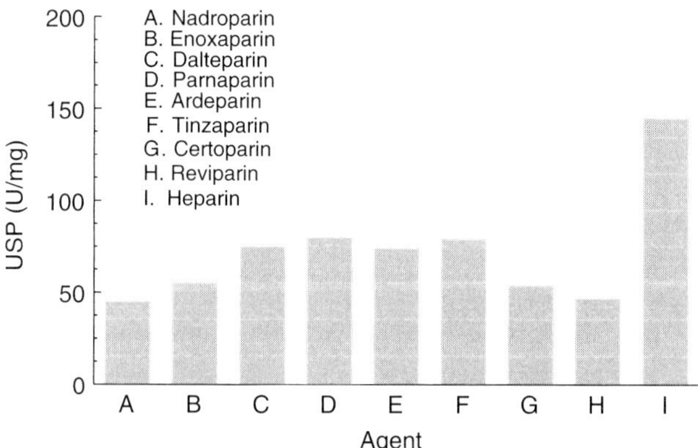

Fig. 3. Comparison of the anticoagulant effects of LMWHs as measured by using the USP method. Initially, these agents were believed to not exhibit any anticoagulant actions; however, each of these agents exhibit anticoagulant effects at concentrations of greater than 5 mg/mL. At higher concentrations, a dose-dependent effect is noted using the USP assays. Thus, the USP method can be used for product differentiation.

Because LMWHs usually are administered in repeated dosages, there is a possibility of these drugs to accumulate. The accumulation profile of each drug also may be product dependent. The effect of repeated administration of various LMWHs on the area under the concentration time curve (AUC) as measured by the anti-Xa and anti-IIa activity is shown in Fig. 4. The AUC of the different LMWHs varies. When the anti-Xa method is used, AUC is higher for tinzaparin (5.4) on day 5 compared with the other LMWHs (range, 3.0–4.6). If the anti-IIa method is used, similar results are obtained for the AUC with the different LMWHs (range, 1.0–1.9). The bioavailability of each LMWH is largely determined by the type of test used to quantitate the pharmacodynamic effects. Therefore, the accumulation profile for each of these drugs may be different, depending on the type of assay used. The bioavailability of each of these drugs also varies, regardless of its in vitro potency.

To show the relative peak concentrations of different LMWHs, rats were administered with different LMWHs and heparin at a 1 mg/kg SC dosage. The LMWH concentration in terms of anti-Xa was measured. As shown in Fig. 5, the different LMWHs showed different peak concentrations. In addition, the enoxaparin peaked at a later time point compared with the other LMWHs. Thus, the pharmacokinetic and pharmacodynamic profile of each LMWH differs widely and will translate into the clinical effects in specific indications.

It has been widely accepted that endogenous protein binding modulates the pharmacologic actions of UFH. The variations in clinical response are attributed to the differential protein binding. Several preclinical and clinical studies have demonstrated the differences in the protein-binding profile of heparin and

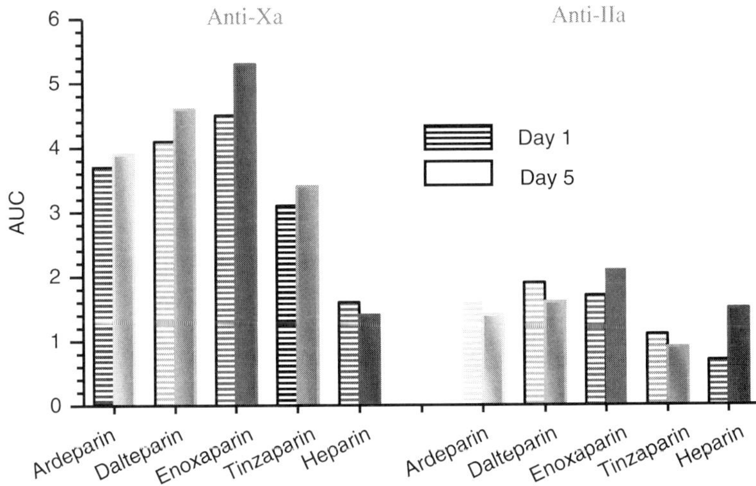

Fig. 4. Effect of repeated administration of various LMWHs on the bioavailability the anti-Xa and anti-IIa actions. Each product exhibits its own variation in the bioavailability of the anti-Xa and IIa effects, which may be proportional to the endogenous availability of oligosaccharides.

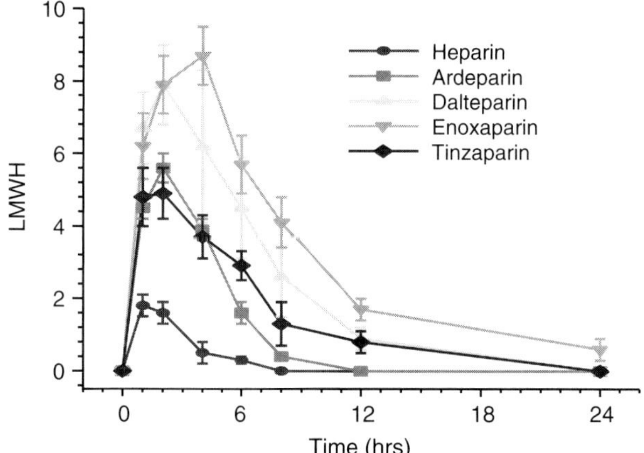

Fig. 5. Differential bioavailability of SC-administered LMWH and heparin. After a 1 mg/kg SC dose, each of the LMWHs exhibited better bioavailability than heparin; however, there are significant differences in the relative bioavailability of each drug.

the LMWHs. Young and colleagues [4], however, were not able show any differences in the protein-binding profile of heparin and LMWHs in normal controls versus patients. Fig. 6 describes the effect of plasma protein binding. At prophylactic and therapeutic dosages of different LMWHs, no effect was observed on the concentrations obtained by the anti-Xa method in plasma from normals versus a cohort of patients.

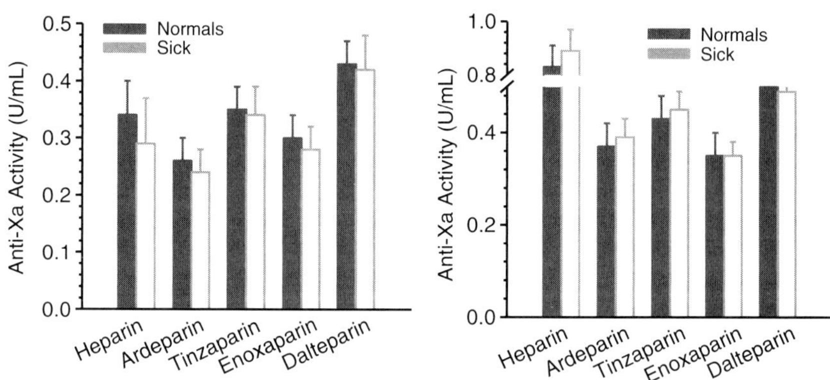

Fig. 6. Influence of protein binding on the anti-Xa activity of various LMWHs in normal and sick individuals. The binding is measured in terms of its influence on the anti-Xa activity. No differences are observed between the sick and normal individuals; however, different products bind differentially to plasma protein. (*From* Young E, Wells P, Holloway S, Weitz J, Hirsh J. Ex vivo and in vitro evidence that low molecular weight heparins exhibit less binding to plasma proteins than UFH. Thromb Haemost 1994;71(3):300; with permission.)

In a study performed by Houbouyan et al [5], the ED 80 for thrombin inhibition was calculated in terms of anti-Xa and anti-IIa activities using chromogenic methods. The ED 80 for the different LMWHs ranged from 0.48 to 1.26 IU/mL for anti-Xa and from 0.19 to 0.35 for anti-IIa. Enoxaparin and nadroparin showed similar Xa/IIa ratios, and dalteparin and tinzaparin showed similar ratios [5]. These results also demonstrate the point that the different LMWHs are distinct drugs.

LMWHs also are capable of producing endogenous release of various substances such as tissue factor pathway inhibitor (TFPI) and von Willebrand Factor. It is expected that various LMWHs will produce differential release of these factors. The effects of various LMWHs on von Willebrand factor release in patients with unstable angina are shown in Fig. 7 [6]. The data reported by Montalescot et al [6] demonstrates that enoxaparin releases less von Willebrand Factor compared with dalteparin or UFH, resulting in reduced platelet aggregation. Thus, each of the LMWHs produces somewhat different effects on vascular function. The release of such substances has an impact on the overall effects of these agent, and is particularly true for LMWH use in surgical and interventional indications.

LMWHs previously have been reported to produce fibrinolytic effects; however, the mechanism or mechanisms of this action are not known. It has been suggested that LMWHs may produce this effect by modulating the fibrinolytic process. Thrombin activatable fibrinolytic inhibitor (TAFI) is a carboxypeptidase

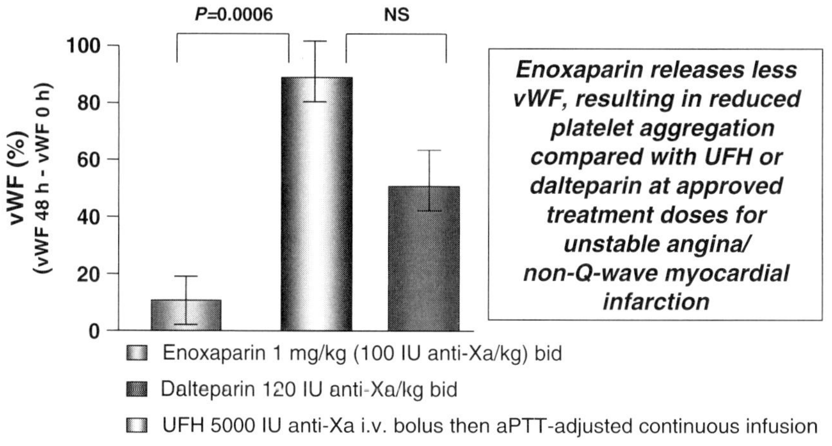

Fig. 7. Differential release of von Willebrand factor (vWF) by enoxaparin and dalteparin. Both drugs exhibit a differential behavior in terms of the endogenous release of vWF. aPTT, activated partial thromboplastin time; i.v., intravenous; NS, not significant. (*From* Montalescot G, Collet JP, Lison L, Choussat R, Anki A. Effects of various anticoagulant treatments on von Willebrand factor release in unstable angina. J Am Coll Cardiol 2000;36(1):110; with permission.)

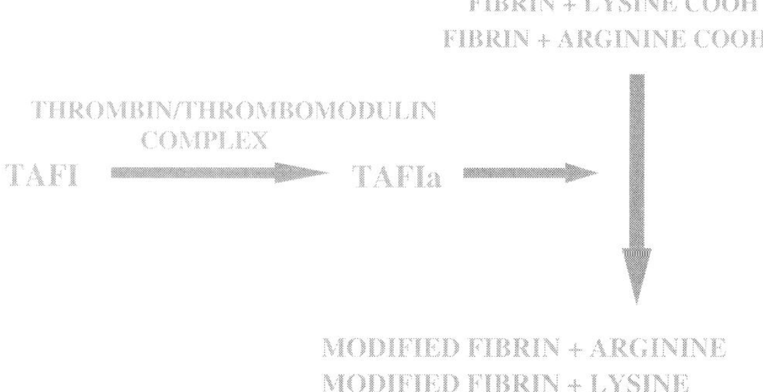

Fig. 8. A diagrammatic representation of mechanism of action of TAFI on the molecular alterations of fibrin. TAFIa converts fibrin to modified fibrin. The modified form of fibrin exhibits impaired binding for plasminogen.

that produces a molecular change in fibrin. This modified fibrin is resistant to the lytic actions of plasmin. Fig. 8 depicts the activation of TAFI to TAFIa (activated) by the thrombin/thrombomodulin complex. LMWHs are capable of inhibiting thrombin and its generation. Accordingly, these agents can modulate the action of TAFI. The different LMWHs produce different effects on the activation of TAFI. It also has been demonstrated that agents with a high anti-Xa/anti-IIa ratio produce weaker inhibition compared with agents with a lower anti-Xa/anti-IIa ratio. This inhibition may play a role in the safety/efficacy of these drugs. Different LMWHs have different anti-Xa/anti-IIa ratios. These agents are expected to modulate the thrombin-mediated activation of TAFI at a different rate. Fig. 9 shows the effects of different LMWHs on the functional levels of TAFI, expressed as the IC_{50}. Different LMWHs produce different effects of the

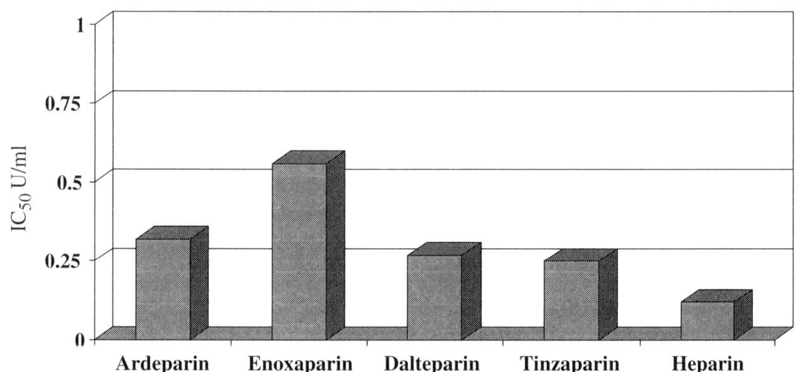

Fig. 9. Effect of various LMWHs on the functional levels of TAFI. The inhibitor effects of each of these agents are expressed in terms of IC_{50} (units per milliliter). Differences in the relative potency of these agents are observed.

activation of TAFI. Thus, the relative antithrombin activity of each of these LMWHs may be proportional to the inhibitory actions on TAFI activation. The profibrinolytic effects produced by different LWMHs may be determined by the composition of these agents. Thus, the bleeding complications and the antithrombotic efficacy of these agents may be related to the modulation of TAFI.

More recently, LMWHs have undergone clinical trials in patients undergoing angioplasty. Marmur and colleagues [7] recently published an article on the successful activated clotting time (ACT)–guided use of dalteparin in interventional cardiology (percutaneous coronary intervention [PCI]). In this study, dalteparin produced a significant increase in the ACT with a small degree of variance compared with UHF. At 80 IU/kg, dalteparin increased the ACT from 125 seconds to 195 seconds. Similarly, the activated partial thromboplastin time (aPTT), Heptest time, anti-IIa activity, and TFPI concentration were increased. These investigators concluded that the ACT and aPTT are sensitive to IV-administered dalteparin at clinically relevant doses. These data suggest that the ACT may be useful in monitoring the anticoagulant effect of IV-administered dalteparin during PCI.

Because of the different anti-Xa and anti-IIa actions, it should be emphasized that each LMWH has its own specific dosage in the interventional cardiovascular indications. Enoxaparin and dalteparin have been used at various dosages in PCI. The comparative anticoagulant effects of various LMWHs as measured by the ACT in patients undergoing PCI are shown in Fig. 10. At a comparative dosage of 100 U/kg IV of various LMWHs, different levels of prolongation of the ACT were measured. Heparin exhibited the strongest prolongation in the ACT. followed by dalteparin, certoparin, and enoxaparin. Thus, the dosing of LMWHs in PCI can be guided by monitoring the ACT.

The effect of dalteparin on the aPTT at two different dosages is depicted in Fig. 11. Dalteparin was administered to patients undergoing PCI at a dosage of 60 or 80 IU/kg IV. Blood samples were drawn at baseline, at 5 minutes, and at

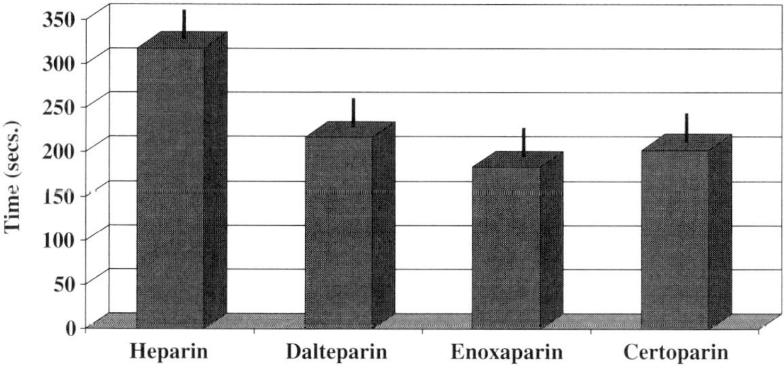

Fig. 10. A comparison of the anticoagulant effect of various LMWHs as measured by ACT in PCI. Heparin produces the strongest anticoagulant effect, whereas the LMWHs produce relatively weaker anticoagulant effects.

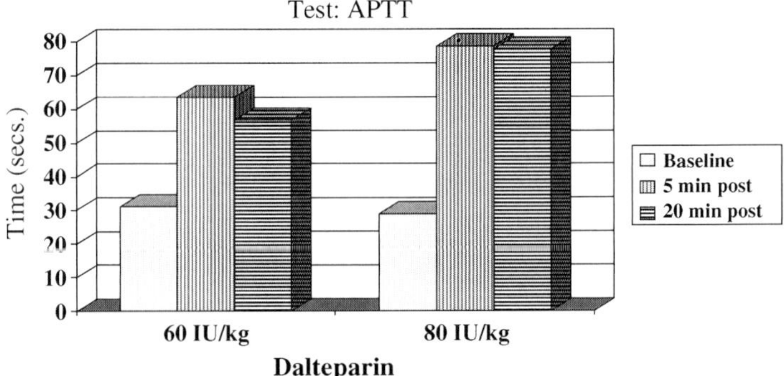

Fig. 11. Comparative anticoagulant effects of dalteparin as measured by aPTT in PCI. Patients were administered 60 and 80 U/kg of dalteparin. A dose-dependent effect is evident.

20 minutes post administration of dalteparin. Fig. 11 shows the prolongation of the aPTT obtained in these patients. A dose response was observed in the aPTT. This study suggested that the aPTT can be used to monitor the anticoagulant effects of dalteparin at these dosages. These data also suggest the view that LMWHs also can be monitored by using the aPTT test. In the same study, the ACT was measured. As shown in Fig. 12, the ACT increased from 125 seconds at baseline to >180 seconds after the administration of 80 IU/kg dalteparin. At the lower dosage, the ACT was prolonged to 170 seconds. Thus, a dose response in the anticoagulant effects of these agents is demonstrable.

The comparative effects of heparin and enoxaparin in PCI as measured by the ACT are shown in Fig. 13. As mentioned before, the prolongation of ACT was more pronounced in the patients treated with heparin (10,000–12,500 U IV) compared with patients treated with enoxaparin (1 mg/kg IV). There was, however, a slight prolongation in the enoxaparin-treated patients, which increased

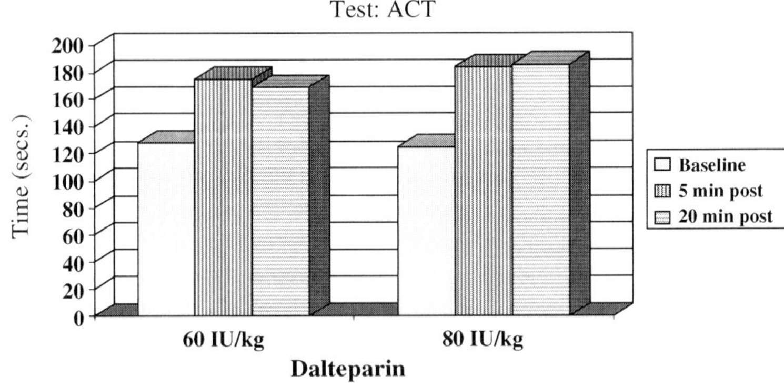

Fig. 12. Comparative anticoagulant effects of dalteparin as measured by ACT in PCI. A dose-dependent effect for 60 and 80 U/kg is observed.

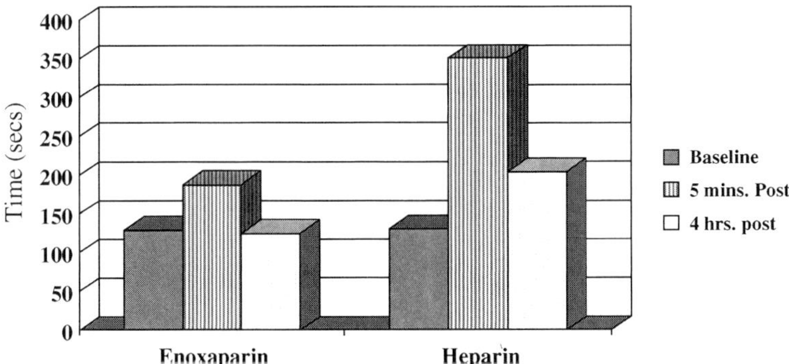

Fig. 13. Comparative anticoagulant effects of UFH and enoxaparin in PCI as measured by ACT. Heparin produced a much stronger effect than enoxaparin.

to 190 seconds. The patients treated with enoxaparin remained anticoagulated throughout the procedure. Although the initial anticoagulant effects of a drug may be stronger, it is likely that the duration of this action may be shorter.

In the same study, the aPTT was measured in the plasma of these patients. As shown in Fig. 14, heparin-treated patients showed a greater prolongation in the aPTT compared with enoxaparin-treated patients. The aPTT value 5 minutes post administration of enoxaparin was >100 seconds. As seen in the previous study using dalteparin, the aPTT can be used at these dosages to monitor the effects of LMWHs. These data suggest that the duration of effects also is dependent on the assay procedure used.

The pharmacokinetics of various LMWHs in terms of biologic half-life as measured by employing the anti-Xa and anti-IIa methods during PCI is depicted in Fig. 15. The half-life of the different LMWHs ranged from 2.3 to 3.4, depending on the LMWH and the method used to determine half-life. Enoxaparin

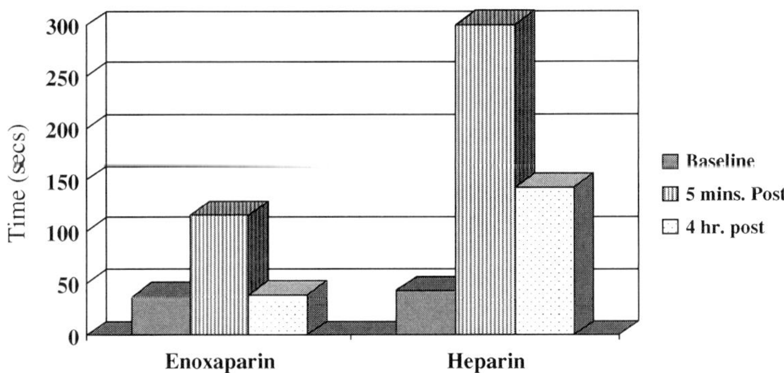

Fig. 14. Comparative anticoagulant effect of heparin and enoxaparin in PCI as measured by aPTT. The relative anticoagulant effect of heparin in this test is much stronger than enoxaparin.

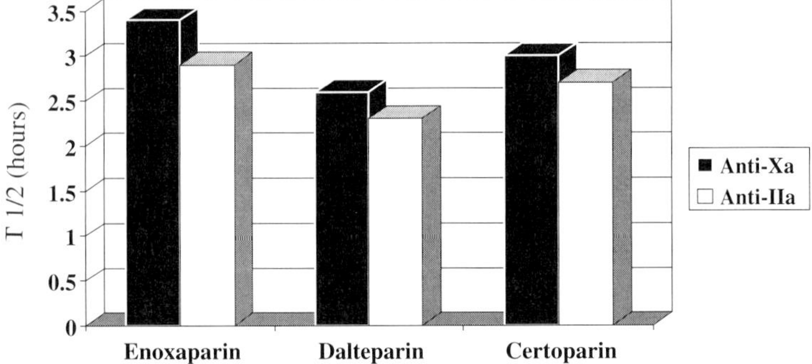

Fig. 15. Pharmacokinetics of three different LMWHs at PCI dosage as measured by anti-Xa and IIa effect. Each drug exhibits interesting effects in terms of the biologic half-life ($T_{1/2}$).

has the longest half-life compared with certoparin and dalteparin. Again, the half-life of this agent is largely dependent on the type of test used.

In addition to the half-life, other pharmacokinetic parameters are equally modulated by individual LMWHs. Each LMWH produces distinct effects and, therefore, may exhibit different profiles. As seen in Fig. 16, different LMWHs gave different clearance rates. Enoxaparin had the highest clearance rate, followed by dalteparin and certoparin. Therefore, the dosing of various LMWHs in interventional cardiology requires individual optimization studies.

One of the drawbacks of the use of LMWHs is that there is no effective antidote to neutralize their effects. Protamine sulfate is only partially effective in the neutralization of LMWHs. More recently, it has been reported that heparinase-1 can neutralize the effects of LMWHs. The digestion of tinzaparin by heparinase-1 is depicted in Fig. 17. Heparinase is an enzyme produced by *Flavobacterium heparinum*. It has been used in several clinical trials and is capable of digesting tinzaparin to form lower molecular weight components

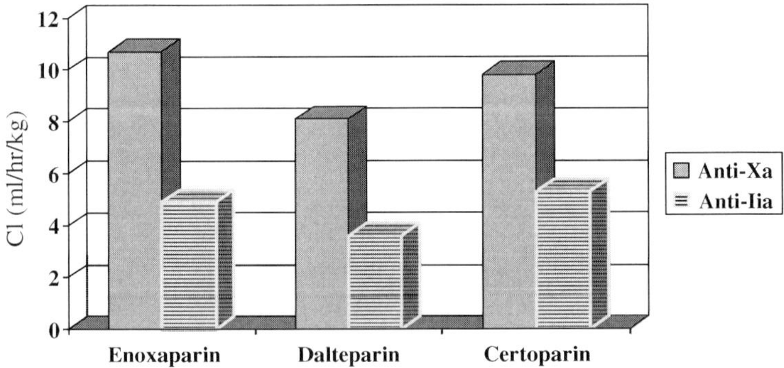

Fig. 16. Pharmacokinetics of various LMWHs during PCI as measured by calculating the clearance rate of the anti-Xa and IIa actions.

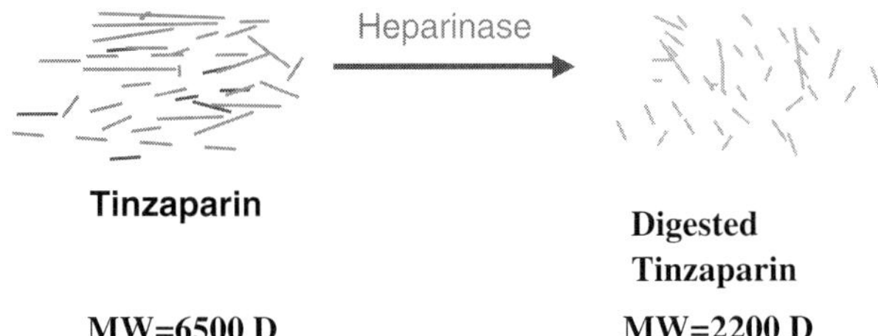

Fig. 17. Heparinase digestion of tinzaparin. Tinzaparin can be digested into various molecular fragments by heparinase. The concentration of heparinase, however, determines the type of oligosaccharides produced. MW, molecular weight.

with a molecular weight in the range of 2200 d. Heparinase is capable of digesting various LMWHs and reducing their anticoagulant actions. This depolymerization is product dependent, and the results show marked variations from one compound to the next. The biologic activities of the resulting products also are different. These data point out that different LMWHs are differentially digested by heparinase-1.

Fig. 18 shows the heparinase digestion of sodium UFH. Heparinase digests UFH and converts it into small molecular weight oligosaccharides. Note the fingerprinting of the digested material. In contrast to heparin, the relative digestion of various LMWHs to heparinase exhibits different profiles. The heparinase digestion of tinzaparin is shown in Fig. 19. Compared with UFH, the fingerprinting of the oligosaccharide profile is different, which clearly suggests that endogenously different LMWHs give rise to different oligosaccharide components. Thus, each LMWH may be digested differentially by endogenous

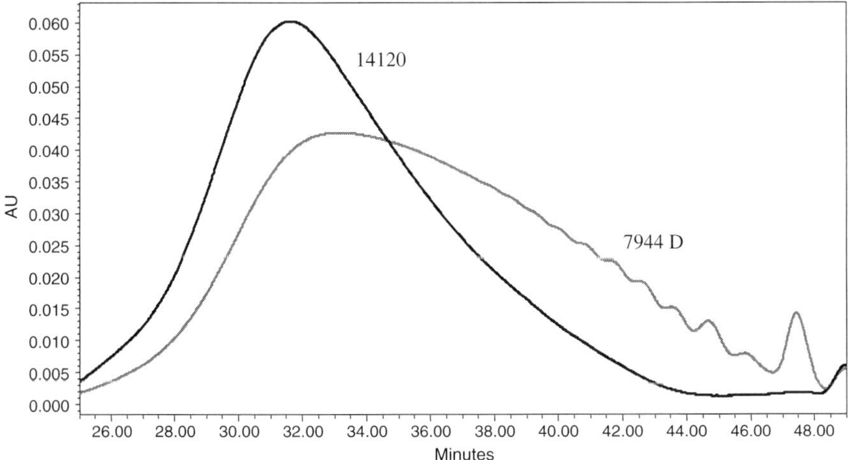

Fig. 18. Heparinase-1 digestion of UFH. A significant reduction in the molecular weight is noted, and the species of oligosaccharides that are formed are visible. UV, ultraviolet.

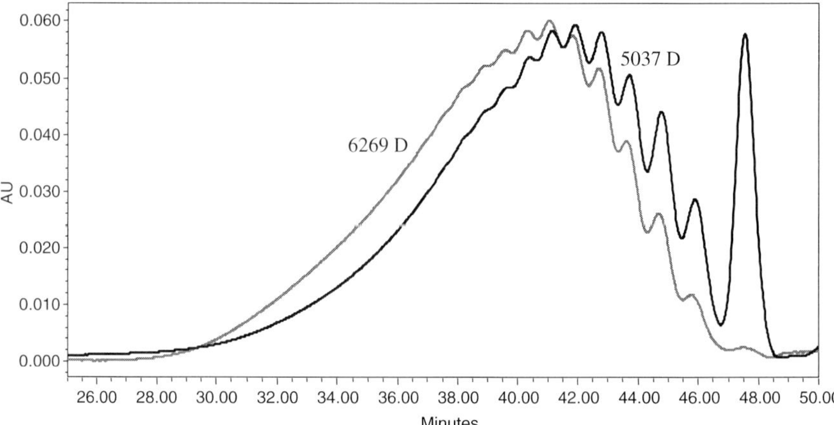

Fig. 19. Heparinase digestion of tinzaparin. At the same heparinase level, tinzaparin is less susceptible to heparinase digestion. UV, ultraviolet.

heparinases. Therefore, the overall pharmacologic action of LMWHs may be dependent on endogenous liver catabolism by heparinase-like enzymes.

Interventional and surgical dosages of LMWHs also can be neutralized by heparinase-1. The effect of heparinase-1 on the interventional dosage of dalteparin as measured by the Heptest is described in Fig. 20. Patients undergoing PCI were treated with 40, 60, or 80 U/kg of dalteparin after heparinase administration. The dalteparin activity, as measured by the Heptest, is completely abolished, which suggests that heparinase is capable of digesting dalteparin. The relative effect of this digestion by heparinase on bleeding and other adverse reactions requires clinical study.

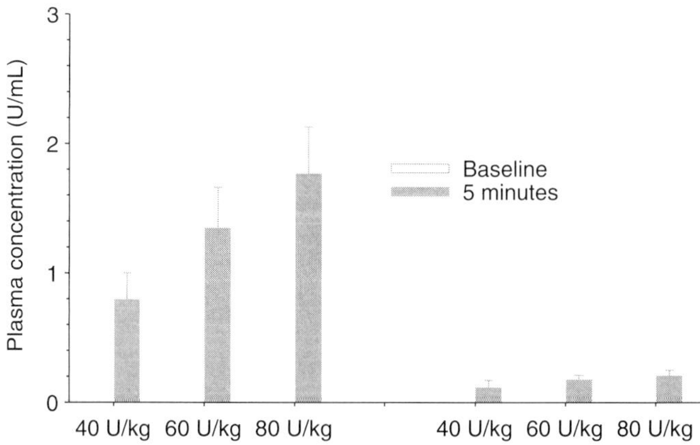

Fig. 20. Effect of heparinase on interventional dosage of dalteparin as measured by Heptest. Samples collected 5 minutes after the administration of 40 to 60 U/kg were completely neutralized by 0.1 U/mL of heparinase in the ex vivo setting.

Although heparin is still the drug of choice for parental anticoagulant therapy, the current data indicate that LMWHs also are capable of producing adequate anticoagulation and antithrombotic effects. Several clinical trials have been completed. At the higher dosages, these drugs can be used for interventional purposes; however, major differences in different products are noted. The following are the current perspectives in parenteral anticoagulant therapy:

- LMWHs currently are being evaluated for surgical and interventional indications.
- Antithrombin drugs are being developed for surgical and interventional use. Unlike heparin, however, there is no antidote for their neutralization.
- Anti-Xa drugs are being developed for various parental indications. Similar to antithrombin drugs, there is no antidote for the neutralization of these agents.
- Major differences in the anticoagulant effects are observed between different LMWHs. Therefore, each drug may produce differential dosing and neutralization approaches.

Based on the published data on the differential behavior of currently available LMWHs, it is clear that each of these drugs is distinct [8–13]. After reviewing the preclinical and clinical data, several regulatory and professional agencies have classified these agents as distinct drugs. The American College of Chest Physicians clearly recommended that LMWHs are different and should not be interchanged. According to American College of Chest Physicians guidelines, the results of clinical trials on LMWHs cannot be generalized to other LMWHs. Thus, the current data on the use of enoxaparin in cardiology are product specific and should only pertain to enoxaparin. The International Cardiology Forum also has the same opinion and has clearly stated that these compounds should be considered as distinct therapeutic agents. Similarly, the American College of Cardiology and American Heart Association have recommended that each drug must be considered individually rather than as interchangeable compounds.

Several other national and international regulatory agencies, along with professional societies, have clearly classified LMWHs as distinct drugs. The US Food and Drug Administration (FDA) has clearly mandated that individual LMWHs cannot be used interchangeably with one another [14]. According to FDA guidelines, LMWHs cannot be used interchangeably, unit for unit, with heparin and one individual LMWH cannot be used interchangeably with another.

The clinical differentiation of LMWHs has been demonstrated in deep vein thrombosis prophylaxis and in treatment for acute coronary syndromes [15–17]. For example, the dosages of enoxaparin and dalteparin are different for acute coronary syndrome [18,19]. Additional data on the clinical differentiation of each of these individual LMWHs are continuously becoming available.

At a higher dosage, such as in surgical use, PCI, and cancer studies, the LMWHs exhibit wide variations in their anticoagulant profile. Similarly, thrombotic stroke and combination treatment protocols have shown the individual effects of LMWHs. It should be emphasized, therefore, that these drugs cannot be interchanged. In the event that interchange is performed, safety and efficacy compromise may be observed, thus risking the welfare of patients.

As shown in Fig. 21, using the depolymerization process, LMWHs, ultra-LMWHs, and heparin-derived oligosaccharides such as pentasaccharides can be prepared. These agents show a progressive change in the anti-Xa/anti-IIa ratio. Therefore, at equivalent anti-Xa activities, these agents exhibit marked differences. It is therefore recommended that these agents should not be considered similar, regardless of potency adjustment. Because most of the commercially available LMWHs are produced by patented manufacturing processes, the resulting products exhibit individual characterization unique to a particular brand of the LMWH. Thus, using patented processes, specific LMWHs can be produced within regulatory guidelines. In addition, generic versions of branded LMWHs can be produced after the expiration of patents. It is important that these generic versions exhibit the same biologic and clinical characterizations.

Although some of the questions on the differentiation of LMWHs have been adequately answered, there may be specific differences that remain unclear at this time. Regardless, the sites of actions of these drugs that contribute to their anticoagulant and antithrombotic actions are known. The mechanisms for the additional actions such as the anti-inflammatory effects, anti-cancer effects, and other regulatory actions, however, remain unclear at this time. Some of these issues have been currently debated in reference to the uniqueness of the commercial product and the claim that the generic versions of LMWHs are not the same as the innovative products.

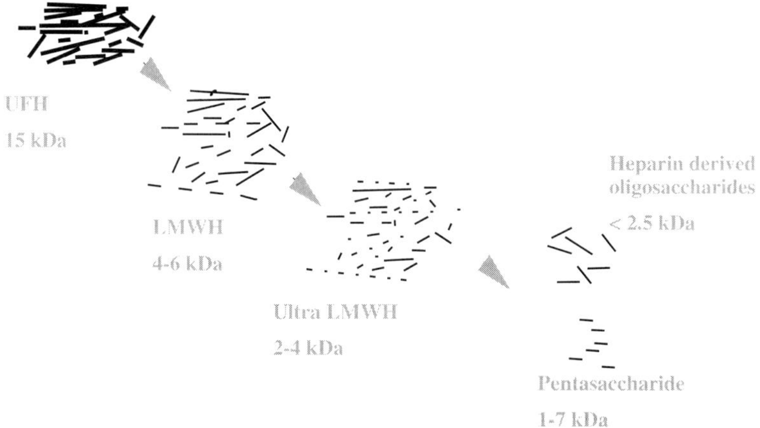

Fig. 21. A diagrammatic illustration of the manufacturing processes for LMWHs and their derivatives. The chemical and the enzymatic depolymerization result in a progress depolymerization of heparins, eventually leading to heparin-derived oligosaccharides. If the depolymerization is exhaustive, then it may result in the generation of heparin-derived disaccharides and trisaccharides.

If a generic version of a branded product is made, then it should use exactly the same process patent and must exhibit physical, chemical, biologic, and clinical equivalence. Therefore, it is very important to make sure that a generic product has a similar profile to the branded product. More important, without regulatory approval, a generic product should not be considered for clinical usage.

A recent communication has addressed several important issues on the possible introduction of generic forms of LMWHs [20]. The investigators argued convincingly in favor of the development of the generic versions of LMWHs and cited certain examples in light of current FDA guidelines. The investigators focused on the equivalence criteria to which the potential manufacturers of generic versions of LMWHs are required to adhere to demonstrate clinical and biologic equivalence of the generic products. They also commented on the nonrequirement for clinical trials of the generic product. The regulatory agency stipulates that a generic drug produced by exactly the same patent/manufacturing conditions is expected to behave similarly to the branded drug. Although this may be true for synthetic drugs such as warfarin and clopidogrel, additional review and discussions in the case of complex mucopolysaccharide-derived agents such as LMWHs will be required.

Because of the complex nature of LMWHs, the adequacy of the current requirements for acceptance of these drugs—be it an original or a generic product—by the regulatory agencies should be questioned. To demonstrate the similarities and differences among various LMWH products, several systematic approaches have been developed [21–23]. The authors recommend that in the case of generic LMWHs, the regulatory bodies have to reconsider their criteria for accepting a generic equivalent. The following lists some of the basic requirements for characterizing a LMWH which should be employed in determining approval of a product as a true generic:

1. Physicochemical equivalence
2. Biological equivalence
3. Pharmacologic and toxicologic equivalence
4. Dosage (for both clinical safety and efficacy) equivalence

In addition to the physicochemical and biologic equivalence, a generic equivalent of a branded drug also should exhibit pharmacologic and toxicologic equivalence at the dosage stipulated in phase I (or equivalent) clinical trials. All studies should be performed over a dosage range at which the branded drug will be used.

Various regulatory agencies such as the FDA, the EMEA, and the World Health Organization consider each of the LMWHs to be a distinct drug. These agencies, however, consider only molecular weight profile and anti-Xa/anti-IIa potency, which may not be adequate for the demonstration of generic product equivalence to the branded product. The branded LMWHs are only partially characterized when these limited specifications are used. A generic version of a branded LMWH not only must be manufactured by exactly the same process as the original drug but also must exhibit physical, chemical, biologic, and clinical equivalence.

The generic pharmaceutical industry has played a key role in providing less expensive equivalents of original branded drugs that otherwise would not be accessible to a large group of patients. Thus, generic drugs have a major public health importance. Recognizing this, President Bush has announced the expansion of the Office of Generic Drugs [24]. Thus, at a federal government level, there is endorsement of the development of generic drugs and to have them accessible to all patients.

There is global pressure to make innovative drug generic versions at a reduced cost. Some regulatory guidelines should be implanted, however, to adjust the operational cost and compensation to companies in the event that a generic version of a branded product is introduced due to the expiration of the patent.

It is now widely agreed that the introduction of generic versions of LMWHs will be approved in the near future. It is important, however, that the generic products are manufactured in strict compliance with the manufacturing specification of the branded product. Furthermore, regulatory agencies should require additional data on the chemical, biologic, pharmacologic/toxicologic, and dose-response relationship in specific settings.

The heparins not only differ substantially in their pharmacodynamics but also in pharmacokinetics. The difficulty in assaying heparins poses another problem because the assays aimed at assessing the pharmacokinetics of UFH or LMWH are based on pharmacodynamic effects such as anti-Xa or anti-IIa activity, rather than direct detection of the molecular species involved [10]. The anti-Xa and anti-IIa activities of UFH correlate well with the concentrations of UFH molecules; however, with enoxaparin, the anti-Xa activity persists for longer than the enoxaparin molecules are detectable [25]. In one study, the anti-Xa activity of enoxaparin persisted for days after discontinuation of SC enoxaparin administered at a dose of 40 mg/d compared with the weak anti-IIa activity during the 7-day treatment period [26]. Enoxaparin is linearly absorbed after SC administration, with peak activity occurring at 2.5 to 4 hours [27–29]. A close relationship also has been shown to exist between the dose of SC-administered enoxaparin and anti-Xa peak activity as measured in plasma using a standardized amidolytic anti-Xa method [30]. LMWHs are absorbed easily from SC tissue and have a lower tendency to bind to endothelial cells [31]. Following the administration of enoxaparin at a dose of 40 mg, more than twice as many heparin molecules of sufficiently high molecular weight to inhibit thrombin were bioavailable than after administration of UFH at a dose of 5000 IU, despite the presence of more than twice the amount of such heparin molecules in the UFH injection [32]. Several studies have shown LMWHs to have greater bioavailability compared with UFH; however, there are significant differences observed among LMWHs following SC administration. The bioavailability of anti-Xa activity varies from 87% with dalteparin to 98% for nadroparin [28]. Bioavailabilities of other LMWHs range from 90% to 98% (90% for tinzaparin,

> 90% for parnaparin and ardeparin) [31]. For anti-Xa activity, enoxaparin (40 mg [4000 IU]) has an AUC of about 3.5 IU · h/mL compared with 3.2 IU · h/mL for dalteparin (5000 IU), 1.35 IU · h/mL for tinzaparin (50 IU/kg), and 1.33 IU · h/mL for UFH (5000 IU). Although the clinical significance is not known, the AUC values for anti-Xa activity are greater than those for anti-II activity [29]. Although laboratory monitoring is required due to high variability in effect following UFH administration [33], the variability with enoxaparin is lower than with UFH [25,34]. The absorption rate of different LMWHs differs in terms of maximal concentration and may or may not be related to bioavailability, which is measurable in terms of AUC. Wide variations in the absorption rate and bioavailability profile are observed with UFH; however, with a given LMWH such as enoxaparin, the absorption rate and bioavailability patterns are consistent and predictable.

The apparent volume of distribution of the anti-Xa activity of enoxaparin and other LMWHs following SC injection is close to plasma or blood volume [29]. The volume of distribution of enoxaparin (5.3 L) has been shown to be significantly lower than dalteparin (7.7 L) and nadroparin (6.8 L) [29]. Significant differences also have been reported for mean residence times. Enoxaparin and nadroparin exhibit significantly longer mean residence times (7 hours) than dalteparin (about 5.3 hours) [29].

UFH and LMWHs are metabolized by depolymerization and desulfation [31,35]. After getting degraded by the liver, they are eliminated by the kidneys in forms retaining their biologic activity [35]. The clearance of enoxaparin and other LMWHs does not change as a function of administered dose (unlike that of UFH, which is dose dependent), which may be attributed to the lower cellular uptake of LMWHs compared with UFH [36]. The average apparent total body clearance of enoxaparin has been shown to be lower than that of UFH [36], and further differences also have been observed between enoxaparin, dalteparin, and nadroparin [28]. In a comparative study between enoxaparin (20 mg and 40 mg; equivalent to 2000 IU and 4000 IU of anti-Xa activity), dalteparin (2500 IU; equivalent to 2500 IU of anti-Xa activity), and nadroparin (7500 IU; equivalent to 3075 IU of anti-Xa activity) injected SC, the average apparent total body clearance of enoxaparin was 1.56 mL/min, which was significantly lower than dalteparin (33 mL/min) and nadroparin (21.4 mL/min) [28]. Dalteparin, therefore, is cleared from the body more rapidly than nadroparin and enoxaparin.

The use of LMWHs has been studied in young and old patients. Its safety has been investigated in a group of very elderly patients (over 80 years, mean age 84) with unstable coronary artery disease. Ninety-eight such patients were randomized to treatment with enoxaparin (1.0 mg/kg SC twice daily) or UFH (1000 IU/h as a continuous IV infusion) for 7 days. There were no significant differences between the groups in the rate of bleeding, cardiac death, angina pectoris, or changes in ECG. This study showed that no obvious adverse events were observed at these doses in the elderly patients recruited in this study. An open study in children who received enoxaparin for a variety of indications showed that a therapeutic anti-Xa activity generally could be obtained after a dose of 1.0 mg/kg twice daily SC. Newborn infants (under 2 months old), however, required a mean dose of 1.6 mg/kg twice daily. The open design of the trial made it difficult to assess the safety of enoxaparin precisely in this population, but no obvious limitations on the safety of enoxaparin were observed. Of interest is a study of 19 children (aged 18 days to 19 years) that showed that a starting dose of 1.0 mg/kg SC enoxaparin twice daily achieved the adult therapeutic target anti-Xa activities. These results, however, should be confirmed, owing to the small number of patients in the study population [37].

Major randomized controlled trials support the use of LMWH as an alternative to UFH in the management of non–ST-segment elevation myocardial infarction [38–41]. The Fragmin in Unstable Coronary Artery Disease Study [39] and the Fraxiparin versus Unfractionated Heparin in Acute Coronary Syndrome [40] trials of dalteparin and nadroparin, respectively, showed equivalence of LMWH with UFH. The Efficacy and Safety of Subcutaneous Enoxaparin in Non-Q-wave Coronary Events (ESSENCE) study and the Thrombolysis in Myocardial Infarction (TIMI) 11B study [41] showed a significant reduction in the composite end points of death, myocardial infarction, and recurrent angina leading to revascularization in patients with unstable angina or non-Q-wave myocardial infarction with enoxaparin versus UFH [40,41]. The Global Registry of Acute Coronary Events is a large prospective study of patients hospitalized with acute coronary syndrome. This study has been launched to improve the quality of care of patients with acute coronary syndrome by providing information about differences or relationships between patient characteristics, treatment practices, and hospital outcomes. In the current Global Registry of Acute Coronary Events report, the use of LMWH and UFH was analyzed in 13,231 acute coronary syndrome patients [42]. The results revealed that patients younger than 60 years receiving antiplatelet therapy, β-blockers, and angiotensin-converting enzyme inhibitors; patients admitted to hospitals with PCI facilities; and patients undergoing invasive procedures received UFH or UFH plus LMWH rather than LMWH alone (80.1% enoxaparin, 19.9% other LMWH). After adjusting for covariables, the use of LMWH was associated with a 37% lower risk of mortality ($P = 0.009$) and 55% lower bleeding rates ($P < 0.0001$) across all acute coronary syndrome categories, and similar results were found in STEMI and UA/NSTEMI subgroups. One of the limitations of the current study is that 80% of patients received enoxaparin; it is cautioned that the results may not be generalized to all LMWHs. This caution is perhaps due to the fact that LMWHs are different entities.

Predictable pharmacodynamic effects after dosing with LMWHs are encouraging and clinical experience has been promising. Two recent trials of enoxaparin in acute coronary syndromes have shown that the theoretic advantages of enoxaparin are indeed realized in terms of important clinical outcomes. The ESSENCE trial compared enoxaparin with UFH in 3171 patients with angina at rest or non-Q-wave myocardial infarction. The risk of death, myocardial infarction, or recurrent angina was significantly lower in the enoxaparin group at 14 days (16.6% versus 19.8%, $P = 0.019$) and at 30 days (19.8% versus 23.3%,

$P = 0.016$), an effect that was maintained until 1 year after initial treatment. The TIMI 11B trial [42] included 3910 patients with unstable angina or non-Q-wave myocardial infarction who were treated with UFH or enoxaparin. The primary end point was death, myocardial infarction, or urgent revascularization in the first 8 days of treatment, which was slightly significantly more common in the UFH group than in the enoxaparin group (14.5% versus 12.4%, $P = 0.048$). Other LMWHs (nadroparin and dalteparin) also have been compared with UFH in unstable angina patients. The results of the major clinical trials have shown that nadroparin and dalteparin are equivalent in terms of efficacy to UFH. Although there are no trials comparing enoxaparin, nadroparin, and dalteparin, the encouraging findings of the ESSENCE and TIMI 11B trials support the use of enoxaparin in unstable angina patients. These findings are further supported by a recent head-to-head trial between enoxaparin and tinzaparin in 438 patients with unstable angina or non-Q-wave myocardial infarction that showed that antithrombotic treatment with enoxaparin for 7 days was more effective than tinzaparin at reducing the incidence of recurrent angina in the early phase and significantly reduced the need for revascularization at 30 days.

Some recent trials in patients undergoing PCI have confirmed that enoxaparin is effective. The Enoxaparin and Ticlopidine after Elective Stenting trial compared a combination of enoxaparin, aspirin, and ticlopidine with UFH, dipyridamole, and warfarin in patients who had undergone coronary stenting. The composite end point of death, myocardial infarction, stent thrombosis, coronary artery bypass graft, and repeat percutaneous transluminal coronary angioplasty at 30 days was significantly lower in the enoxaparin group (4 of 79 patients) than in the UFH group (9 of 44 patients). The National Investigators Collaborating on Enoxaparin 1 and 4 (NICE-1 and NICE-4) trials treated patients undergoing PCI with enoxaparin alone (NICE-1) or in combination with abciximab (NICE-4). Both trials were open label. The incidence of major non–coronary artery bypass graft–related bleeding was 0.5% of 828 patients in the NICE-1 trial and only 0.2% of 818 patients in the NICE-4 trial. There seemed to be a synergistic effect of enoxaparin and abciximab, the combination being more effective than either drug alone.

As an illustration of the differences that can occur between LMWHs, enoxaparin (40 mg once daily) was compared with UFH (5000 IU three times a day) as prophylaxis against venous thrombosis in patients undergoing hip surgery. The incidence of deep vein thrombosis was 25% in a group of 113 patients receiving UFH and 12.5% in a group of 124 patients receiving enoxaparin ($P = 0.03$). This benefit is important for enoxaparin, particularly in view of the more convenient dosing regimen. In contrast, a trial with a similar design that compared nadroparin with UFH found very similar rates of deep vein thrombosis in both treatment groups (33% of 137 nadroparin patients versus 34% of 136 UFH patients). Although this trial clearly cannot be regarded as a direct comparison of enoxaparin and nadroparin in this indication, it appears that LMWHs have the advantage over UFH of reducing the incidence of deep vein thrombosis, whereas nadroparin does not.

Pentasaccharide (fondaparinux) versus low molecular weight heparins

Fondaparinux (Arixtra; Sanofi-Synthélabo/Organon) is the first of a new class of antithrombotic agents. Like the originally investigated heparin pentasaccharide, this synthetic selective factor Xa (FXa) inhibitor mimics the site of heparin that binds to ATIII; however, there are several minor structural differences between these two agents. Fondaparinux has several potentially important advantages over other antithrombotic agents (Box 1). It proved to be an effective antithrombotic through numerous animal model investigations, now confirmed through four phase III clinical trials in orthopedic surgery [44–48]. The FDA has approved fondaparinux for the prevention of venous thromboembolic events following orthopedic surgery. Although a 55% relative risk reduction of venous thrombosis was found in clinical trials, the bleeding risk with fondaparinux was not reduced compared with LMWHs.

A comparison of the original heparin pentasaccharide and various LMWHs is given in Table 4. LMWHs show wide variations in their physicochemical, biochemical, and pharmacologic actions; pentasaccharide exhibits markedly different properties in comparison to these drugs. It has a homogenous molecular weight distribution and exhibits high anti-Xa activity, low USP activity, and strong antithrombotic and bleeding actions. The relative release of TFPI is much lower with the pentasaccharide. The reported incidence of heparin-induced thrombocytopenia (HIT II) is surprisingly high, as depicted in Table 5. Because pentasaccharide does not show any anti-IIa activity, its anti-Xa/IIa ratio is ∞ compared with the LMWHs (1.5–4.0), as shown in Fig. 22. The anti-Xa activities of LMWHs range from 140 to 160 U/mg in contrast to the specific activity of pentasaccharide, which is around 650 U/mg. Although the anti-IIa activities of various LMWHs range from 59 to 26 U/mg, pentasaccharide does not show any anti-IIa actions.

Although solely dependent on ATIII to inhibit FXa and, therefore, thrombin generation, fondaparinux is distinct from heparin and LMWH, with a unique therapeutic profile apparently based on the sole targeting of FXa. The synthetic nature of fondaparinux provides for a pure material of one known chemical

Box 1. Potential advantages of fondaparinux

- Synthetic
- No viral or other animal contaminants
- Well-defined pure, homogenous molecular structure
- Relatively long half-life
- Superior bioavailability
- Predictable dose effect
- Does not interact with platelet factor 4
- Does not cross-react with heparin antibody

Table 4
Low molecular weight heparin versus heparin pentasaccharide

LMWH	Heparin pentasaccharide
Polycomponent drug composed of oligosaccharide chains ranging in composition (4–14 hexose units)	Synthetic oligosaccharide composed of five hexose units
Prepared by the depolymerization of porcine mucosal heparin by various processes	Synthesized by organic chemical methods
Oligosaccharide chains exhibit affinity to ATIII and heparin cofactor II	Sole affinity to ATIII, exhibits high affinity
Exhibits anti-Xa and anti-IIa activities	Exhibits only anti-Xa activity
Releases TFPI from vascular endothelium	Does not release TFPI from the vascular endothelium
Partially neutralizable by protamine sulfate	Not neutralized by protamine sulfate
Does not pass through the placental or blood-brain barrier	Partially able to pass the blood-brain barrier
Capable of forming complexes with platelet factor 4	Does not form complexes with platelet factor 4
Polytherapeutic actions	Monotherapeutic actions

structure with no biologic and pharmacologic differences between batches. It is characterized by complete bioavailability when administered SC, rapid onset of action, no evidence of metabolism, and renal excretion. To date, no drug interactions or nonspecific protein binding has been reported with fondaparinux. Based on the 14- to 20-hour half-life and predictable pharmacokinetics in healthy volunteer studies, once-a-day dosing and no monitoring currently are being recommended for clinical use. This drug does not affect the aPTT, prothrombin time, or ACT assays. Drug levels can be determined only by anti-Xa assays. There is no established antidote for this agent.

Fondaparinux continues to be studied in additional clinical settings such as interventional cardiology procedures and as an adjunct to thrombolysis. The pharmacokinetic profile makes this drug optimal for long-term thrombosis prophylaxis such as in-home therapy. Long-term safety studies, however, are required.

Synthetic oligosaccharides mimicking the ATIII binding site in heparin have been the focus of intense research directed toward the understanding of the

Table 5
Incidence of heparin-induced thrombocytopenia with low molecular weight heparins

Heparin	Incidence of HIT II
UFH (American College of Chest Physicians meta-analysis)	1%
Dalteparin (meta-analysis)	0.3%
Enoxaparin (Adventis documents)	1.9%
Tinzaparin [43]	1%
Pentasaccharide	3.9%

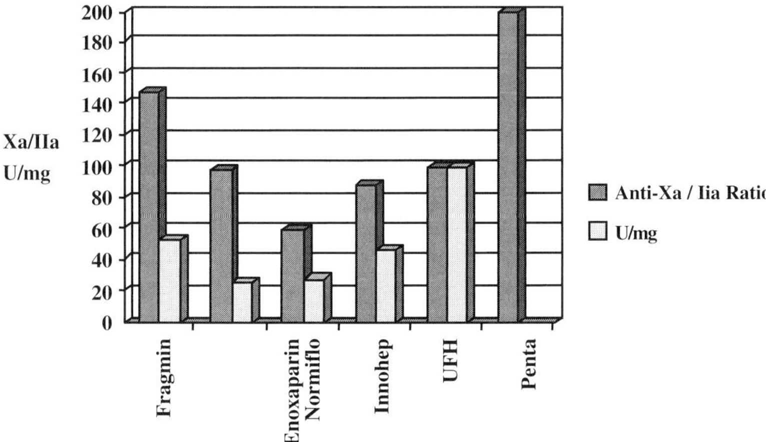

Fig. 22. Comparison of anti-Xa/anti-IIa ratios of LMWHs and pentasaccharide. Penta, pentasaccaride.

mechanisms of action of heparins. Hypersulfated oligosaccharides with specific sulfated hexose units have been developed to study the interaction of heparin cofactor II with heparin-related drugs. The synthetic heparin pentasaccharide (fondaparinux) represents a sole anti–FXa agent and is devoid of inhibiting any other proteases in contrast to heparins; however, fondaparinux provides a novel approach to designer drug development. It also provides insight into the mechanism of action of heparin and LMWH. The synthetic nature of this agent offers the possibility to produce structurally designed derivatives and analogs that can provide unique tools for defined structure–activity relationship studies related to heparin and ATIII. In the case of fondaparinux, the high potency compared with other heparins accounts for its effectiveness in contrast to other oligosaccharides. In addition, conjugated forms with other agents, such as peptides, can be produced to create more effective antithrombotic drugs. Such conjugates have been prepared and tested in limited studies.

The availability of a synthetic antithrombotic drug may prove to be timely. There is an increased demand for LMWHs and other glycosaminoglycans and there are stricter regulatory controls due to the increase in viral contaminants such as bovine spongiform encephalopathy and other biologic contaminants. It is projected that the supply of animal-source tissue eventually will become limited, reinforcing the development of synthetic drugs [1,49].

As with any new drug, there are certain developmental issues to be considered for fondaparinux. The reported predictable pharmacokinetics are based on studies in normal volunteers and in relatively healthy orthopedic patients. These parameters may not be comparable in pathologic states in which, for example, variations in patient weight occurs, ATIII levels fluctuate with the disease process or with interventional procedure/surgery, and renal dysfunction or liver disease is common. Therefore, the FDA has alerted physicians to not use this drug at fixed dosage in underweight patients [49].

The lack of dose-efficacy response in different clinical trials deserves further investigation because there is no clear explanation for these observations with fondaparinux [49]. In addition, the interpretation of the bleeding and thrombosis rates observed with fondaparinux and LMWH in the VTE prevention trials already has been questioned in several public forums [49]. Are the differences between the two drugs due to the drug itself or the regimen of the study designs (LMWH starting 12–24 hours after surgery compared with 6 ± 2 hours after surgery for fondaparinux)? The clinical trial study designs for this agent did not allow for a valid comparison from a pharmacologic standpoint. If fondaparinux and the comparator LMWH are given at identical times, the outcome results may be different.

The observed bleeding questions the appropriateness of the fixed dosing regimen without monitoring. The clinical bleeding events reported in several trials with fondaparinux were somewhat unexpected. From the structure–activity relationship standpoint, it was predicted that oligosaccharides such as pentasaccharide should not produce any bleeding effects. The long half-life may have an effect on drug accumulation, especially in patients with impaired clearance. Unlike heparin, the effects of fondaparinux cannot be neutralized by conventional methods. There may be subpopulations of patients who will require monitoring for safety and efficacy reasons. It also should be considered that the traditional clot-based assays for monitoring heparin cannot be used to monitor fondaparinux at high or low doses [49].

Fondaparinux represents a small molecular weight oligosaccharide that can cross placental and blood-brain barriers. Therefore, its use in pregnant women and in elderly patients with compromised blood-brain barrier is questioned. Prolonged usage of this agent may result in drug accumulation, with projected bleeding complications. Similarly, this agent can pass through various membranes, suggesting that its efficacy in hemodialysis and in other indications in which membranes are used is questionable [48].

Although fondaparinux is a heparinomimetic, it only exhibits a monotherapeutic pharmacologic action of heparin; namely, the anti-FXa effect on binding to ATIII. It is devoid of the other therapeutic effects of heparins, such as the release of TFPI, antithrombin, profibrinolytic actions, and anti-inflammatory targets. Thus, the safety/efficacy profile of this agent in specific indications is likely distinct from that of heparins. It may be possible, however, to combine fondaparinux with other anticoagulant/antithrombotic agents to achieve desired therapeutic actions, as in the case of clopidogrel and aspirin.

How and when fondaparinux is used clinically and how it will compete with LMWHs, direct thrombin inhibitors, and direct FXa inhibitors to combat the various types of clinical thromboses remain to be determined. The indirect nature of the therapeutic action of this drug and sole dependence on ATIII, along with only anti-Xa actions make this drug a somewhat-narrow therapeutic efficacy agent. In addition, the cost for fondaparinux has not yet been established except in the recommended use for prophylactic indications. Nevertheless, synthetic agents have certain advantages over naturally derived products, not the least of which is their specific chemical design to target desired biologic effects.

Fondaparinux essentially represents the oligosaccharide consensus sequence of heparin, which is capable of binding to ATIII, facilitating FXa/thrombin generation inhibition actions [49]. The discovery of oligosaccharides with the ATIII binding consensus was based on the isolation of ethanol-precipitated oligosaccharides from fractionated or depolymerized LMWHs. Such oligosaccharides are present in varying proportions in the available LMWH preparations. Thus, fondaparinux represents a purified and concentrated homogenous oligosaccharide with strong affinity to ATIII; however, it lacks the other functional components of heparin that express additional pharmacologic activities. Thus, the other actions of LMWHs, such as the anti-inflammatory, profibrinolytic, anticancer, and antiproliferative actions may not be observed with pentasaccharide [49].

To compare fondaparinux to LMWHs, several fundamental and biologic considerations may be taken into account. Fondaparinux is a synthetic homogenous oligosaccharide with defined chemical characteristics, whereas LMWHs represent a diverse group of drugs that are prepared after digestion of porcine mucosal heparin. Not only do these oligosaccharides vary in their molecular composition but they also exhibit diverse pharmacologic actions including interactions with ATIII and heparin cofactor II, release of TFPI, interactions with growth factors, modulation of adhesion molecules, and endothelial cell effects. It is unlikely that fondaparinux will exhibit all these biologic actions based on its structure–activity relationships. The interplay between various oligosaccharide components of LMWHs and a dynamic balance with these drugs make the LMWHs a unique group of drugs [49].

Because thrombogenesis is a polypathologic process in which multiple targeting of cellular and plasmatic sites may be important, fondaparinux may only have a narrow spectrum compared with LMWHs. Although in reported clinical trials, fondaparinux (at a relatively lower dosage) exhibited a superior therapeutic efficacy compared with a specific LMWH, the relative hemorrhagic effects of fondaparinux were, in several instances, higher than the comparator drug. Based on the current data, the therapeutic index of fondaparinux is relatively narrow compared with LMWHs. Additional clinical trials and comparisons with LMWHs are warranted to validate the claim that fondaparinux is superior to LMWH. The results of other indications such as acute coronary syndromes do not show any superiority over LMWHs. The relative hemorrhagic risks at a low dose (without having any antidote) and the absence of a clear-cut dose therapeutic response in different clinical trials require additional basic studies to understand these observations [49].

Due to their polypharmacologic actions, LMWHs are now proved to be effective at their optimized dosages in expanded indications in thrombotic and cardiovascular disorders. Whether fondaparinux will exhibit a similar expanded therapeutic spectrum is unknown at the present time. Based on current biochemical and pharmacologic knowledge, it is reasonable to speculate that a comparable clinical spectrum for this designer synthetic heparin analog may not be achievable. It must be stressed, however, that there may be certain endogenous biologic actions of fondaparinux independent of its interaction with ATIII that may be responsible for some of the effects of this drug. Whether fundamental research will clarify this hypothesis is unknown. From a developmental standpoint, it is unlikely that the polypharmacologic actions and the expanded clinical spectrum of LMWHs can be equated by fondaparinux [49]. The development of oligosaccharide conjugates that express additional actions such as antithrombin and TFPI release may eventually provide a drug with a comparable pharmacologic and clinical profile [49].

Fondaparinux is an indirect-acting drug that requires endogenous ATIII for it actions. In contrast to other synthetic peptide/peptidomimetic agents that can directly inhibit FXa, this agent is limited in its antiprotease spectrum. Furthermore, it does not exhibit any antiprotease actions on its own, which may be one of the reasons why this agent does not exhibit a clear dose dependence in most of the clinical trials. The synthetic anti-FXa agents also possess additional antiprotease actions, whereas fondaparinux is devoid of these effects. The relative half-life of fondaparinux is long, probably due to its interactions with ATIII; however, the biologic half-life of non–ATIII-affinity pentasaccharides is found to be short. Thus, the prolonged half-life of fondaparinux is due to its binding to ATIII. The synthetic anti-FXa agents exhibit varying degrees of anti-FXa effects, and the relative biologic actions also may differ. Thus, the pharmacokinetic and pharmacodynamic behavior of these drugs may be quite variable; however, because of their direct anti-FXa actions, the biologic actions may be predictable. Because the synthetic anti-FXa agents do not have any affinity to ATIII, their interactions with ATIII at vascular sites and other cell membranes may be unpredictable [49].

It is important to know that the development of pentasaccharide is basically due to the understanding of the oligosaccharide composition of LMWHs. The discovery of pentasaccharide was based on the identification of the ATIII binding consensus region in the LMWHs. In these drugs, oligosaccharides of similar molecular weight without any affinity to ATIII also are present. To compare LMWHs in a stepwise fashion, some of the characteristics of these drugs are directly listed along with pentasaccharide in Table 6. This agent represents only a portion of the polycomponent pharmacologic actions of LMWHs. It is generally assumed that nearly all of the pharmacologic actions of LMWHs are dependent on the interaction of ATIII. In reality, this assumption is not valid. Many of the pharmacologic effects of heparins are mediated by way of non-ATIII processes. Pentasaccharide also is incapable of releasing TFPI and other biologic mediators from the vascular sites. This is in contrast to LMWHs, which are capable of releasing several mediators from the vascular sites. The presence of non–ATIII-affinity oligosaccharide components also influences the biologic actions of ATIII-affinity components of LMWHs. Such is not the case with pentasaccharide.

Table 6
Comparison of fondaparinux with various low molecular weight heparins

Agent	MW <2500 d	MW >7500 d	Anti-Xa (U/mg)	USP (U/kg)	ATIII activity	Bleeding index (IV)	Bleeding index (SC)	TFPI release
Fragmin	4%	25%	148	75	14	0.3	45	110
Lovenox	15%	37%	98	53	9	0.5	68	120
Normiflo	6%	35%	60	70	5	0.9	35	130
Innohep	8%	31%	89	60	14	0.8	71	168
Pentasaccharide	100%	0%	650	<5	3	0.3	27	24

Abbreviation: mw, molecular weight.

Side effects and adverse reactions to heparin, low molecular weight heparin, and pentasaccharide

Heparin has been the most important anticoagulant in clinical use over the past half century. It is effective, relatively inexpensive, and readily available. Even today, it represents the most common agent for the treatment of acute thrombosis. Its extensive clinical use has commonly led to complacency and even disregard of the potential complications that relate to its use in the therapeutic setting. Although bleeding is the most obvious potential complication of heparin therapy, a common sequela is HIT II, which further can be complicated by the advent of thrombosis. Less common complications include osteoporosis, skin reactions, eosinophilia, alopecia, liver dysfunction, and hyperkalemia. The following review characterizes these potential, often serious sequelae (Box 2).

Heparin-induced thrombocytopenia

Although immune-mediated HIT II was first described by Fedlar and Jacques in 1948 [50], the characterization of clinical manifestations associated with this finding, definition of the potential sequelae, delineation of laboratory features, and recognition of the related therapeutic concepts have largely evolved only during the past decade [51–66].

Two clinical forms of HIT II are now recognized. The first, now commonly termed *HIT II type I* (HIT I), is a nonidiosyncratic, nonimmunologic form (Box 3). The thrombocytopenia occurs early in the exposure: within the first few

Box 2. Side effects of heparin therapy

Potentially severe

Bleeding
Acute heparin ''anaphylaxis''
HIT II

Generally mild

Heparin-associated osteoporosis
Skin reactions: urticaria, erythematous papules, skin necrosis
Abnormal liver function tests
Eosinophilia
Hyperkalemia
Hypoaldosteronism
Priapism
Alopecia

Box 3. Heparin-induced thrombocytopenia type I (non-immune; non-idiosyncratic)

Episode of thrombocytopenia occurs early in exposure: generally, in the first few days in naïve patients and in the first hours in previously exposed patients
Mild thrombocytopenia: 10% to 30% decrease in platelet numbers
Clinical manifestations: none
Mechanism: heparin-induced platelet aggregation.
True incidence: uncertain (but common)
Biologic issues: episode transient—counts normalize even with continued therapy
Therapy: none
Relationship to HIT II: unclear, but probably none

days of therapy in the heparin naïve patient and within hours in the patient previously exposed to heparin. The decline in platelet numbers is modest (10%–30%) and not associated with any clinical manifestations. The decline in platelet numbers is the result of platelet aggregation by a mechanism or mechanisms that are currently uncertain; nevertheless, the aggregation is associated with platelet sequestration and increased consumption. Higher molecular weight heparins have the greatest likelihood of producing this change. Of particular interest is that the episodes are transient and platelet counts normalize by unknown mechanisms, despite continued exposure to heparin. Presently, there is no evidence that this clinical laboratory event is related to the more serious immune form of HIT II (commonly termed *HIT II-II*).

By contrast, HIT II is an immune-mediated lesion with serous clinical sequelae and significant morbidity and mortality [56,58,62,64,66]. Some have considered this lesion to have two subtypes, HIT II-II and HITT, the later serving to recognize the presence of thrombosis that is often the important clinical result of immune HIT II. Box 4 lists the common clinical characteristics of this lesion. Although recognition of the decreased number of platelets generally takes place after several days of therapy (3–14 days, with the median day being day 10), prior exposure to heparin can result in precipitous declines in circulating platelet numbers, even within hours. Also, most instances of HITT involve antibodies to the multimolecular heparin/platelet factor 4 complex (IgG, IgA, or IgM idiotypes); however, rarer antibodies appear to be against platelet membrane interleukin (IL)-8 or platelet membrane neutrophil activating peptide-2 (protein) receptors; these rarer forms may not behave typically with respect to temporal relationships with heparin delivery or degree of decrease in platelet count.

Historically, the parameter of diagnostic recognition was a decrease in platelets to below 100×10^9/L. It is now clear that clinical sequelae can occur

Box 4. Clinical features of heparin-induced thrombocytopenia type II

1. Usual onset at day 3 to day 14 (median day 10)
2. Nadir platelet count: usually 30,000 to 60,000 but may be as low as 5000. The most appropriate definition is a 50% decrease in platelet numbers from the baseline values.
3. Risk factors:
   a. Can occur with all methods of administration:
      Most common: continuous infusion of UFH
      Seen: heparin flushes at 500 U/d; heparin-coated catheters at 3 U/h
      Higher with IV than SC administration
      Greater: bovine > porcine > LMWHs
   b. Can occur within hours in previously treated patients
   c. Increased incidence with recent surgery (primarily venous problems)
   d. Increased incidence with pre-existing cardiovascular disease (primarily arterial).
   e. Absent risks:
      Equal in men and women
      Age not a factor
      No relation to inherited deficiency or founder defects of clotting factors

when a significant decline in platelet numbers occurs, even when the usual parameter of true thrombocytopenia is not present [66]. Therefore, there is no specific platelet number that should be used to trigger suspicion of the presence of HIT II. Currently, the best-working rule is that the diagnosis must be suspected when the platelet count falls by 30% from the baseline and should be strongly considered or ruled out when the platelet count has declined to 50% of baseline levels [66,67]. This rule infers that the thrombocytopenia may be relative rather than absolute because the patients' baseline values may be in the 250 to 400 $\times$ 10^9/L range, a circumstance that is particularly true in surgical patients. Postoperative patients who have undergone cardiac surgery (particularly bypass procedures) have special criteria because most such patients have platelet counts in the 100 to 150 $\times$ 10^9/L range during the first postoperative day. In such circumstances, the diagnosis of HIT II should be based on a platelet count that is reduced 50% from the day 1 postoperative platelet count [66]. An appropriate postoperative clinical parameter is that for any patient whose platelet count declines 20% to 30% from a day 1 postoperative value, the physician should suspect HIT II and follow such individuals with daily platelet counts.

When suspecting HIT II in any medical or surgical patient, it is extremely important to graph out the platelet count, noting the rate of decline and temporal relationships to heparin administration. The rate of decline, as with other immune-mediated thrombocytopenias, typically is rapid, generally even more rapid than other immune thrombocytopenias and typically much more rapid than nonimmune causes of thrombocytopenia (disseminated intravascular coagulation; marrow suppressive mechanisms including medications, sepsis, and other causes).

An important clinical rule is that HIT II can occur with any amount and any type of heparin that is administered by any route. Although HIT II is most common with the continuous infusion of UFH, it has occurred with heparin flushes as low as 500 U/d and even with heparin-coated catheters in which the delivery can be as low as 3 U/h [68,69].

An important component of HIT II is the development of thrombotic lesions, which is ominous and associated with significant morbidity and mortality. Its threat, therapeutic urgency, and treatment complexities are such that the term *HIT-thrombosis* (often abbreviated HITT) has been applied to highlight this sequence, and considerable effort has been expended to attempt to define risk factors for this occurrence [70,71]. Indeed, it is of interest that even with severe thrombocytopenia (counts $< 10 \times 10^9$/L), thrombosis is a more common sequela than bleeding. It merits noting that in earlier literature regarding HIT II, the event of vascular thrombosis was almost entirely correlated with large vessel arterial occlusions. Indeed, the term *white clot syndrome* had been used to highlight the event of a massive arterial occlusion of the lower extremity [70,72,73]. Clinical experience now has identified thrombotic sequelae in arterial and venous circulation [68,73,74]. It is unfortunate that in a given patient who has developed HIT II, the clinician cannot predict the subsequent advent of thrombosis; however, it is now evident that in patients who develop HIT II in juxtaposition to recent surgery, the thrombosis occurs most commonly in the venous circulation. By contrast, the occurrence of HIT II in patients with pre-existing cardiovascular disease commonly results in arterial occlusions [68,71,75]. Also, pulmonary emboli are quite common in medical and surgical patients developing HITT. In attempts to better characterize the risks, it has been noted that the incidence of HIT II is similar in men and women and age is not a factor. Therefore, when strongly suspecting HITT, not only must the heparin be immediately withdrawn but also a careful search for evidence of thrombosis must be initiated. Also, the presence of inherited deficiencies of clotting factors (ie, antithrombin, protein C, or protein S) or founder mutations (ie, factor V Leiden, Prothrombin G20210A) does not correlate with the occurrence of HIT II or the thrombotic sequelae (ie, HITT).

The diagnostic criteria for HIT II are shown in Box 5. Although past definitions have included a definable platelet number to denote the degree of thrombocytopenia, these parameters no longer apply, as discussed previously. Classically, one would expect that another cause of the thrombocytopenia has been excluded. It is unfortunate that the temporal events in HIT II often are so

Box 5. Heparin-induced thrombocytopenia type II (immune-idiosyncratic)

Common diagnostic criteria

1. Thrombocytopenia: decrease of 50% or more from baseline platelet numbers
2. Absence of other cause
3. Confirmation by a heparin-associated antibody assay
4. Return to normal platelet numbers when heparin is stopped

abrupt that a long-agonizing clinical evaluation of other potential mechanisms to explain the thrombocytopenia often can contribute to severe clinical sequelae [66,67]. Therefore, these criteria are interpreted to mean that clinical judgment has eliminated other causes (including noting the rate of platelet count decrease, temporal relationships with heparin, and evaluation of comorbid conditions and medications) and that HIT II is the most likely responsible diagnosis. Similarly, a delay in diagnosis and therapy to await a serologic confirmation is, in general, no longer acceptable. From the studies of Walenga and Bick [66,67], the multiplicity of tests and lack of an absolute "gold standard" further emphasizes the importance of clinical judgment. An important basis for such a conclusion is related to some of the complex temporal relationships in the clinical features of HIT II. Thus, as many as 45% of the thrombotic episodes of HIT II occur in the first 48 hours after identification of the thrombocytopenia. A delay in diagnosis to await laboratory confirmation can, therefore, result in serious clinical risk to the patient. It also must not be assumed, as discussed previously, that other comorbid conditions or medications are automatically responsible for the thrombocytopenia.

A second issue relates to comorbid diseases. Concurrent illness can alter the pattern and severity of onset of HIT II. An even more difficult aspect of HIT II is the circumstance of "delayed onset of HIT II." Clinical features and thrombocytopenia have been seen to develop 7 to 14 days after discontinuing the heparin therapy, and thrombosis has been described up to 1 month after heparin discontinuation [64]. Although uncommon, the clinician must be aware of such potential, which further complicates the role of confirmatory testing. A related caveat is of clinical concern. The comorbid condition of the patient can have a significant effect on this pattern of development and, similarly, can affect the expected temporal pattern of repair of circulating platelet numbers after cessation of the heparin.

Several clinical laboratory features are characteristic. Thus, although thrombocytopenia is the cardinal laboratory feature, bleeding is uncommon. Thrombosis, by contrast, is the clinical event that primarily results in morbidity and mortality in HIT II. As mentioned earlier, the classic descriptions defined the white clot syndrome with an associated abrupt occlusion of a major artery. Although this represents a dramatic event of an acutely emergent care requirement, it is now clear that more common are thrombi in small arterial and arteriolar beds and venous occlusive lesions; the latter are estimated to occur with threefold frequency over arterial lesions [56,58,61,62,65–67,70,72]. Pulmonary emboli also are common. Important clinical clues to the potential occurrence of HIT II include the recognition of "relative" heparin resistance during induction of heparin therapy or the presence of unexplained chills, fever, and constitutional symptoms. Four other rare clinical events can occur as part of the evolution of HIT II, and these should alert the physician to the development of the syndrome: (1) skin necrosis, (2) transient global amnesia, (3) thrombosis on a present prosthetic value, or (4) bleeding into the adrenal glands with the abrupt development of adrenal insufficiency.

The true incidence of HIT II is not certain, although an occurrence in 3% to 5% of all heparin-treated individuals is a reasonable figure. The diagnostic parameters are not absolute. In the past, significant or severe thrombocytopenia was the initial and, frequently, only identifying marker. The recent clinical observations have more clearly defined a 50% decrease from baseline platelet levels, although a 30% decrease should arouse strong suspicion unless another highly plausible explanation is found [66,67]. Also, it has been common to demand a "confirmatory" laboratory test. As has been well defined, no single laboratory test recognizes all clinical cases of HIT II and many medical centers lack the ability to perform such assays [66,67]. Therefore, if the incidence data require absolute confirmatory testing, then the number of cases identified would be greatly reduced. In addition, the absolute incidence is affected by comorbid conditions so that patients who present with a thrombosis for heparin therapy or who are given heparin for thrombosis prophylaxis during an orthopedic surgical procedure have a higher incidence than general hospital populations [76–80]. Incidence figures also relate to the mode of heparin therapy; it is well established that continuous infusion is more commonly associated with HIT II than intermittent UFH, and each is more common than therapy with LMWHs.

Even more difficult is the delineation of the incidence of the most important clinical sequela of HIT II: thrombosis. Estimates of thrombosis in a patient with HIT II are as high as 35%, and in those patients who develop such a thrombosis, amputation rates of 25% and mortality of 25% to 30% have been reported [56,58,63,64,66,67,74]. The incidence of HITT appears to be about 1% (1/100 patients) of patients receiving UFH for at least 5 days [81,82]. All such data must be considered tentative until firm diagnostic criteria are more widely accepted and prospective studies are done in which the comorbid conditions are well documented. Although the current incidence data may be "soft," it is clear that morbidity and mortality in HIT II are significant; therefore, the clinical recognition of the syndrome and proper therapy are critical. Finally, it merits noting that data from a variety of centers have suggested that the occurrence of HIT II predicts future significant thrombotic events, further emphasizing the importance of clinical awareness.

Several controversies still exist in the emerging clinical understanding of HIT II. First, the level of platelet numbers or the level of change in platelet numbers from baseline that serves as the clinical parameter of diagnosis and thereby provides the parameter to perform other laboratory studies and alter therapy is not yet absolutely established. Second, the issue of whether incidence can be defined only by a specific serologic assay continues to be controversial and will probably always be so as long as no single absolute assay defines all cases. The authors believe that the clinical evidence that shows that up to 45% of the thrombotic episodes occur in the first 48 hours of recognition of HIT II strongly interdicts "waiting for laboratory confirmation" before therapeutic action, particularly in the current era when excellent alternatives to heparin are available. Third, the exact incidence of thrombosis in HIT II is not well defined but is thought to be 1% of those receiving UFH for 5 days. Fourth, the clinical sense that an HIT II thrombosis is clinically more dangerous in circumstances in which the patient is being treated with heparin for a present thrombosis and the true role of comorbid conditions are not settled issues. Fifth, the relationship of an uncommonly described event, that is, the paradoxic thrombotic complication of venous limb gangrene in patients on heparin during their transition to oral anticoagulant therapy with coumadin, is not fully clarified; however, many of these patients are now known to harbor an acquired protein C deficiency that may accentuate or precipitate this problem [83].

Pentasaccharide- and heparin-induced thrombocytopenia

An unexpected finding in clinical trials with pentasaccharide was the reported higher prevalence of HIT II [49]. In these studies, moderate HIT II (was found to be present at a rate of 2.9%). The incidence of HIT II with thrombotic events was found to be 0.9%, which is comparable to the LMWHs [49]. In the earlier preclinical studies, pentasaccharide was not found to produce any thrombocytopenia. Why, then, was pentasaccharide reported to produce a rather unexpected effect on platelets in the clinical trial? [49]. The reason may be that many of the patients treated with pentasaccharide were also treated with heparin. These patients exhibited HIT/HITT [49]. Although pentasaccharide is not thought to be capable of mobilizing platelet factor 4, it may displace heparan sulfate from vascular sites and remain bound to these sites for an extended period of time [49]. Such displacement of heparan sulfate may be able to mobilize platelet factor 4 from endogenous sites and form the complexes. These may trigger the generation of antiheparin platelet factor 4 antibodies [49]. An alternate hypothesis for the thrombocytopenia effects may be related to the generation of thrombin and direct thrombocytopenic effect without the generation of antiheparin platelet factor 4 antibodies. The thrombin-induced thrombocytopenic effects of pentasaccharide probably represent an indirect effect of this agent [49]. Because pentasaccharide has a high affinity to ATIII, other oligosaccharides are unable to bind to ATIII in the presence of pentasaccharide. Although the pentasaccharide represents the consensus sequence of heparin, which binds to the ATIII, it exhibits markedly distinct physiochemical, biochemical, and pharmacologic actions compared with LMWHs [49].

Treatment of heparin-induced thrombocytopenia/heparin-induced thrombocytopenia–thrombosis

Several immediate measures must be undertaken as soon as a clinical diagnosis of HIT/HITT is made. The first imperative measure is to immediately stop heparin; like any immune-mediated adverse reaction, the "antigen" (heparin) must be promptly removed. Next, the clinician must make a decision regarding the need for rapid institution of alternative antithrombotic therapy. In many patients, the underlying thrombosis or hypercoagulable condition for which the patient was initially placed on heparin will still be present; in this case, rapid institution of alternate antithrombotic therapy is needed. Also, when making a diagnosis of HIT, the clinician must immediately suspect the possibility of thrombosis/thromboembolism (HITT) and institute a diligent search for thrombosis, such as color flow Doppler of the lower extremity deep veins, ventilation/perfusion lung scan, magnetic resonance agiography of abdominal vasculature, and other studies. Obviously, if this search is positive for clinical or occult thrombosis, then rapid institution of antithrombotic therapy is indicated. The only agents currently FDA approved for this purpose are recombinant hirudin (lepirudin) and argatroban. If no thrombosis is present and the clinical condition for which the patient was initially heparinized has abated, then rapid or routine warfarinization may be considered. Before embarking on this approach, however, it is mandatory that functional protein C and protein S levels are measured. For those patients needing rapid warfarinization, a protocol for quick warfarinization, within 24 hours, recently has been published [84]. If the patient only requires prophylactic therapy with heparin and has a prior or current history of HIT/HITT, then lepirudin (10 to 20 mg SC every 12 hours) has been advocated [85]. Box 6 provides a practical summary of treatment for HIT/HITT.

Bleeding

The most common and more regularly anticipated complication of heparin therapy is bleeding [80,86–91]. The true incidence of major bleeding is not known, but estimates commonly range between 6% and 14% [87,88]. Hirsh and colleagues [68,88,89] emphasized important variables relative to heparin-related bleeding: (1) the dose of heparin administered; (2) the method of administration (ie, continuous versus intermittent, and so forth); and (3) the comorbid and concomitant therapy administered. Thus, heparin therapy is more commonly associated with bleeding when given to chronic alcoholics [86]. More complex and not completely resolved is the consideration that bleeding is more commonly

Box 6. Management of heparin-induced thrombocytopenia type II

1. Stop heparin immediately
2. Alternate rapid-onset antithrombotic therapy if original condition persists
   a. Lepirudin: 0.4 mg/kg bolus followed by 0.15 mg/kg infusion and adjust to maintain the aPTT at 1.5 to 3.0 times medial of normal aPTT
   b. Argatroban: investigational, pending FDA approval
   c. Ancrod: investigational, pending FDA approval
3. Assess immediately for evidence of occult thrombosis; rapid-onset antithrombotic if suspected or found
4. If heparin/LMWH needed for prophylaxis, may use lepirudin at 20 to 30 mg SC every 12 hours

seen in patients on aspirin [86,89,91]. Because this is not an uncommon treatment combination in patients with arterial vascular disease, clinical vigilance for bleeding is the only intelligent approach.

Bleeding activity of pentasaccharide

It is rather surprising that patients treated with a relatively small dosage of pentasaccharide (2.5 mg) exhibited a relatively higher incidence of bleeding in recent clinical trials [46,49]. In phase II trials, the bleeding effects of pentasaccharide were significant [46,49], which is highly suggestive of the role of ATIII in the mediation of the bleeding actions. LMWH at a 30 mg or 40 mg dosage produced comparable or relatively less bleeding. One possible explanation of the pentasaccharide-induced bleeding is related to the high affinity of this agent to the ATIII that is bound to vascular endothelium. Because pentasaccharide forms a strong complex with the ATIII, it most likely produces a strong localized inhibition of thrombin generation for an extended time. Because localized generation of thrombin is important in the mediation of the hemostatic function of platelets, its extended and relatively potent inhibition can easily compromise the platelet function. Thus, at the surgical sites/lesions, this important generation of thrombin compromises the hemostatic function of patients treated with pentasaccharide. It would be important to find the bleeding incidence of pentasaccharide in the therapeutic trials that currently are ongoing. In addition, pentasaccharide also may have some direct effects on vasculature and, thus, may compromise hemostatic function. One such mechanism is the inhibition of ATPase at the surgical site. Such an inhibition is reported with the LMWHs.

In May 2000, the FDA released a MedWatch warning regarding certain doses of enoxaparin in elderly patients; clinicians using enoxaparin (Lovenox) need to be aware of this report [92] that states the following:

> Over 2800 patients, 65 years and older, have received enoxaparin sodium in pivotal clinical trials. The incidence of bleeding complications was similar between elderly and younger patients when 30 mg every 12 hours or 40 mg once a day doses of Lovenox Injection were employed. The incidence of bleeding complications was higher in elderly patients as compared with younger patients when Lovenox Injection was administered at doses of 1.5 mg/kg once a day or 1 mg/kg every 12 hours. The risk of Lovenox Injection-associated bleeding increased with age. Serious adverse events increased with age for patients receiving Lovenox Injections. Other clinical experience (including postmarketing surveillance and literature reports) has not revealed additional differences in the safety of Lovenox Injection between elderly and younger patients. Careful attention to dosing intervals and concomitant medications (especially antiplatelet medications) is advised. Monitoring of geriatric patients with low body weight (<45 kg) and those predisposed to decreased renal function should be considered. [92]

Acute heparin reaction (anaphylaxis?)

A rare but potentially lethal acute reaction to heparin can occur. The event is abrupt and clinically dramatic [93]. It has been seen only in patients previously treated with heparin. It again merits emphasis that the heparin exposure does not need to be quantitative because reaction has occurred with heparin exposure as minimal as heparin flush or with the use of a heparin-coated catheter. Symptoms occur dramatically within 5 to 10 minutes of institution of the heparin bolus and include abrupt onset of chills and fever, tachycardia, diaphoresis, and nausea. Hypotension may be noted, although most patients have become abruptly and transiently hypertensive. Retrosterned chest pain with the pattern of an acute myocardial infarction is common. Finally, a global amnesia syndrome has been linked to the crises event. This anaphylaxis-like reaction has all of the features of an IgE-stimulated response. Immediate cessation of the heparin is critical. Other nonheparin antithrombotic agents should be used to treat the patient. One of the authors (R.L. Bick) has seen four different patient episodes of anaphylaxis with enoxaparin; these have been reported to the FDA.

Heparin-associated osteoporosis

Prolonged heparin exposure has been correlated with the development of osteoporosis [94,95]. The clinical findings that led to the evaluation of this finding were the unexpected development of bone pain or the identification of vertebral body or rib or fractures. The clinical correlate was that the patient had been on long-term heparin (in excess of 6 months) and usually at daily doses in excess of 15,000 anti-Xa units [67]. Limited epidemiologic and controlled studies are available to define the incidence of heparin-associated osteoporosis. In addition, many of the studies have focused on pregnant patients because such patients represent a group likely to have a long duration of therapy. Because pregnancy itself is commonly associated with osteoporosis, however, such data must be interpreted cautiously. Howell et al [96], in randomized trials, identified a 5% incidence of vertebral fractures in women treated with UFH during their pregnancy. Monreal et al [97], in a randomized study of 40 men and 40 women (mean age of 68) on long-term heparin therapy, identified a 10% incidence of vertebral fractures. Six of the seven occurred with UFH, the seventh with LMWH (Fragmin). An interesting finding in this study was that there was no difference in bone density between the group developing fractures and the group without fractures. These investigators could not show a correlation between the lumbar bone density and the dose or duration of therapy [97].

Barbour and associates [98] evaluated the subclinical occurrence of heparin-associated osteoporosis in pregnancy by means of bone densitometry in a prospective, consecutive cohort of 14 pregnant women requiring heparin therapy and 14 pregnant controls matched for age, race, and smoking status. Proximal femur bone density measurements were taken at baseline, immediately postpartum, and 6 months postpartum in the cases and controls. Vertebral measurements also were obtained on both groups immediately postpartum and 6 months postpartum. Bone density relative to heparin dose and duration was examined. Five of 14 cases (36%) had a 10% decrease from their baseline proximal femur measurements to their immediate postpartum values, whereas no decreases occurred in the 14 matched controls ($P = 0.04$). Mean proximal femur bone density measurements also decreased, and this difference was still statistically significant 6 months postpartum ($P = 0.03$). This study concluded that no clear dose-response relationship could be demonstrated and that UFH adversely affected bone density in about 33% of exposed patients [99].

Dahlman [99] studied the effect of long-term heparin treatment during pregnancy and the incidence of osteoporotic fractures and thromboembolic recurrence. Long-term SC prophylaxis with heparin twice daily in pregnancy was used in 184 individuals. The dose of heparin was adjusted to anti-FXa activity or aPTT, and different regimens were given depending on risk stratification. Symptomatic osteoporotic fractures of the spine occurred postpartum in 4 women (2.2%). Their mean dosage of heparin ranged from 15,000 to 30,000 IU per 24 hours (mean, 24,500 IU per 24 hours) and their duration of treatment was from 7 to 27 weeks (mean, 17 weeks). It is of interest that despite prophylaxis with heparin, thromboembolic complications occurred in 5 women. Thus, osteoporotic vertebral fractures were found in 2.2%, and these correlated with the amount of heparin administered. There were no thromboembolic events, thrombocytopenias, or excessive hemorrhage. Hunt et al [100], during a study of LMWH (Fragmin) for thromboprophylaxis in 34 high-risk pregnancies, identified 1 woman who developed an osteoporotic vertebral collapse post partum. This woman had no other risk factors for osteoporosis. Parenthetically, this study supported the efficacy of LMWH in preventing recurrent thromboembolic disease in pregnant women at high risk. In this study, the incidence of osteoporotic fracture was 3%; however, bone density studies to assess asymptomatic osteoporosis were not reported.

Douketis et al [101], in a prospective, matched cohort, studied the effects of long-term (>1 month) UFH therapy on lumbar spine bone density. Twenty-five women who received heparin during pregnancy and 25 matched controls underwent dual photon absorptiometry of the lumbar spine in the postpartum period. None of 25 heparin-treated patients developed fractures. Heparin-treated patients had a 0.082 g/cm^2 lower bone density compared with untreated controls, which was statistically significant ($P = 0.0077$). There were six matched pairs in which only the heparin-treated patient had a bone density below 1.0 g/cm^2 compared with only one pair in which only the control patient had a bone density below this level ($P = 0.089$). The duration of heparin therapy, the mean daily dose, and the total dose of heparin were not at levels of independent significance. These investigators concluded that long-term heparin therapy was associated with a significant reduction in bone density, although fractures are uncommon. They could not show a correlation between the lumber bone density and the dose or duration of heparin therapy. This finding is in contradistinction to the generally held views that heparin-induced osteoporosis is related to the dose and duration of therapy [66,67].

A variety of studies have focused on the mechanism whereby heparin affects bone metabolism and structure. Muir et al [102] treated rats with once-daily SC injections of UFH or saline for 8 to 32 days and monitored the effects on bone histomorphometrically and measured urinary type 1 collagen cross-linked pyridinoline and serum alkaline phosphatase as surrogate markers of bone resorption and formation. Biochemical markers of bone turnover showed that heparin produced a dose-dependent decrease in serum alkaline phosphatase and a transient increase in urinary pyridinoline, thus confirming the histomorphometric data. They concluded that heparin decreases trabecular bone volume by decreasing the rate of bone formation and by increasing the rate of bone resorption [102]. In a subsequent study, this group evaluated the effect of LMWH in a similar model system [103]. It was found that UFH and LMWH decreased cancellous bone volume in a dose-dependent fashion, but UFH caused significantly more bone loss than the LMWH. The biochemical markers of bone turnover demonstrated that both heparins produced a dose-dependent decrease in serum alkaline phosphatase, consistent with reduced bone formation, whereas only the UFH caused an increase in urinary pyridinoline, consistent with increased bone resorption. They concluded that UFH decreases cancellous bone volume by decreasing the rate of bone formation and by increasing the rate of bone resorption; in contrast, LMWH causes less osteopenia because it only decreases the rate of bone formation [103].

Panagakos et al [104] demonstrated that heparin induces osteoporosis by enhancing the effects of other bone-resorbing factors, particularly parathyroid hormone. Shaughnesy et al [105] further examined the issue of calcium loss by an in vitro calcium release assay and demonstrated that size and sulfation of the heparins were the major determinants of the promotion of bone resorption. Their extrapolation was that LMWH preparations would therefore reduce the risk of the expected heparin-associated osteoporosis.

Murray and associates [106] examined bone density in a rabbit model. A reduction in cortical and trabecular bone density was seen with UFH ($P < 0.05$) and high molecular weight heparin ($P < 0.01$) but not with LMWH.

Thus, heparin-associated osteoporosis is a clinically uncommon event occurring in less than 5% of long-term heparin-treated patients. The evidence supports a lesser risk with LMWH than with UFH. The mechanisms appear related to impaired bone deposition and formation plus enhanced bone resorption with UFH. A change in new bone deposition appears to be the major mechanism with LMWH. Most clinical evidence supports the view that a long duration of therapy (ie, greater than 6 months) and a higher dose of heparin increase the risk of bone changes.

From these observations, the authors currently recommend that bone density studies be done in patients whose duration of therapy will be greater than 6 months at an equivalent of 20,000 anti-Xa U/d or at 3 months if the dose will exceed 20,000 anti-Xa U/d. In addition, the authors encourage calcium supplements. If the patient is going to be on low-dose SC UFH or LMWH for 1 year or more, then baseline bone density studies are recommended and repeat comparative studies should be done yearly; if a significant change occurs and continued heparin is required, then alendronate should be started [107].

Heparin-related dermal reactions

Three general types of skin reactions can occur with heparin therapy [66,67,108]. The most common are those seen in patients being treated with SC heparin. These are small ecchymotic or erythematous papular or nodular lesions that are slightly tender and generally less than 1 cm. These lesions occur at the sites of injection. Although at times, these are the result of violated sterile technique and, therefore, represent infections, most are sterile and require no change in therapy except the selection of an alternate site. The exact mechanism is not certain, but local cytokine release is the current working concept.

A second skin reaction is that of urticarial, often pruritic, lesions; again, largely at the sites of SC injection. These allergic reactions commonly have been associated with the vehicle for the heparin and often can be avoided by either a change in the brand of heparin or the use of an antihistamine at the time of the injections.

Heparin-induced skin necrosis is the most serious form of dermal reaction and, fortunately, the least common [108–113]. These lesions have many features similar to warfarin (Coumadin) necrosis, but the pathophysiology is distinctly different. The route and form of heparin is unrelated to this occurrence. Commonly, these lesions begin 5 to 10 days into the heparin therapy and are manifest on the extremities, abdominal wall, or nose, and several of the case reports highlight their occurrence on the dorsum of the hand [111–113]. The onset is abrupt, with a dusky or erythematous plaquelike lesion that can rapidly evolve into a hemorrhagic bullae with necrosis. The exact pathophysiologic basis for these necrotic lesions is not clear. The antibodies found in HIT II have been seen in many patients, yet only about 25% of them will develop HIT II. These lesions signal an acute need to discontinue the heparin therapy and select an appropriate alternative agent.

Altered liver function tests

Abnormal liver function studies, primarily a transaminasemia of minimal degree, have been correlated with long-term heparin administration [66,67]. The finding is uncommon and the pathophysiologic mechanisms have never been defined. These changes revert to normal when heparin is discontinued.

Heparin and eosinophilia

Eosinophilia occurs in 5% to 10% of patients receiving UFH or LMWH therapy [66,67,114]. The eosinophilia is asymptomatic. In almost all of the patients, it is unrelated to systemic allergic reactions, dermal allergic reactions, skin necrosis, or any other evident symptom complex. It is not associated with any physiologic changes or sequelae. The eosinophilia abates 4 to 8 weeks after cessation of the heparin therapy. The current hypothesis relative to this occurrence is the activation of CD4 cells, with the subsequent release of granulocyte-macrophage colony–stimulating factor, IL-3, and IL-5, which can induce eosinophilia [115].

Hyperkalemia, hypoaldosteronism, and related metabolic disorders

Prolonged heparin therapy has been recognized to be associated with functional hypoaldosteronism, hyperkalemia, and correlate metabolic abnormalities [68,116,117]. Although rare, the evidence supports heparin suppression of synthesis of aldosterone [66]. Cessation of heparin results in resolution of the metabolic abnormalities and return to normal.

Priapism

Priapism has been considered to be a possible complication of heparin therapy [68]. In the few reports available, it is not clear whether specificity of a vascular occlusive event is present or whether this simply represents thrombosis as part of an HIT II event. The authors favor the latter pathophysiologic explanation.

Alopecia

Alopecia has been related to long-term heparin therapy [66–68]. Its occurrence and its potential pathophysiologic mechanisms have not been well defined.

Other adverse reactions

In January 2002, the FDA issued a MedWatch drug alert regarding enoxaparin and maternal hemorrhage, fetal hemorrhage, birth defects, and dangers associated with use of enoxaparin (Lovenox) in patients with prosthetic cardiac valves [118]. Clinicians must be aware of this report that states the following:

WARNINGS:

Prosthetic Heart Valves: The use of Lovenox Injection is not recommended for thromboprophylaxis in patients with prosthetic heart valves. Cases of prosthetic heart valve thrombosis have been reported in patients with prosthetic valves who have received enoxaparin for thromboprophylaxis. Some of these cases were pregnant women in whom thrombosis led to maternal deaths and fetal deaths. Pregnant women with prosthetic heart valves may be at higher risk for thromboembolism (see PRECAUTIONS: Pregnancy).

PRECAUTIONS

Pregnancy

Teratogenic effects

[Second paragraph added]:

There have been reports of congenital anomalies in infants born to women who received enoxaparin during pregnancy including cerebral anomalies, limb anomalies, hypospadias, peripheral vascular malformation, fibrotic dysplasia, and cardiac defect. A cause and effect relationship has not been established nor has the incidence been shown to be higher than in the general population.

Non-Teratogenic Effects

[First paragraph revised (ITALICS)*]:

*Non-Teratogenic Effects: *There have been a few spontaneous post-marketing reports of fetal death when pregnant women received enoxaparin. Causality of the cases has not been determined. In one case, placental hemorrhage and detachment were found in association with the fetal death. If enoxaparin is used during pregnancy, or if the patient becomes pregnant while taking this drug, the patient should be apprised of the potential hazard to the fetus.**
(* = changed to):

There have been post-marketing reports of fetal death when pregnant women received Lovenox Injection. Causality for these cases has not been determined. Pregnant women receiving anti-coagulants, including enoxaparin, are at increased risk for bleeding. Hemorrhage can occur at any site and may lead to death of mother or fetus. Pregnant women receiving enoxaparin should be carefully monitored. Pregnant women and women of child-bearing potential should be apprised of the potential hazard to the fetus and the mother if enoxaparin is administered during pregnancy.

[Second paragraph added]:

In a clinical study of pregnant women with prosthetic heart valves given enoxaparin (1 mg/kg bid) to reduce the risk of thromboembolism, 2 of 7 women developed clots resulting in blockage of the valve and leading to maternal and fetal death. There are postmarketing reports of prosthetic valve thrombosis in pregnant women with prosthetic heart valves while receiving enoxaparin for thromboprophylaxis. These events resulted in maternal death or surgical interventions. The use of Lovenox Injection is not recommended for thromboprophylaxis in pregnant women with prosthetic heart valves (see WARNINGS: Prosthetic Heart Valves).

ADVERSE REACTIONS

Ongoing Safety Surveillance: Since 1993, there have been over *(79 reports)* 80 reports of epidural or spinal hematoma formation with concurrent use of Lovenox Injection and spinal/epidural anesthesia or spinal puncture. [118]

References

[1] Fareed J, Ma Q, Florian M, Maddineni J, Iqbal O, Hoppensteadt D, et al. Unfractionated and low-molecular-weight heparins basic mechanisms of action ad pharmacology. Semin Cardiothorac Vascu Anesth 2003;7:357.

[2] Linhardt J, Gunay SN. Production and chemical processing of low molecular weight heparins. Semin Thromb Hemost 1999;25(Suppl 3):5.

[3] Casu B, Torri G. Structural characterization of low nolecular weight heparins. Semin Thromb Hemost 1999;25(Suppl 3):17.

[4] Young E, Wells P, Holloway S, Weitz J, Hirsh J. Ex vivo and in vitro evidence that low molecular weight heparins exhibit less binding to plasma proteins than unfractionated heparin. Thromb Haemost 1994;71(3):300.

[5] Houbouyan L, Padilla A, Gray E, Longstaff C, Barrowcliffe TW. Inhibition of thrombin generation by heparin and LMW heparins: a comparison of chromogenic and clotting methods. Blood Coag Fibrinolysis 1996;7:24.

[6] Montalescot G, Collet JP, Lison L, Choussat R, Anki A. Effects of various anticoagulant treatments on von Willebrand factor release in unstable angina. J Am Coll Cardiol 2000; 36(1):110.

[7] Marmur JD, Anand SX, Bagga RS, Fareed J, Pan CM, Sharma SK, et al. The activated clotting time can be used to monitor the low molecular weight heparin dalteparin after intravenous administration. J Am Coll Cardiol 2003;41:394.

[8] Kaiser B, Kirchmaier M, Breddin KH, Fu K, Fareed J. Preclinical biochemistry and pharmacology of low molecular weight heparins in vivo—studies of venous and arterial thrombosis. Semin Thromb Hemost 1999;25(Suppl 3):35.

[9] Dietrich CP, Shinjo SK, Moraes FA, Richardo AB, Castro R, Mendes A, et al. Structural features and bleeding activity of commercial low molecular weight heparins: neutralization by ATP and protamine. Semin Thromb Hemost 1999;25(Suppl 3):43.

[10] Cornelli U, Fareed J. Human pharmacokinetics of low molecular weight heparins. Semin Thromb Hemost 1999;25(Suppl 3):57.

[11] Nader HB, Walenga JM, Berkowitz SD, Ofosu F, Hoppensteadt DA, Cella G. Preclinical differentiation of low molecular weight heparins. Semin Thromb Hemost 1999;25(Suppl 3):63.

[12] Fareed J, Fu L, Yang LH, Hoppensteadt DA. Pharmacokinetics of low molecular weight heparins in animal models. Semin Thromb Hemost 1999;25(Suppl 3):51.

[13] Mammen EF, Arcelus J, Messmore H, Altman R, Nurmohamed M, Eldor A. Clinical differentiation of low molecular weight heparins. Semin Thromb Hemost 1999;25(Suppl 3):135.

[14] Nightingale SL. From the Food and Drug Administration. JAMA 1993;270(14):1672.

[15] McCart GM, Kayser S. Therapeutic equivalency of low molecular weight heparins. Ann Pharmcother 2002;36:1042.

[16] Nenci G. Low molecular weight heparins: are they interchangeable? No. J Thromb Hemostasis 2003;1:12.

[17] Merli G, Vanscoy G, et al. Applying scientific criteria to therapeutic interchange: a balanced analysis of low molecular weight heparins. J Thromb Thrombolysis 2001;11(3):247.

[18] Cohen M. Low molecular weight heparins in the management of unstable angina/non-Q-wave myocardial infarction. Semin Thromb Hemost 1999;25(Suppl 3):113.

[19] Gulba D. Differentiation of low molecular weight heparins in acute coronary syndromes: an interventionalist's perspective. Semin Thromb Hemost 1999;25(Suppl 3):123.

[20] Leong W, Hoppensteadt DA. Generic forms of low molecular weight heparins. Some practical issues. Clin Appl Thromb Hemost, in press.

[21] Fareed J, Haas S, Sasahara A, editors. Differentiation of low molecular weight heparins: applied and clinical considerations [special issue]. Semin Thromb Hemost 1999;25(3).

[22] Fareed J, Walenga JM, Hoppensteadt D, Huan X, Racanelli A. Comparative study on the in vitro and in vivo activities of seven low-molecular-weight heparins. Haemostasis 1988; 18(Suppl 3):3.

[23] Fareed J, Walenga JM, Williamson K, Emanuele RM, Kumar A, Hoppensteadt D. Studies on the antithrombotic effects and pharmacokinetics of heparin fractions and fragments. Semin Thromb Hemost 1985;11(1):56.

[24] Abboud L. Bush acts to speed generics to market. In: Wall Street Journal, vol. CCXLI 114. June 12, 2003. p. A3.

[25] Dawes J. Comparison of the pharmacokinetics of enoxaparin (Clexane) and unfractionated heparin. Acta Chirur Scand 1990;156(Suppl 556):68.

[26] Fareed J, Walenga JM, Hoppensteadt DA, et al. Laboratory studies on the intravenous and subcutaneous adminstration of PK 10169 in man. Haemostasis 1986;16:123.

[27] Azizi M, Veyssier-Belot C, Alhenc-Gelas M, et al. Comparison of biological activities of two low molecular weight heparins in 10 healthy volunteers. Br J Clin Pharmacol 1995; 40:577.

[28] Collignon F, Frydman A, Caplain H, et al. Comparison of pharmacokinetic profiles of three low molecular mass heparins: dalteparin, enoxaparin and nadroparin: adminstered subcutaneously in healthy volunteers (doses for prevention in thromboembolism). Thromb Haemost 1995;73:630.

[29] Eriksson BI, Soderberg K, Widlund L, et al. A comparative study of threee low molecular weight heparins (LMWH) and Unfractionated heparin (UH) in healthy volunteers. Thromb Haemost 1995;73:398.

[30] Frydman AM, Bara L, Le Roux Y, et al. The antithrombotic activity and pharmacokinetics of enoxaparine, a low molecular weight heparin, in humans given single subcutaneous doses of 20 to 80 mg. J Clin Pharmacol 1988;28:609.

[31] Samama MM, Gerotziafas GT. Comparative pharmacokinetics of LMWHs. Semin Thromb Hemost 2000;26(Suppl 1):31.

[32] Bendetowicz AV, Beguin S, Caplain H, et al. Pharmacokinetics and pharmacodynamics of a low molecular weight heparin (enoxaparin) after subcutaneous injection, comparison with unfractionated heparin: a three way cross-over study in human volunteers. Thromb Haemost 1994;71:305.

[33] Hirsh J, Warkentin TE, Raschke R, et al. Heparin and low molecular-weight heparin: mechanisms of action, pharmacokinetics, dosing considerations, monitoring efficacy and safety. Chest 1998;114(Suppl 5):489S.
[34] Bara L, Bloch MF, Zitoun D, et al. Comparative effects of enoxaparin and unfractionated heparin in healthy volunteers on prothrombin consumption in whole blood during coagulation and release of tissue factor pathway inhibitor. Thromb Res 1993;69:443.
[35] Frydman A. Low-molecular-weight heparins: an overview of their pharmacodynamics, pharmacokinetics and metabolism in humans. Hemostasis 1996;26(Suppl 2):24.
[36] Bara L, Samama MM. Pharmacokinetics of low molecular weight heparins. Acta Chir Scand Suppl 1988;543:65.
[37] Fareed J, Hoppensteadt DA, Walenga JM, Iqbal O, Ma Q, Jeske W, et al. Pharmacodynamic and pharmacokinetic properties of enoxaparin. Implications for clincial practice. Clin Pharmacokinet 2003;42(12):1043.
[38] Fragmin during Instability in Coronary Artery Disease (FRISC) Study Group. Low-molecular-weight heparin during instability in coronary artery disease. Lancet 1996;347:561.
[39] Klein W, Buchwald A, Hillis SE, et al, for the FRIC Investigators. Comparison of low molecular weight heparin with unfractionated heparin acutely and with placebo for six weeks in the management of unstable coronary artery disease: Fragmin in Unstable Coronary Artery Disease Study (FRIC). Circulation 1997;96:61.
[40] The FRAXIS Study Group. Comparison of two treatment durations (6 days and 14 days) of a low molecular weight heparin with a 6-day treatment of unfractionated heparin in the initial management of unstable angina or non-Q-wave myocardial infarction: FRAX.I.S. FRAXiparine in Ischemic Syndrome. Eur Heart J 1999;20:1553.
[41] Cohen M, Demers C, Gurfinkel EP, et al. A comparison of low molecular weight heparin with unfractionated heparin for unstable coronary artery disease. N Engl J Med 1997;337:447.
[42] Klein W, Kraxner W, Hodl R, Steg PG, et al, for the GRACE Investigators. Patterns of use of heparins in ACS correlates and hospital outcomes: the Global Registry of Acute Coronary Events. 2003;90:519.
[43] Hull RD, Raskob GE, Brant RF, Pineo GF, Elliott G, Stein PD, et al. Low-molecular-weight heparin vs heparin in the treatment of patients with pulmonary embolism. American-Canadian Thrombosis Study Group. Ann Intern Med 2000;160(2):229.
[44] Walenga JM, Jeske WP, Bara L, Samama MM, Fareed J. State-of-the-art article. Biochemiccal and pharmacologic rationale for the development of a heparin pentasaccharide. Thromb Res 1997;86(1):1.
[45] Walenga JM, Jeske WP, Samama MM, Frapaise VF, Bick RL, Fareed J. Fondaparinux: a synthetic heparin pentasaccharide as a new antithrombotic agent. Expert Opin Investig Drugs 2002;11(3):1.
[46] Turpie AGG, Gallus AS, Hoek JA, for the Pentasaccharide Investigators. A synthetic pentasaccharide for the prevention of deep vein thrombosis after total hip replacement. N Engl J Med 2001;344:619–25.
[47] Eriksson BI, Bauer KA, Lassen MR, Turpie AGG, for the Steering Committee of the Pentasaccharide in Hip-Fracture Surgery Study. Fondaparinux compared with enoxaparin for the prevention of venous thromboembolism after hip-fracture surgery. N Engl J Med 2001;345:1298.
[48] Hoppensteadt DA, Jeske WP, Walenga JM, Fu K, Yang LH, Ing T, et al. Efficacy of pentasaccharide in a dog model of hemodialysis. Thromb Res 1997;88(2):159.
[49] Hoppensteadt D, Walenga JM, Fareed J, Bick RL. Heparin, low molecular weight heparins and heparin pentasaccharide: basic and clinical differentiation. Hematol Oncol Clin N Am 2003;17:313.
[50] Fedlar E, Jacques LB. The effect of commercial heparin on the platelet count. J Lab Clin Med 1948;33:1410.
[51] Nelson JC, Lerner RG, Goldstein R, Cagin NA. Heparin-induced thrombocytopenia. Arch Intern Med 1978;138:548.

[52] Ansell J, Slepchuk Jr N, Kumar R, Lopez A, Southard L, Deykin D. Heparin induced thrombocytopenia: a prospective study. Thromb Haemost 1980;43:61.
[53] King DJ, Kelton JG. Heparin associated thrombocytopenia. Ann Intern Med 1984;100:535.
[54] Chong BH, Ismail F. The mechanism of heparin-induced platelet aggregation. Eur J Haematol 1989;43:245.
[55] Warkentin TE, Kelton JG. Heparin and platelets. Hematol Oncol Clin N Am 1990;4:243.
[56] Boshkov LK, Warkentin TE, Hayward CPM, Andrew M, Kelton J. Heparin induced thrombocytopenia and thrombosis: clinical and laboratory studies. Br J Haematol 1993;84:322.
[57] Chong BH. Heparin induced thrombocytopenia. Brit J Haematol 1995;89:431.
[58] Aster RH. Heparin-induced thrombocytopenia and thrombosis. N Engl J Med 1995;332:1374.
[59] Kelton JG, Warkentin TE. Diagnosis of heparin-induced thrombocytopenia: still a journey, not yet a destination [editorial]. Am J Clin Path 1995;104:611.
[60] Schmitt BP, Adelman B. Heparin associated thrombocytopenia: a critical review and pooled analysis. Am J Med Sci 1993;305:208.
[61] Mumer R, Schulman IC, Wolf DJ, Rosengart TK. Heparin induced thrombocytopenia thrombosis after cardiopulmonary bypass. Ann Thorac Surg 1994;14:1764.
[62] Shorten GD, Comunale ME. Heparin induced thrombocytopenia. J Cardiothorac Vasc Anesth 1996;10:521.
[63] Kibbe MR, Rhee RY. Heparin induced thrombocytopenia: pathophysiology. Semin Vasc Surg 1996;9:284.
[64] Warkentin TE, Kelton JG. A 14 year study of heparin induced thrombocytopenia. Am J Med 1996;101:502.
[65] Jackson MR, Krishnamurti C, Aylesworth CA. Diagnosis of heparin induced thromboctypenia in the vascular surgery patient. Surgery 1997;121:419.
[66] Walenga JM, Bick RL. Heparin-induced thrombocytopenia, paradoxical thromboembolism, and other side effects of heparin therapy. Cardiol Clin Ann Drug Ther 1998;2:123.
[67] Walenga JM, Bick RL. Heparin-induced thrombocytopenia, paradoxical thromboembolism, and other side effects of heparin therapy. Med Clin N Am 1998;82:635.
[68] Hirsh J, Raschke R, Warkentin TE, Dalen JE, Deykin D, Poller L. Heparin: mechanism of action, pharmacokinetics, dosing considerations, monitoring, efficacy, and safety. Chest 1995;108:259S.
[69] Moberg P, Geary V, Sheikh M. Heparin-induced thrombocytopenia: a possible complication of heparin-coated pulmonary artery catheters. J Cardiothorac Anesth 1990;4:266.
[70] Weismann RE, Tobin RW. Arterial embolism occurring during systemic heparin therapy. Arch Surg 1958;76:219.
[71] Abhyankar V, Kouides P, Phatak P. Heparin-induced thrombocytopenia is a cause of thromboembolism following coronary by-pass surgery [abstract]. Blood 1995;86:846.
[72] Towne JB, Bernhard VM, Hussey C, Garancis JC. White clot syndrome: peripheral vascular complications of heparin therapy. Arch Surg 1979;114:372.
[73] Stanton Jr PE, Evans JR, Lefemine AA, Vo NM, Rannick GA, Morgan Jr CV, et al. White clot syndrome. South Med J 1988;81:616.
[74] Battey PM, Salam AA. Venous gangrene associated with heparin-induced thrombocytopenia. Surgery 1985;97:618.
[75] Kappa JR, Risher CA, Todd B. Intraoperative management of patients with heparin-induced thrombocytopenia. Ann Throac Surg 1990;49:714.
[76] Green D, Martin GJ, Shoichet SH, DeBacker N, Bomalski JS, Lind RN. Thrombocytopenia in a prospective, randomized, double blind trial of bovine and porcine heparin. Am J Med Sci 1984;288:60.
[77] Powers PJ, Kelton JG, Carter CJ. Studies on the frequency of heparin-associated thrombocytopenia. Thromb Res 1984;33:439.
[78] Ansell JE, Price JM, Beckner RR. Heparin induced thrombocytopenia: what is its real frequency? Chest 1985;88:878.
[79] Warkentin TE, Levine MN, Hirsch J, Horsewood P, Roberts RS, Gent M, et al. Heparin-induced

thrombocytopenia in patients treated with low-molecular-weight heparin or unfractionated heparin. N Engl J Med 1995;332:1330.
[80] Thomas DP. Heparin prophylaxis and treatment of venous thromboembolism. Semin Hematol 1978;15:1.
[81] Hirsh J, Warkentin TE, Raschke R, Granger C, Ohman EM, Daslen JE. heparin and low molecular weight heparin: mechanisms of action, pharmacokinetics, dosing considerations, monitoring, efficacy and safety. Chest 1988;114(Suppl):489.
[82] Warkentin TE. Clinical presentation of heparin-induced thrombocytopenia. Semin Hematol 1998;35(Suppl):9.
[83] Warkentin TE. Limitations of conventional treatment options for heparin-induced thrombocytopenia. Semin Hematol 1998;35(Suppl):17.
[84] Neverre DR, Digiovanni A. Hypercoagulability and the management of anticoagulant therapy in surgical patients: review and recommendations. J Endovasc Surg 1998;5:282.
[85] Eriksson BI, Ekman S, Kalebo P. Prevention of deep-vein thrombosis after total hip replacement: direct thrombin inhibition with recombinant hirudin CGP 39393. Lancet 1996; 347:635.
[86] Walker AM, Jick H. Prediction of bleeding during heparin therapy. JAMA 1980;244:1209.
[87] Salzman EW, Deykin D, Shapiro RM, Rosenberg R. Management of heparin therapy. N Engl J Med 1975;292:1046.
[88] Levine M, Hirsh J. Hemorrhagic complications of anticoagulant therapy. Semin Thromb Hemost 1986;12:39.
[89] Hirsh J. Heparin. N Engl J Med 1991;327:1565.
[90] Morabia A. Heparin doses and major bleedings. Lancet 1986;1:1278.
[91] Yett HS, Skillman JJ, Salzman EW. The hazards of aspirin plus heparin. N Engl J Med 1978;298:1092.
[92] Food and Drug Administration. Lovenox (enoxaparin sodium) injection [May 30, 2000: Aventis Pharmaceuticals] PRECAUTIONS: Geriatric use: new subsection. Available at: http://www.fda.gov/medwatch/safety/2000/may00.htm#lovenox. Accessed June 2000.
[93] Warkentin TE, Soutar RL, Panju A. Acute systemic reactions to intravenous bolus heparin therapy: characterization and relationship to heparin induced thrombocytopenia [abstract]. Blood 1992;80:160.
[94] Jaffe MD, Willis PW. Multiple fractures associated with long-term sodium heparin therapy. JAMA 1965;193:152.
[95] Levine M. Non-hemorrhagic complications of anticoagulant therapy. Semin Thromb Hemost 1986;12:63.
[96] Howell R, Fidler J, Letsky E, DeSwiet M. The risks of antenatal subcutaneous heparin prophylaxis: a controlled trial. Br J Obstet Gynaecol 1983;90:1124.
[97] Monreal M, Lafoz E, Olive A, del Rio L, Vedia C. Comparison of subcutaneous unfractionated heparin with low molecular weight heparin (Fragmin) in patients with venous thromboembolism and contraindications to coumarin. Thromb Haemost 1994;71:7.
[98] Barbour LA, Kick SD, Steiner JF, LoVerdeme ME, Heddleston LN, Lear JL, et al. A prospective study of heparin-induced osteoporosis in pregnancy using bone densitometry. Am J Obstet Gynecol 1994;170:862.
[99] Dahlman TC. Osteoporotic fractures and the recurrence of thromboembolism during pregnancy and the puerperium in 184 women undergoing thromboprophylaxis with heparin. Am J Obstet Gynecol 1993;168:1265.
[100] Hunt BJ, Doughy H, Majumdar G, Copplestone A, Kerslake S, Buchanan N, et al. Thromboprophylaxis with low molecular weight heparin (Fragmin) in high risk pregnancies. Thromb Haemost 1997;77:39.
[101] Douketis J, Ginsberg JS, Burrows RF, Duku EK, Webber CE, Brill-Edwards PL. The effects of long-term therapy during pregnancy on bone density. A prospective matched cohort study. Thromb Haemost 1996;75:254.
[102] Muir JM, Andrew M, Hirsh J, Weitz JI, Young E, Deschamps P, et al. Histomorphometric analysis of the effects of standard heparin on trebular bone in vivo. Blood 1996;88:1314.

[103] Muir JM, Hirsh J, Weitz JI, Andrew M, Young E, Shaughnessy SG. A histomorphometric comparison of the effects of heparin and low-molecular-weight heparin on cancellous bone in rats. Blood 1997;89:3236.

[104] Panagakos FS, Jandinski JJ, Feder L, Kumar S. Heparin fails to potentiate the effects of IL-1 beta-mediated bone resorption of fetal rat long bones in vitro. Biochimie 1995;77:915.

[105] Shaughnesy SG, Young E, Deschamps P, Hirsh J. The effects of low molecular weight and standard heparin on calcium loss from fetal rat calvoria. Blood 1995;86:1368.

[106] Murray WJ, Lindo VS, Kakkar VV, Melissari E. Long term administration of heparin and heparin fractions and osteoporosis in experimental animals. Blood Coag Fibrinolys 1995; 6:113.

[107] Bick RL. Heparin therapy and monitoring: guidelines and practice parameters for clinical and laboratory approaches. J Clin Appl Thromb Hemost 1996;2(Suppl):12.

[108] Warkentin TE. Heparin-induced skin lesions. Br J Haematol 1996;92:494.

[109] Hill J, Caprini JA, Robbins JL. An unusual complication of minidose heparin therapy. Clin Orthop 1976;118:130.

[110] White PW, Sadd JR, Wensel RE. Thrombotic complications of heparin therapy. Ann Surg 1979;190:595.

[111] Kelly RA, Gelfand JA, Pincus SH. Cutaneous necrosis caused by systemically administered heparin. JAMA 1981;246:1582.

[112] Hall JC, McConahay D, Gibson D, Crockett J, Conn R. Heparin necrosis an anticoagulation syndrome. JAMA 1980;244:1831.

[113] Levine LE, Bernstein JE, Soltani K. Heparin-induced cutaneous necrosis unrelated to injection sites. Arch Derm 1983;119:400.

[114] Bircher AJ, Itin PH, Buchner SA. Skin lesions, hypereoinophilia and subcutaneous heparin. N Engl J Med 1994;343:861.

[115] Giustolisi R, Guglielmo P, di Raimondo F, Cacciola E, Stagno F. Hypereosinophilia and subcutaneous heparin. N Engl J Med 1993;342:1371.

[116] Lechy D, Gantt C, Linn V. Heparin-induced hypoaldosteronism. JAMA 1981;246:2189.

[117] Aull L, Chao H, Coy K. Heparin-induced hyperkalemia. Ann Pharmacother 1990;24:244.

[118] Food and Drug Adminstration. Lovenox (enoxaparin sodium) injection [January 9, 2002: Aventis Pharmaceuticals]: WARNINGS. FDA MedWatch 1/9/2002. Available at: http://www.fda.gov/medwatch/SAFETY/2002/jan02.htm#lovenox. Accessed January 2002.

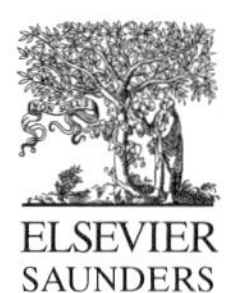

ELSEVIER
SAUNDERS

Hematol Oncol Clin N Am
19 (2005) 53–68

HEMATOLOGY/
ONCOLOGY
CLINICS OF
NORTH AMERICA

Development of Generic Low Molecular Weight Heparins: A Perspective

Jawed Fareed, PhD[a,b,*],
Wendy Leong, Pharm D, MCPS, MBA[c],
Debra A. Hoppensteadt, PhD[a], Walter P. Jeske, PhD[a,d],
Jeanine Walenga, PhD[a,d], Rodger L. Bick, MD, PhD[e]

[a]*Department of Pathology, Loyola University Chicago, 2160 South First Avenue, Maywood, IL 60153, USA*
[b]*Department of Pharmacology, Loyola University Chicago, 2160 South First Avenue, Maywood, IL 60153, USA*
[c]*Burnaby Research, University of British Columbia, Box 425, 141-6200 McKoy Avenue, Burnaby BC, VSH 4M9, Canada*
[d]*Department of Thoracic and Cardiovascular Surgery, Loyola University Chicago, 2160 South First Avenue, Maywood, IL 60153, USA*
[e]*Departments of Medicine and Pathology, University of Texas Southwestern Medical School, 2201 Inwood Road, Dallas, TX 75235-8852, USA*

There is a considerable debate over the development of generic versions of branded low molecular weight heparins (LMWHs) such as dalteparin, enoxaparin, tinzaparin, and others. Because the patents of some of these drugs have expired or are reaching term, there is considerable interest in the major suppliers of generic drugs to introduce generic versions of the branded products at a lower cost. LMWHs are unique because these products are of biologic origin yet there is significant chemical processing that makes each drug unique. The current pharmacopial descriptions of LMWHs are oversimplistic and do not take into account their unique molecular structural and biologic features. Not having proper guidelines, the generic drug industry has introduced products with the molecular profile specifications and biologic activity in terms of anti-Xa U/mg,

* Corresponding author. Department of Pathology, Loyola University Chicago, 2160 South First Avenue, Maywood, IL 60153.
E-mail address: jfareed@lumc.edu (J. Fareed).

doi:10.1016/j.hoc.2004.09.005

but this is inadequate, and products manufactured by different chemical processes are claimed to be equal to generic versions of products of distinct characteristics. Thus, these products cannot be interchanged on the basis of the claimed generic equivalence.

The primary aim of drug interchangeability is to reduce costs without compromising patient care (ie, drug acquisition cost) [1]. There are two types of drug interchangeability: therapeutic and generic. Therapeutic interchangeability is the substitution of chemically distinct drugs that exhibit therapeutic equivalence [1]. Therapeutically equivalent drugs may be interchanged or used as substitutes because they are expected to produce almost identical therapeutic outcomes and adverse reactions [2]. Guidelines usually are provided to assist with therapeutic interchangeability (substitutions) for specific medical conditions.

There are six criteria for scientifically justifiable and pharmacoeconomically beneficial therapeutic interchangeability [1]. If chemically unique drugs fail to meet any one of the following six criteria, then therapeutic interchangeability is not accepted [1]:

1. Pharmacologic equivalence
2. Clinical evidence supporting the therapeutic interchange in a given indication
3. Cost/availability
4. Thorough evaluation process (eg, Pharmacy and Therapeutics Committee)
5. Regular monitoring of patient outcomes
6. Response variations

There are heated debates about the therapeutic interchangeability for LMWHs [1,3–5]. The brand-name LMWH products of dalteparin (Fragmin), enoxaparin (Lovenox), nadroparin (Fraxiparin), and tinzaparin (Innohep) are chemically and biologically unique drugs [6–8]. These drugs are not interchangeable.

Pharmacologic equivalence between LMWHs has not been established [1]. Furthermore, there may be medicolegal implications for the indiscriminate interchange of the branded LMWHs for specific indications; this is particularly true of the LMWHs for which a dosage for a given indication is objectively established based on valid clinical trials.

On the other hand, generic LMWH interchangeability with the branded products may be more acceptable in the future. It appears that the manufacturing process for LMWHs must be preserved to produce an identical antithrombotic with similar clinical outcomes. The bioequivalence or pharmacodynamic data for LMWHs will need to include antithrombotic markers such as anti-Xa activity, anti-IIa activity, anti-Xa/anti-IIa ratio, partial thromboplastin time, international normalized ratio, and so forth. In addition, head-to-head clinical trials in specific indications will prove the safety and efficacy of a generic LMWH compared with the branded LMWH.

If a generic drug company is able to imitate the original manufacturing process, then it is likely that the regulatory bodies will grant generic LMWH approval. One must remember that other complex antithrombotics such as unfractionated heparin sodium (injection) and warfarin sodium (tablets) are now available as generic products. Numerous versions of aspirin have been available as generic products in North America for several years.

Generic interchangeability clearly refers to the substitution of a drug chemically identical and bioequivalent to the branded, native (original, pioneer, innovative) drug. For example, warfarin is the name of a widely used oral anticoagulant drug that commonly is sold under its branded name, Coumadin. An approved generic product, namely, Taro-warfarin also is sold. Taro Pharmaceuticals USA obtained US Food and Drug Administration (FDA) approval for generic warfarin (Abbreviated New Drug Application [ANDA]-40-301) in June 1999. In Canada, there is another generic version of warfarin named Apo-warfarin.

Unfractionated heparin is a complex mixture of sulfated mucopolysaccharide that is yet to be fully characterized. This widely used anticoagulant not only is polycomponent but also has polypharmacologic effects not yet fully understood. A generic unfractionated heparin sodium injection produced by American Pharmaceutical Partners was approved by the FDA in March 2002 (ANDA 17-029/S-099).

More recently, Apotek and Dr. Reddy have filed applications with the FDA seeking to market a generic version of the antiplatelet drug clopidogrel (Plavix) before all of the applicable patents expire. The active ingredient is clopidogrel bisulfate for which the innovator company Sanofi-Synthelabo holds several United States and foreign patents. Clopidegrel bisulfate is the bisulfate salt of the d-enantiomer of a chemical compound abbreviated MATTPCA. In the disputed patent, Sanofi-Synthelabo asserts that the d-enantiomer of MATTPCA is substantially separate from the e-enantiomer. The patent of MATTPCA's d-enantiomer is disputed by Apotek and Dr. Reddy. Thus, even before the patent expiration, Apotek and Dr. Reddy have challenged the validity of the 265 patent. If the efforts of Apotek and Dr. Reddy are successful, then it may allow the generic conversion of clopidogrel in the United States.

In 1984, the US Congress passed the Drug Price Competition and Patent Term Restoration Act (www.fda.gov). The Act expanded the number of drugs eligible to be manufactured as generics by eliminating the need for duplicate safety and efficacy testing, saving the pharmaceutical company producing the generic version of branded drugs time and money. It is stipulated that a bioequivalent generic drug would produce safety and efficacy benefits similar to the brand-name product.

Currently, the FDA approves approximately 300 generic drugs per year. The Generic Drug Review Process (ie, ANDA) has been clearly defined by the US Dept of Health and Human Services, the FDA, and the Center for Drug Evaluation and Research (June 2002 www.fda.gov/cder/handbook/anda.htm). The process includes the following:

- Bioequivalence review (human pharmacokinetics)
- Chemistry, manufacturing, and controls review

- Plant inspection
- Labeling review

According to the FDA, bioequivalency is a mandatory requirement for generic drugs. Bioequivalency is a demonstration of acceptable parameters established for bioavailability (ie, the extent and rate of drug absorption). Bioequivalency does not require the replication of clinical trials by generic drugs that were originally established by the brand-name drug. Bioequivalence studies usually include assay validation, dissolution studies, and in vitro and in vivo testing of the generic drugs. Pharmacokinetic profile in terms of the bioavailability and area under the curve for the drug's effect also is considered.

A generic drug manufacturer must provide the product's pharmacokinetic data for comparison with the original brand-name product. Traditionally, the pharmacokinetic profile of a drug includes the following:

- Absorption (eg, oral bioavailability)
- Distribution (eg, plasma protein binding)
- Metabolism (eg, active metabolites, cytochrome P450 enzymes)
- Elimination (eg, renal/hepatic, other)

LMWHs represent the depolymerized products obtained from porcine mucosal heparin by employing chemical, enzymatic, and physical methods. As shown in Fig. 1, these drugs are complex in molecular and structural composition and are

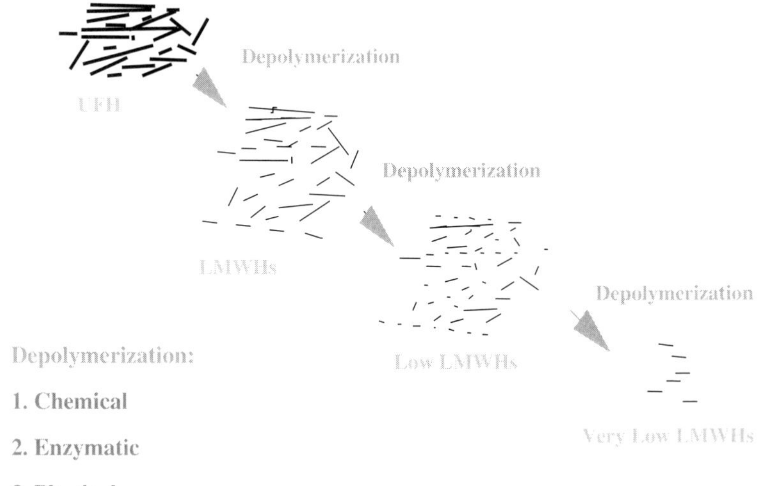

Fig. 1. Manufacturing process for LMWHs and ultra- LMWHs. Depolymerization of porcine mucosal heparin is accomplished by chemical, enzymatic, and physical methods. Newer depolymerization products include "low LMWHs" and "very low LMWHs."

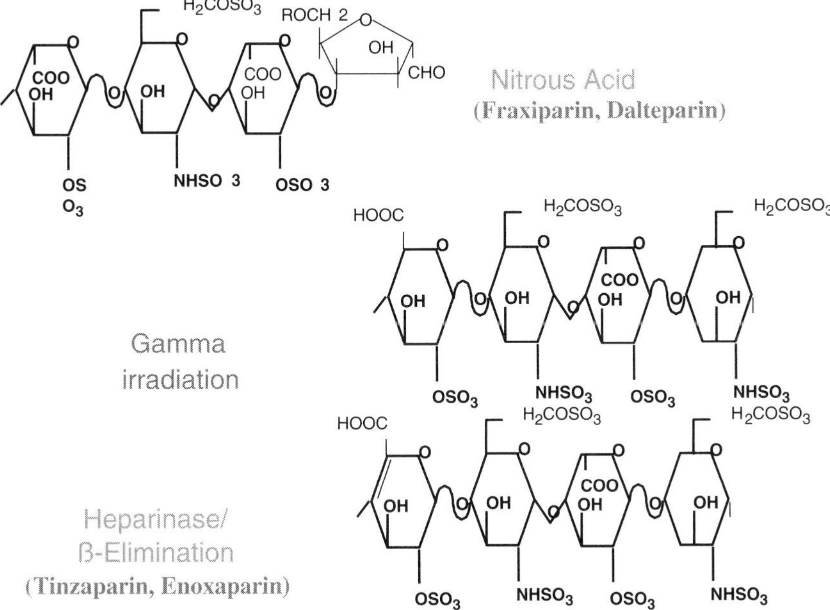

Fig. 2. Structural differences in the oligosaccharide are present in various LMWHs. These minor chemical changes are specific for each distinct depolymerization process. Although LMWHs may have similar molecular profiles, they can differ in their chemical composition.

heterogeneous. Different LMWHs are produced by specific patented procedures, resulting in compositional variations that strongly influence their biologic properties [9]. Fig. 2 shows a comparison of the oligosaccharide components of various LMWHs. Nadroparin (Fraxiparin) and dalteparin (Fragmin) are produced by nitrous acid digestion and are characterized by the presence of a sulfated pentose at the reducing end. No major structural changes result from γ radiation–mediated cleavage. Heparinase and β elimination result in the generation of a double bond that is characteristic of tinzaparin and enoxaparin.

Table 1
Molecular and chemical characteristics of various low molecular weight heparins

LMWH	Characteristics
Nadroparin	Presence of 2,5-anhydro-D-mannose at reducing terminus
Enoxaparin[a]	Presence of 4,5 unsaturated uronic acid at nonreducing terminus
Dalteparin	Presence of 2,5-anhydro-D-mannose at reducing terminus
Certoparin	Presence of 2,5-anhydro-D-mannose at reducing terminus
Tinzaparin	Presence of 4,5 unsaturated uronic acid at nonreducing terminus
Reviparin	Presence of 2,5-anhydro-D-mannose at reducing terminus
Ardeparin	Labile glycosidic bonds

[a] 1,6-Anhydromanno and anhydrogluco groups.

Table 1 depicts the structural and chemical characteristic of various LMWHs. Table 1 shows that different depolymerization processes produce specific structural alterations in these LMWHs. Aventis recently claimed that enoxaparin also contains specific 1,6-anhydromanno and anhydrogluco groups that are characteristic of this particular LMWH. Fig. 3 depicts the structure of the 1,6-anhydro ring of the enoxaparin fragment at the reducing end. Therefore, enoxaparin can be differentiated from tinzaparin due to the presence of the anhydro sugars at the reducing end. Thus, in addition to the molecular profile differences, specific minor chemical changes in different LMWHs can be used to differentiate these agents. It is not known, however, to what extent these changes influence the biologic actions of these agents.

The currently developed LMWHs include the following:

- Enoxaparin (Aventis, France)
- Dalteparin (Pfizer, USA)
- Tinzaparin (Leo/Pharmion, USA)
- Parnaparin (Opocrin, Italy)

Generic versions of these agents have been produced in various countries; some versions also have become available for clinical use in India, South American countries, and the Middle East.

The class of LMWHs has not received status as a therapeutically non-interchangeable drug, although it is recommended that they not be used interchangeably, at least on a unit-for-unit basis. Examples of traditional non-interchangeable drugs in North America include L-thyroxine and digoxin.

Is each LMWH a chemically and therapeutically unique antithrombotic agent that may not be interchanged? In 1993, the World Health Organization (WHO) acknowledged that each LMWH is a distinct entity. LMWH noninterchangeability also has been supported by the FDA, the American College of Chest Physicians, the American College of Cardiology, and the American Heart Association [10–13].

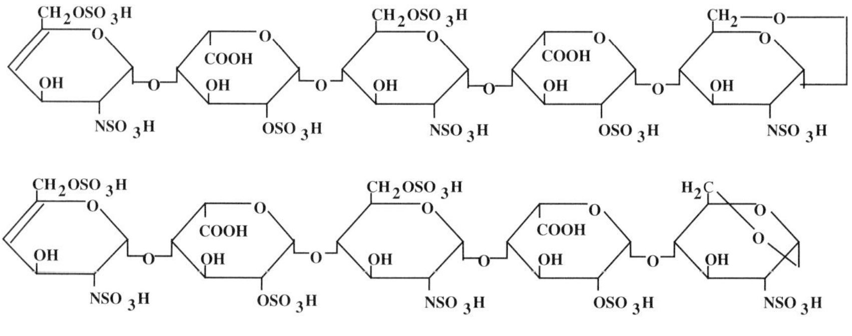

Fig. 3. The generation of a 1,6-anhydromanno group at the reducing terminus of oligosaccharides in enoxaparin represents a unique structural feature in the LMWH that initially was thought to be an artifact but now is considered an attribute.

Pharmacologic equivalence between LMWHs has not been proved because direct LMWH comparison studies are not readily available [14]. For example, the Efficacy and Safety of Subcutaneous Enoxaparin in Non-Q wave Coronary Events study established the enoxaparin dose of 1 mg/kg subcutaneously twice a day for the management of acute coronary syndrome [15]. In contrast, the studies on dalteparin demonstrated its efficacy in this syndrome at a 120 U/kg twice-daily dose, which amounts to a lower dosage in milligrams per kilogram (0.8 mg/kg) in this patient population (Fragmin in Unstable Coronary Artery Disease and Fragmin during Instability in Coronary Artery Disease studies) [16,17]. Thus, the dosages of the two different LMWHs were different in these studies. Regardless of the debates, LMWHs are not therapeutically interchangeable according to the WHO, the FDA, the American College of Cardiology, and the American Heart Association [10–13].

Generic interchangeability between a brand name and a generic LMWH has yet to be established. Clearly, the data must extend beyond basic bioequivalence due to the complex pharmacodynamic profile of these agents [13,18]. At this time, there are no clear guidelines for regulatory bodies such as the FDA and the European Medicines Agency to compare the generic version of these drugs.

A major focus of generic conversion is enoxaparin. This LMWH was one of the first widely used drugs prescribed for various indications including deep vein thrombosis prophylaxis and treatment, acute coronary syndrome, and several other indications. Enoxaparin is made by using benzylation followed by alkaline depolymerization of porcine mucosal heparin. One of the patents covering this drug has expired; the second patent will expire in December 2004. Knowing this, several manufacturers of LMWHs have produced generic versions of enoxaparin with claimed equivalence in accordance to the available specifications. Although the generic products may have similar molecular weight and anti-Xa potency, their biochemical and pharmacologic behavior may not be the same and requires further characterization is required. Enoxaparin represents a LMWH with wide clinical indications including arterial, venous, and cardiovascular use throughout the world. The dosage range varies widely for different indications. In addition, minor compositional differences in the generic version may impact the pharmacokinetic/pharmacodynamics of these agents. The generic versions of enoxaparin, therefore, must exhibit all physicochemical and biologic attributes to mimic the clinical performance of the innovator product.

On June 26, 2003 the FDA accepted the application for a generic version of Aventis's enoxaparin (Lovenox) from Amphastar (USA) who filed a certification against one of two patents for enoxaparin. The FDA, however, cannot approve the generic version before the drug's second patent expires December 24, 2004. Teva Pharmaceutical (USA), submitted an ANDA against the same enoxaparin patent on June 30, 2003. Gland Pharma (India) introduced the Cutenox brand of generic enoxaparin in India. The same generic version of enoxaparin also is available in Brazil. Several other companies throughout the world are considering the development of generic versions of the branded LMWHs. It is important, therefore, to have specific guidelines for the acceptance of generic LMWHs.

The history of LMWH development reveals current practice of the approval process. It is interesting that both the FDA and several European agencies have allowed manufacturers of branded LMWHs to substitute considerably changed products for the original product, merely controlling the molecular weight or a specified biologic activity.

The first LMWH, nadroparin (Fraxiparin, Sanofi-Synthelabo), originally was produced by ethanolic precipitation of porcine heparin followed by chromatographic separation. Due to limited yield, it was not possible to manufacture this drug in amounts large enough to meet the market demand. The manufacturer then produced a nitrous acid depolymerized product that exhibited a molecular weight profile and anti-Xa/anti-IIa ratio similar to that of the ethanolic-derived product [19,20]. The European regulatory agency approved the equivalence of the natural and depolymerized versions of this drug without requiring any chemical data. Eventually, the company replaced the original nadroparin with the chemically depolymerized version. The currently available nadroparin, therefore, represents a nitrous acid depolymerized product with a five-member sugar at the reducing end.

The currently marketed version of tinzaparin (Logiparin, Leo/Pharmion) is a product with considerably higher molecular weight than the originally introduced product (6400 versus 4300 d). The manufacturer refined the initial process by eliminating the ultra–low molecular weight fractions (<1500 d) from this drug. Thus, the resulting mean molecular weight was higher. The biologic activity in terms of anti-Xa activity, however, was not modified. Despite this major change, the regulatory agencies accepted the modification of the final processing and required only phase I bioequivalence data in terms of anti-Xa and anti-IIa to approve the modified product [21]. Therefore, the currently available tinzaparin is considerably different in molecular composition than the originally accepted product on which most of the clinical trials for approval were based.

These examples attest to the flexibility of the regulatory bodies to accept products with similar but not exactly the same molecular and biologic characteristics and call them the same. It would thus appear that if a process patent is used by a generic manufacturer, then it is relatively assured that the resulting product would be approved by the regulatory bodies.

Because of the complex nature of LMWHs, one should question the adequacy of the current requirements for acceptance of these drugs—be it an original or a generic—by the regulatory agencies. To demonstrate the similarities and differences among various LMWH products, several systematic approaches have been developed [22–24]. It is recommended that in the case of generic LMWHs, the regulatory bodies reconsider their criteria for accepting a generic equivalent. The following lists some of the basic requirements for characterizing a LMWH that should be employed in determining approval of a product as a true generic:

1. Physiochemical equivalence
2. Biological equivalence

3. Pharmacologic and toxicologic equivalence
4. Dosage (for both clinical safety and efficacy) equivalence

In addition to the physicochemical and biologic equivalence, a generic equivalent of a branded drug also should exhibit pharmacologic and toxicologic equivalence at the dosage stipulated in phase I (or equivalent) clinical trials. All studies should be performed over a dosage range at which the branded drug will be used.

Various regulatory agencies such as the FDA, European Medicines Agency, and WHO consider each of the LMWHs to be a distinct drug [10–13]. These agencies, however, only consider molecular weight profile and anti-Xa/anti-IIa potency, which may not be adequate for the demonstration of generic product equivalence to the branded product. The branded LMWHs are only partially characterized when these limited specifications are used. A generic version of a branded LMWH not only must be manufactured by exactly the same process as the original drug but also must exhibit physical, chemical, biologic, and clinical equivalence.

It is well known that each of the branded LMWHs exhibits product specific pharmcodynamic and pharmacokinetic differences. Such data as the molecular weight distribution of the components, structural characteristics, interactions with endogenous proteins, biologic actions such as the anti-Xa and anti-IIa, and other specific actions should be identical. Physiochemical methods such as nuclear magnetic resonance and oligosaccharide profiling such as the structural distribution of various components and the heparinase digestion signature profile can be used to prove the identity of a generic drug.

Current regulatory requirements do not consider all of these specifications, making it very likely that a generic product would not behave in a fashion similar to the original drug if the required characterization is not undertaken. Generic versions of each branded product can be manufactured by using methodology described in each of the individual patents of the branded products. Certain specific differences may still exist, however, that can be demonstrated only in biologic assays and dosage optimization studies in clinical trials.

Initially, wide lot-to-lot variations were observed between batches of the same branded product. It is expected that the generic-equivalent agents also may exhibit similar variations. The impact of these batch variations on each product should be documented on the clinical outcome. Some regulatory stipulations on the batch-to-batch variations also should be addressed.

Aventis submitted a Citizen's Petition on February 19, 2003 to the FDA stipulating the following:

- The product is unique. The product is not fully characterized. Not until full characterization has been completed, can a generic product be authorized.
- Clinical trials are needed to prove the clinical equivalence of the generic product.

The first argument of the Citizen's Petition also holds true for unfractionated heparin. Heparin is obtained from various natural sources, different salts are prepared, and impurities are known to exist within the products. Heparin has never been fully characterized in terms of its molecular and biologic actions. Using new techniques, we are still learning about this drug. Heparin initially was used as an antithrombotic in the 1930s. Owing to the physiochemical heterogeneity of this complex drug, a standard was established in 1942 [25]. The standardization practices at regulatory levels used the concept "like versus like" to standardize this drug.

On February 12, 2004, a supplement to the Citizen's Petition was filed by Aventis that claimed additional new discoveries in support of the petition. The following summarizes these claims:

- The antithrombin binding sequences are highly dependent on the manufacturing process of LMWHs.
- Additional, new anticoagulant effects due to the 1,6-anhydromanno reducing structure contribute to the overall pharmacologic actions of enoxaparin.

This supplement to the petition also contained several other sets of data on the structural characterization of the product, inhibition of thrombin generation, and potential heparin-induced thrombocytopenic actions as studied in an in vitro screening assay. Although the information provided additional attributes to enoxaparin, the relevance of these data to product uniqueness is not clear.

Furthermore, the Citizen's Petition and its supplement submitted to the FDA asserted that the bicyclic 1,6-anhydro ring structure may exert significant anticoagulant and nonanticoagulant pharmacologic effects with potential impact on its clinical efficacy. Oligosaccharide fingerprinting also is exemplified as a process-dependent antithrombin binding site. It should be clarified that enoxaparin represents a complex mixture of sulfated oligosaccharides and polysaccharide components that, on a comparative basis in a complex vascular environment, may produce polypharmacologic effects that are different from the studies reported on the purified/isolated oligosaccharides in simplified reaction conditions. Thus, any interpretation of the data on this matter may not be valid. It is likely that oligosaccharides attributed from other LMWHs also may behave in identical fashion in isolated systems. The relevance of some of these newer findings in the supplement such as the anticoagulant activity of oligosaccharide fractions, fibroblast growth factor differentiation, smooth muscle cell proliferation screening of individual oligosaccharides for potential cross-reactivity with antiheparin platelet factor 4 antibodies, P-selectin–mediated platelets/neutralization interactions is unclear. These types of studies may provide product-based variations; however, regardless of the 1,6-anhydromanno groups' presence, all sulfated oligosaccharides derived from different LMWHs may behave in a similar manner. Thus, the supplementary information in the Citizen's Petition extension does not add to the product individuality; however, the supplement's request for the following points may be partially valid:

- The manufacturing process for generic enoxaparin should be equivalent to Aventis's manufacturing process for enoxaparin.
- The statement "generic enoxaparin should contain 15% to 25% of the anhydromanno ring structure at the reducing end of the polysaccharide chain" may require further clarification and the range of the 1,6-anhydromanno groups may vary from 5% to 50% in the branded product.

The content of the two Citizen's Petitions should be evaluated objectively, a unilateral acceptance of the requested stipulations may not be consistent with generic drug regulatory guidelines.

Similarly, LMWH standards for the molecular profile and potency in terms of anti-Xa potency have been used to standardize various LMWH preparations [26,27]. These standards are useful only in the molecular weight profile and anti-Xa/anti-IIa potency evaluation. The standardization and cross-referencing methods described in various publications and the European Pharmacopoeia represent conventional methods that have been used for the characterization of unfractionated heparin and LMWHs may not be adequate for the specific characterization of generic versions of LMWHs. To demonstrate the equivalence of the generic products to the branded products, additional analytic and pharmacologic data may be needed. Several reports on the differences in the pharmacokinetic and pharmacodynamic profiles of various LMWHs have clearly shown discordance between the anti-Xa activity and the overall biologic actions of these agents [28]. Thus, the standardization of the biologic actions of LMWHs is of limited value in terms of establishing equivalence not only for different branded LMWHs but also for the characterization of the generic LMWHs. An integrated profile may be more relevant for this process.

The Citizen's Petition and its supplement submitted on behalf of Aventis to the commissioner of the FDA requesting the agency to withhold approval of ANDA for a generic version of enoxaparin until the arbitrary conditions stated in this petition are satisfied may not be consistent with the accepted scientific and regulatory guidelines set forth by the agency and manufacturers of drugs. Enoxaparin represents a depolymerized heparin that has been characterized by physical, chemical, and biologic terms. The characteristics of the final product are described publicly by the company and by the scientific community using the originally published procedure and the information in the patent. Therefore, enoxaparin-equivalent products with chemical and pharmacologic equivalence can be produced. The chemical process of depolymerization using benzylation of porcine mucosal heparin followed by alkaline hydrolysis results in the formation of oligosaccharide chains that contain the 1,6-anhydro ring structure at the reducing ends. This chemical moiety easily can be adjusted between 15% and 25% of total poly/oligosaccharide components, which therefore, may not be a unique feature of the branded product.

On the other hand, it is conceivable that each of the branded LMWHs may have some unique microchemical or physical feature that may not be reproducible by merely using the process described in the patent. Additional guidelines requiring specific structural information are needed to reinforce the requirements for molecular and structural characterizations. Because some of these unique features or attributes may not have been described in the original patent, the manufacturer of the generic version may contest the addition of such previously unreported characteristics. In the authors' opinion, however, although these characteristics were not reported in the patent, they previously existed but were not revealed because the technology and knowledge to do so did not exist at the time of the patent filing. When revealed, these characteristics need to be accepted as defining the original product. Manufacturers may therefore provide additional information on the product characterization as it becomes available. A generic product should only be approved, however, when it complies with existing specifications for a given product.

Regarding the second argument of the Citizen's Petition, in reference to the requirement for clinical equivalence trials, the authors currently point to the Drug Price Competition and Patent Term Restoration Act (www.fda.gov). This Act waived the requirement for the duplicate safety and efficacy testing in humans for comparing generic equivalent products to the branded drug. The generic drug review process is clearly outlined by the FDA in which bioequivalency is a mandatory requirement. Because of the multiple biologic actions of LMWHs, specific guidelines may be needed to demonstrate bioequivalency. Furthermore, because of their use in critical clinical settings such as acute coronary syndrome and pulmonary embolism, specific guidelines should be developed to obtain data on clinical equivalence for generic LMWHs. The FDA has granted only product- and indication-specific approval for these drugs. Thus, a generic version of a branded LMWH can be considered only for the approved indications for the branded product.

At the present time, there are no specific guidelines for the assessment of generic-equivalent LMWHs. The existing guidelines from the Bureau of Generic Drugs may not be adequate for generic LMWHs. Because LMWHs represent a hybrid drug product of biologic and chemical entities, there is a need to develop specific guidelines for the acceptance of individual generic versions of branded LMWHs. Technologic advances have provided newer tools to characterize the LMWHs by chemical and biologic methods. In addition to the molecular profile, oligosaccharide composition, depolymerization profile, and structural analysis including sophisticated methods may provide additional unique features that can be used to characterize the branded LMWHs. The generic product manufacturers have to prove that their product exhibits similar characteristics.

The regulatory bodies eventually may allow the generic versions of LMWHs and apply the same (or expanded) guidelines as for other biologics. Doing so may result in generic products that will meet these guideline specifications but may not be identical and, therefore, may behave differently in clinical settings. It is important, therefore, to have additional requirements to provide supplementary chemical and biologic data to support the filing of a generic version of a branded drug. Whether clinical trials are required for specific products for approved indications depends on the filing process to evaluate data for the FDA review.

The generic pharmaceutical industry has played a key role in providing less expensive equivalents of original branded drugs that otherwise would not be accessible to a large group of patients. Thus, generic drugs have a major public health importance. Recognizing this, President Bush has announced the expansion of the Office of Generic Drugs [29]. Thus, at a federal government level, there is endorsement of the development of generic drugs and to have them accessible to all patients.

In the case of generic versions of the LMWHs, it is clear that the manufacturers of the generic versions may not have adequate expertise to compare these different LMWHs in refined methods to assure clinical, biologic, and pharmacologic equivalence. Such studies should be performed by independent research groups following the establishment of specific guidelines.

It is now clear that the introduction of generic versions of LMWHs is inevitable; however, it is important that the generic products are manufactured in strict compliance with the manufacturing specification of the branded product. Furthermore, regulatory agencies should require additional data on the chemical biologic, pharmacologic/toxicologic, and dose-response relationship in specific settings.

The following are several important questions and brief answers regarding the development of generic versions of LMWHs.

1. Are the differences between the branded LMWHs significant enough to consider each of these drugs to be classified as different? Yes, there are significant differences between most of the branded LMWHs. Although the potency of these agents can be adjusted in anti-Xa units per milligram, because these drugs are polycomponent, their therapeutic and toxicologic profile can vary widely. Various agencies have considered each of these drugs as distinct.
2. Using the patents for each of these agents, is it possible to manufacture the generic versions of such branded LMWHs as dalteparin, enoxaparin, nadroparin, tinzaparin, certoparin, parnaparin, and bemiparin? Yes, it is possible to manufacture generic versions of various branded LMWHs. Several generic versions of enoxaparin have been manufactured by different companies, and generic versions of dalteparin and nadroparin also have become available.
3. Are there additional unique features in each of these LMWHs that attribute additional uniqueness to these products that are not covered in the patent and can be described only as product art and manufacturing refinements? In the original product description, there was a limited description of these LMWHs; however, with the advances in analytic and biologic methods, each of these products can be characterized further in structural and biologic terms. Such features, however, also can be attributed to the generic process.

4. Are the batch differences within a branded product significant enough to suggest that within a brand-name LMWH, marked variations in product profiles can be observed? Significant batch-to-batch variations can be observed within one brand; however, the current guidelines only require the adjusted anti-Xa per milligram potency, which is specified for each of the different branded products. There are several other biologic actions and clinical characteristics not readily detectable that may influence the product profile.
5. It is claimed that branded products are unique and only partially characterized. This claim suggests that individual LMWHs are unique and the patent-described process may not provide sufficient information to make a generic version of each drug. Therefore, additional physiochemical analyses using newer technology have provided specific data that can be used to characterize different products. This also is true for unfractionated heparin. Even with simple drugs such as aspirin and warfarin, we are learning new information on the biologic actions and pharmacodynamic interactions. Thus, it is conceivable that additional characteristics and biologic actions will be discovered for each product. The generic manufacturers should be required to prove that these products are similar.
6. Are there any guidelines from regulatory bodies or professional societies to evaluate the generic versions of LMWHs and to set up acceptance or rejection criteria? At the present time, there are no specific guidelines for the acceptance of generic versions of various LMWHs. The FDA has received several requests for the approval of generic versions of enoxaparin. The Citizen's Petition and its supplement filed by Aventis and submitted to the FDA stipulated that several requirements must be met before the FDA will give any consideration to the generic LMWHs.
7. Who are the manufacturers of the generic versions of enoxaparin? Do they have adequate knowledge to produce comparable products? The generic versions of LMWHs are manufactured by several different companies, some of which have wide experience developing these drugs. Some of the generic LMWH manufacturers also represent large, ethical drug companies who have interest in marketing the generic versions of these agents. Not all of the companies capable of manufacturing generic LMWHs have adequate knowledge of the characterization of these drugs. Therefore, clear guidelines regarding the manufacturing and product specifications for generic LMWHs may be helpful in introducing drug-comparable pharmacologic and clinical properties.

There is a strong move to introduce generic versions of branded LMWHs and a strong opposition to stop the introduction of these drugs. Development of these generic drugs, however, will reduce cost and permit availability to all patients who need them. Thus, some objective guidelines for the proper development of these drugs are needed. Only expert groups and advisory panels to the regulatory bodies can develop these guidelines.

References

[1] Merli G, Vanscoy G, Rihn TL, et al. Applying scientific criteria to therapeutic interchange: a balanced analysis of low molecular weight heparins. J Thromb Thrombolysis 2001;11(3): 247–59.

[2] American Society of Hospital Pharmacists. ASHP statement on the formulary system. Am J Hosp Pharm 1988;43:2839–41.

[3] McCart GM, Kayser S. Therapeutic equivalency of low molecular weight heparins. Ann Pharmcother 2002;36:1042–57.

[4] Prandoni P. Low molecular weight heparins: are they interchangeable? Yes. J Thromb Hemostasis 2003;1:10–1.

[5] Nenci G. Low molecular weight heparins: are they interchangeable? No. J Thromb Hemostasis 2003;1:12–3.

[6] Bick RL, Fareed J. Low Molecular weight heparin: differences and similarities in approved preparations in the United States. Clin Appl Throm Hemost 1999;5(Suppl 1):S63–6.

[7] Fareed J, Hoppensteadt D, Jeske W, et al. Low molecular weight heparins. Are they different? Can J Cardiol 1998;14(Suppl E):28E–34E.

[8] Fareed J, Haas S, Sasahara A. Past, present and future considerations on low molecular weight heparins differentiation: an epilogue. Sem Thromb Hemost 1999;25(Suppl 3):145–7.

[9] Linhardt RJ, Gunay NS. Production and chemical processing of low molecular weight heparins. Semin Thromb Hemostas 1999;25(Suppl 3):5–16.

[10] Nightingale SL. From the Food and Drug Administration. JAMA 1993;270(14):1672.

[11] Hirsch J, Warkentin TE, Shaughnessy SG, et al. Heparin and low molecular weight heparin: mechanisms of action, pharamcokinetics, dosing considerations, monitoring, efficacy, and safety. Chest 1998;114(Suppl 5):489S–510S.

[12] Ryan TJ, Antman EM, et al. 1999 update. ACC/AHA guidelines for the management of patients with acute myocardial infarction. J Am Col Cardiol 1999;34(3):890–911.

[13] Fareed J, Fu K, Hoppensteadt D, et al. Pharmacokinetics of low molecular weight heparins in animal models. Semin Thromb Hemost 1999;25(Suppl 3):51–5.

[14] Kaiser B, Kirchmaier CM, Breddin HK, et al. Preclinical biochemistry and pharmacology of low molecular weight heparins in vivo. Semin Thromb Hemost 1999;25(Suppl 3):35–42.

[15] Cohen M, Demers C, Gurfinkel EP, et al. A comparison of low molecular weight heparin with unfractionated heparin for unstable coronary artery disease. Efficacy and safety of subcutaneous enoxaparin in non-Q wave coronary events study group (ESSENCE). N Engl J Med 1997;337(7):447–52.

[16] Klein W, Buchwald A, Arnd MD, et al. Fragmin in unstable angina pectoris or in non-Q wave acute myocardial infarction. Fragmin in unstable coronary artery disease (FRIC). Am J Cardiol 1997;80(5A):30E–4E.

[17] FRISC study group. Low molecular weight heparin during instability in coronary artery disease. Fragmin during instability in coronary artery disease (FRISC). Lancet 1998;347(9001): 561–8.

[18] Mousa S, Fareed J. Overview: from heparin to low molecular weight heparins: beyond anticoagulation. Curr Opin Invest Drug 2001;2(8):1077–80.

[19] Fareed J, Kumar A, Walenga JM, et al. Antithrombotic actions and pharmacokinetics of heparin fractions and fragments. Nouv Rev Fr Hematol 1984;26:267–75.

[20] Fareed J, Walenga JM, Racanelli A, et al. Validity of the newly established low-molecular-weight heparin standard in cross-referencing low-molecular-weight heparins. Haemostasis 1988; 18(Suppl 3):33–47.

[21] Barrett JS, Hainer JW, Kornhauser DM, et al. Anticoagulant pharmacodynamics of tinzaparin following 175 IU/kg subcutaneous administration to healthy volunteers. Thromb Res 2001;101: 243–54.

[22] Fareed J, Haas S, Sasahara A, editors. Differentiation of low molecular weight heparins. Applied and clinical considerations [special issue]. Semin Thromb Hemost 1999;25(3).

[23] Fareed J, Walenga JM, Hoppensteadt D, et al. Comparative study on the in vitro and in vivo activities of seven low-molecular-weight heparins. Haemostasis 1988;18(Suppl 3):3–15.
[24] Fareed J, Walenga JM, Williamson K, et al. Studies on the antithrombotic effects and pharmacokinetics of heparin fractions and fragments. Semin Thromb Hemost 1985;11(1):56–74.
[25] Memorandum on a provisional international standard for heparin. Bull Health Organ League Nations 1942;151–4.
[26] Barrowcliffe TW, Curtiss AD, Johnson EA, et al. An international standard for low molecular weight heparin. Thromb Haemost 1988;60:1–7.
[27] Mulloy B, Gee C, Wheeler SF, et al. Molecular weight measurements of low molecular weight heparins by gel permeation chromatography. Thromb Haemost 1997;77(4):668–74.
[28] Cambus JP, Saivin S, Heilmann JJ, et al. The pharmacodynamics of tinzaparin in healthy volunteers. Br J Hematol 2002;116:649–52.
[29] Abboud L. Bush acts to speed generics to market. Wall Street Journal. June12, 2003;A3, vol. CCXLI 114.

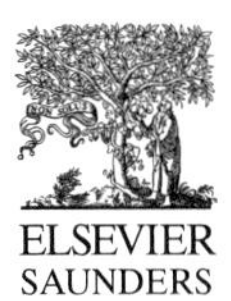

ELSEVIER
SAUNDERS

Hematol Oncol Clin N Am
19 (2005) 69–85

HEMATOLOGY/
ONCOLOGY
CLINICS OF
NORTH AMERICA

Vitamin K Antagonists and Direct Thrombin Inhibitors: Present and Future

Graham F. Pineo, MD*, Russell D. Hull, MBBS, MSc

Department of Medicine, University of Calgary, Foothills Hospital, 601 South Tower, 1403 29 Street Norhtwest, Calgary, AB T2N 2T9, Canada

Warfarin and related compounds have been shown to be efficacious and safe in a wide variety of clinical thrombotic disorders including venous thromboembolism, stroke prevention in nonvalvular atrial fibrillation, and prevention of systemic emboli in patients who have myocardial infarction or prosthetic heart valves. Also, in North America, vitamin K antagonists (VKAs) are commonly used for the prevention of venous thromboembolism following orthopedic surgery. With these drugs having a narrow therapeutic window with respect to international normalized ratio (INR), inadequate therapy is associated with an increased thrombotic risk, whereas overanticoagulation is associated with bleeding. For these reasons, attempts have been made to develop alternatives to warfarin. Low molecular weight heparin (LMWH) provides an alternative for the long-term treatment of venous thromboembolism but must be given by injection. Ximelagatran, an oral direct thrombin inhibitor, has been shown to be of equal efficacy and safety compared with warfarin for the prevention and treatment of number of different thrombotic disorders. This article reviews the pharmacology of the coumarins, the most commonly used VKAs, and the practical aspects regarding the use of these agents in the management of thrombotic disorders. The future role of the oral direct thrombin inhibitor ximelagatran also is reviewed.

* Corresponding author.
E-mail address: pineo@ucalgary.ca (G.F. Pineo).

0889-8588/05/$ – see front matter
doi:10.1016/j.hoc.2004.09.006 ***hemonc.theclinics.com***

Pharmacology

The vitamin K cycle

Vitamin K induces the post-translational conversion of glutamate residues into γ-carboxyglutamate in a limited number of proteins, the best known of which are the blood coagulation factors II, VII, IX, X, protein C, protein S, and protein Z [1–4].

γ-Carboxyglutamic acid enhances the binding of calcium by these proteins, and in the presence of calcium, the coagulation factors undergo a conformational change that is required for their binding to various active cofactors on cell surfaces [2,3]. The reduced form of vitamin K (KH_2) acts as a coenzyme for carboxylase. The vitamin K cycle is demonstrated in Fig. 1. The oxidation of vitamin KH_2 by oxygen into vitamin K epoxide (KO) provides energy to fix

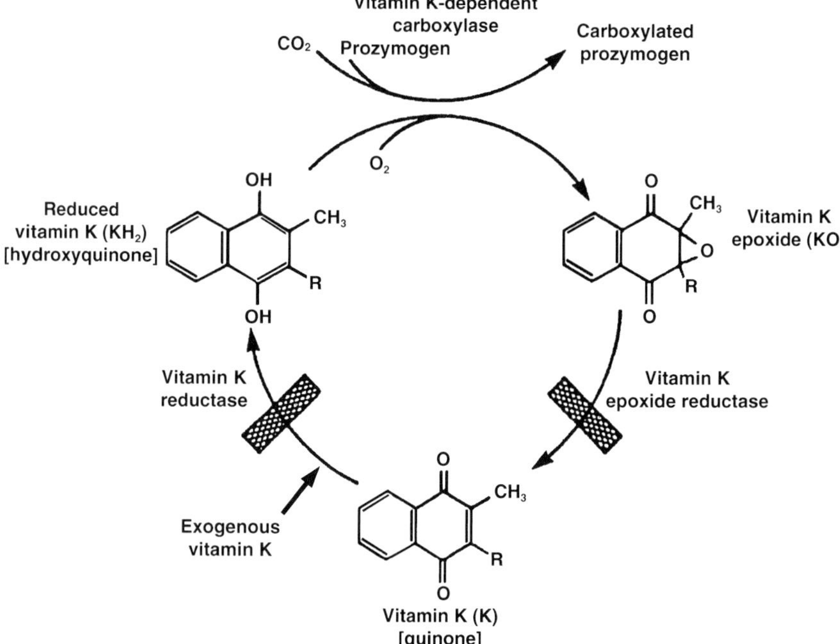

Fig. 1. The vitamin K cycle: the effect of warfarin and exogenous vitamin K (phytomenadione). Vitamin K (quinone) is converted to reduced vitamin K (KH_2, hydroxyquinone) by vitamin K reductase. Vitamin KH_2 is the substrate for the carboxylation of prozymogens (eg, factors II, VII, IX, and X) to active enzymes. Carbon dioxide (CO_2) and oxygen are required for this reaction, and vitamin KH_2 is converted to vitamin K epoxide (KO). Vitamin K is regenerated for vitamin KO by vitamin KO reductase. Warfarin inhibits vitamin KO reductase and, to some extent, vitamin K reductase (*hatched areas*). Exogenous vitamin K in large doses overcomes the blockage by warfarin presumably because vitamin K reductase is less sensitive to warfarin than vitamin KO reductase (*straight arrow*). (*From* Furie B, Furie BC. Molecular basis of vitamin K–dependent gamma-carboxylation. Blood 1990;75:1754; with permission.)

carbon dioxide at the γ-position of a glutamate residue [3]. The vitamin KO is then recycled, first by vitamin KO reductase to vitamin K (quinone) and then by vitamin K reductase to vitamin KH_2 (hydroquinone). It is essential that each molecule of vitamin K be recycled several hundred times before being metabolized. The VKAs inhibit vitamin KO reductase and possibly vitamin K reductase, thereby depleting vitamin KH_2 and causing the build-up of vitamin KO in tissues such as the liver and plasma [5–7].

The two forms of vitamin K are phylloquinones (vitamin K_1) and menaquinones (vitamin K_2) [2]. Phylloquinones are found in green, leafy vegetables such as spinach, cabbage, and broccoli. Deficiencies of these vegetables in the diet can cause vitamin K deficiency, whereas excessive amounts can reverse the effects of oral anticoagulants. The menaquinones occur in various foods such as yogurt and organ meats and are produced by the bacterial flora of the colon and, possibly, the small intestine. Factors interfering with the production or absorption of these menaquinones (eg, broad-spectrum antibiotics), may lead to vitamin K deficiency [8–10] and interference with anticoagulant control. In addition, certain cephalosporins containing an N-methyl-thiotetrazole side chain may interfere directly with vitamin KO reductase in the liver [9], thereby leading to vitamin K deficiency. Most of the vitamin K stores in the liver are menaquinones and it is thought that most of these originate from the diet rather than intestinal flora [11,12].

Large doses of vitamin K can overcome the blockade of vitamin KH_2 by VKAs presumably because vitamin K reductase is less sensitive to the coumarins than vitamin KO reductase [2] (see Fig. 1). This reversal of VKAs applies to the first-generation agents such as warfarin but not to the second-generation rodenticides known as the "super warfarins," which have an extremely long half-life [13]. Accidental consumption of these agents requires repeated injections of vitamin K and fresh frozen plasma for up to 1 or 2 years to completely overcome their effects [13,14]. Hereditary resistance to VKAs has been described; individuals with resistance may require extremely high doses of warfarin to achieve adequate anticoagulation [15,16].

Pharmacokinetics and pharmacodynamics of warfarin

There are two distinct chemical groups of VKAs: the 4-hydroxycoumarin derivatives (eg, warfarin sodium, acecoumarin) and the indane-1,3-dione derivatives (eg, phenindione) [17]. The coumarin derivatives are the VKAs of choice because they are associated with fewer nonhemorrhagic side effects than the indanedione derivatives. In North America, the most commonly used agent is warfarin sodium (Coumadin) but in recent years, various generic forms of warfarin sodium have been introduced.

Warfarin is a racemic mixture of stereoisomers (R and S forms); the S form is the most potent [17,18] and is highly water soluble and highly bioavailable [17]. Peak absorption occurs at around 90 minutes and the half-life is between 36 and

42 hours [19–21]. Warfarin is highly protein bound (primarily albumin), and only the non–protein-bound material is biologically active [19]. Any drug or chemical that also is bound to albumin may displace warfarin from its protein binding sites and thereby increase the biologically active material [18]. The S form of warfarin is metabolized in the liver by the P450 (CYP2C9) system of enzymes [22–24]. Interference with the CYP2C9 enzymes by various drugs or a mutation in the gene coding for one of the common CYP2C9 enzymes can markedly interfere with the metabolism of warfarin [24]. In recent years, a genetic mutation of the factor IX propeptide has been described. Subjects with this mutation may have a precipitous fall in factor IX concentration with VKA therapy, leading to a prolonged activated partial thromboplastin time but without excessive prolongation of the INR, and they may experience excessive bleeding [25]. It is fortunate that this defect is rare.

The anticoagulant effect of warfarin is mediated by the inhibition of the vitamin K–dependent γ-carboxylation of coagulation factors II, VII, IX, and X [1–3,26,27]. This inhibition results in the synthesis of immunologically detectable but biologically inactive forms of these coagulation proteins. Warfarin also inhibits the vitamin K–dependent γ-carboxylation of proteins C and S [27] and protein Z [26]. Protein C circulates as a proenzyme that is activated on endothelial cells by the thrombin/thrombomodulin complex to form activated protein C. Activated protein C in the presence of protein S inhibits activated factor VIII and activated factor V activity [28]. Therefore, VKAs such as warfarin create a biochemical paradox by producing an anticoagulant effect due to the inhibition of procoagulants (factors II, VII, IX, and X) and a potentially thrombogenic effect by impairing the synthesis of naturally occurring inhibitors of coagulation (proteins C and S) [28]. For this reason, heparin or LMWH and warfarin treatment should overlap by 4 to 5 days when warfarin treatment is initiated in patients who have thrombotic disease [28,29]. The role of protein Z in the coagulation process is less definite [26].

The anticoagulant effect of warfarin is delayed until the normal clotting factors are cleared from the circulation, and the peak effect does not occur until 36 to 72 hours after drug administration [30–32]. During the first few days of warfarin therapy, the prothrombin time reflects mainly the depression of factor VII, which has a half-life of 5 to 7 hours. There is now good evidence that this decrease in the level of factor VII does not provide antithrombotic protection [33,34]. Equilibrium levels of factors II, IX, and X are not reached until about 1 week after the initiation of therapy [31,34]. The dose-response relationship to warfarin therapy varies widely between individuals and, therefore, the dose must be carefully monitored to prevent overdosing or underdosing.

Many factors influence the anticoagulant response of warfarin in individual patients. These factors include inaccuracies in laboratory testing, noncompliance of patients, and abnormal liver function but, more important, reflect the influence of dietary changes or the influence of drugs that interfere with the metabolism of warfarin. The availability of vitamin K can be influenced by dramatic changes in dietary intake [35,36] or by drugs such as antibiotics that interfere with the synthesis of vitamin K in the gastrointestinal tract [8–10]. Many drugs may interact with warfarin [37]; however, a critical appraisal of the literature reporting such interactions indicates that the evidence substantiating many of the claims is limited [38]. The interactions of drugs and food with warfarin are reviewed in detail in the recent publication by Hirsh et al [18]. Aspirin is particularly problematic because it interferes with platelet function and displaces warfarin from its protein binding, augmenting its biologic activities and possibly causing gastric erosions (as with the nonsteroidal anti-inflammatory drugs), thus creating a site for bleeding. The newer cyclooxygenase-2 inhibitors may have less of a tendency to cause gastrointestinal bleeding in patients on VKA, but at this time, there is little evidence to support this. Acetaminophen in small doses can be used as an analgesic in patients on long-term VKA treatment, but high doses (eg, 9100 mg/week or more) may cause excessive warfarin anticoagulation [39]. In certain patients, the use of aspirin and warfarin is indicated to improve efficacy even though bleeding may be somewhat increased [18,40]. It is important that patients be warned against taking any new drugs without the knowledge of their attending physician, and it is prudent to monitor the INR more frequently when any drug (including natural compounds or food supplements) is added or withdrawn from the regimen of the patient being treated with a VKA.

Laboratory monitoring and therapeutic range

The laboratory test most commonly used to measure the effects of warfarin is the one-stage prothrombin time [18,41]. The prothrombin time is sensitive to reduced activity of factors II, VII, and X but insensitive to reduced activity of factor IX. To promote standardization of the prothrombin time for monitoring oral anticoagulant therapy, the World Health Organization developed an international reference thromboplastin from human brain tissue and recommended that the prothrombin time ratio be expressed as the INR [18,41,42].

Warfarin usually is administered in an initial dose of 5 mg/day for the first 2 days, and then the daily dose is adjusted according to the INR [37,43,44]. Heparin or LMWH therapy is discontinued on the fifth day following initiation of warfarin therapy, provided the INR is prolonged into the recommended therapeutic range (INR 2.0–3.0) for at least 2 consecutive days [18]. Frequent INR determinations are required initially to establish therapeutic anticoagulation.

After the anticoagulant effect and the patient's warfarin dose requirements are stable, the INR should be monitored every 1 to 3 weeks throughout the course of warfarin therapy [37]. If there are factors that may produce an unpredictable response to warfarin (eg, concomitant drug therapy) [18], then the INR should be monitored more frequently to minimize the risk of complications due to poor anticoagulant control [37,44].

The long-term use of VKAs has been shown to be efficacious and safe for the prevention of (1) recurrent venous thromboembolism in patients who present with deep vein thrombosis or pulmonary embolism, (2) stroke in patients related to atrial fibrillation, (3) thrombotic events in patients who have prosthetic heart valves, (4) systemic embolism in patients who have acute myocardial infarction or valvular heart disease, and (5) venous thromboembolism following total hip replacement surgery (up to 30 days). For these conditions, the target INR is 2.5, with a range of 2.0 to 3.0 [18].

There have been attempts to improve the safety of warfarin therapy by using a lower INR target, but this can result in an increased thrombotic risk [45]. Although long-term treatment with warfarin to a target INR of 1.5 to 2.0 in patients who have venous thromboembolism proved to be more effective than placebo treatment [46], a similar study that compared a target INR of 1.5 to 2.0 to the standard INR of 2.0 to 3.0 showed significantly lower recurrence rate with the standard treatment, with no added risk of bleeding [47]. A number of other studies using less-intense warfarin (eg, for the prevention of thrombosis in central venous catheters) showed such treatment to be ineffective [48–50]. In some cases, the target INR is greater than 3.0. For example, based on retrospective studies, patients who have mechanical heart valves have been treated with a target INR of 2.5 to 3.5 [51]. In patients who have bioprosthetic heart valves or in low-risk patients who have bileaflet mechanical valves in the aortic position, the target INR is still 2.0 to 3.0 [28]. Although retrospective studies suggested that patients who have antiphospholipid antibodies and recurrent thrombosis required an INR of greater than 3.0 [52–54], a randomized study comparing an INR of 2.0 to 3.0 with an INR of 3.1 to 4.0 showed that the incidence of recurrent thrombosis and major bleeding was comparable in the two groups [55].

Adverse effects of vitamin K antagonists

Bleeding and vitamin K antagonist therapy

The major side effect of VKA therapy is bleeding. Bleeding that occurs during well-controlled oral VKA therapy usually is due to surgery or other forms of trauma or to local lesions such as peptic ulcer or carcinoma [42,56]. Spontaneous bleeding may occur when warfarin is given in an excessive dose that results in a marked prolongation of the INR, and this bleeding may be severe or even life threatening [57–61]. The risk of bleeding may be substantially reduced by carefully adjusting the warfarin dose to maintain a therapeutic INR range (usually 2.0–3.0) [18,37,59]. Management in anticoagulant management clinics [62–65] or the use of point-of-care INR testing [66–68] has been shown to be more effective than routine management for maintaining patients in their desired therapeutic range.

Numerous attempts have been made to estimate bleeding risks for patients being treated with oral anticoagulants. One such risk is age greater than 65 years [69–73]. In a large administrative database, White et al [70] analyzed the risk factors for rehospitalization for bleeding among patients initially hospitalized for venous thromboembolism. The rate of bleeding was highest during the first month of treatment and then fell to a stable rate over the next 2 months. As in previous studies, risk factors for major bleeding that required intervention included age 65 or older, female gender, previous gastrointestinal bleeding, alcoholism, chronic renal failure, and cancer [70,72,73].

Management of overanticoagulation

The approach to the patient who has an elevated INR depends on the degree of elevation and the clinical circumstances [37]. Options available to the physician include temporary discontinuation of VKA treatment, administration of vitamin K, or administration of blood products such as fresh frozen plasma or prothrombin concentrate to replace the vitamin K–dependent clotting factors. If the increase is mild and the patient is not bleeding, then no specific treatment is necessary other than reduction in the warfarin dose [60]. The INR can be expected to decrease during the next 24 hours with this approach. With more marked increase of the INR in patients who are not bleeding, treatment with small doses of vitamin K_1 (eg, 1 mg), given orally or by subcutaneous injection could be considered [74–76]. With very marked increase of the INR, particularly in a patient who is actively bleeding or at risk for bleeding, the coagulation defect should be corrected. If ongoing anticoagulation with warfarin is planned, then repeated small doses of vitamin K should be given so that there is no problem with warfarin resistance [74–76].

When bleeding occurs in a patient on a VKA, it is important to consider the site of bleeding. Bleeding from the upper gastrointestinal tract commonly is seen in patients on VKAs; concomitant use of other medications often is an association. When the bleeding is controlled, it is important to carry out the necessary investigations to identify bleeding lesions in the gastrointestinal or genitourinary tract, which often are unsuspected [18,77].

Nonhemorrhagic adverse effects

Coumarin-induced skin necrosis is a rare but serious complication that requires immediate cessation of therapy [78–81]. It usually occurs between 3 and 10 days after therapy has commenced, is more common in women, and most often involves areas of abundant subcutaneous tissues such as the abdomen, buttocks, thighs, and breasts. The mechanism of coumarin-induced skin necrosis, associated with microvascular thrombosis, is uncertain but appears to be related, at least in some patients, to depression of protein C levels [81]. Patients who have congenital deficiencies of protein C or protein S may be particularly prone to the development of coumarin skin necrosis. Combination use of VKA treatment with heparin for 10 to 14 days has been reported to be successful for anticoagulation in patients who have severe protein C deficiency [81,82].

Management of patients on long-term oral anticoagulants requiring surgical intervention

Physicians commonly are confronted with the problem of managing VKA therapy in individuals who require temporary interruption of treatment for surgery or other invasive procedures. In the absence of data from randomized clinical trials, recommendations based only on cohort studies, retrospective reviews, and expert opinions can be made. The most common conditions requiring long-term anticoagulant therapy are atrial fibrillation, mechanical or prosthetic heart valve replacement, and venous thromboembolism [83–85]. For each of these conditions, the risk of arterial or venous thromboembolism after anticoagulants have been discontinued must be weighed against the risk of bleeding if intravenous heparin is applied before or after the surgical procedure or if VKA therapy is continued at the therapeutic level. The possible choices based on the risk/benefit assessment in the individual patient (based on a previous American College of Chest Physicians consensus conference [84] on anththrombotic therapy) include the following:

1. Discontinuing warfarin for 3 to 5 days before the procedure to allow the INR to return to normal, and then restarting therapy shortly after surgery
2. Lowering the warfarin dose to maintain an INR in the lower or subtherapeutic range during the surgical procedure
3. Discontinuing warfarin and treating the patient in-hospital with intravenous heparin or LMWH before and after the surgical procedure until warfarin therapy can be reinstituted

LMWH, which can be given by once- or twice-daily subcutaneous injection, offers a convenient alternative to intravenous unfractionated heparin for patients requiring temporary interruption of warfarin therapy for invasive procedures [86]. Data from cohort studies supports the use of LMWH in such circumstances [86–89]. Furthermore, LMWH is cost-effective when compared with unfractionated heparin for this purpose [90].

Alternatives to vitamin K antagonists for long-term treatment

Long-term treatment of venous thromboembolism with low molecular weight heparin

LMWH has been compared with warfarin therapy for the long-term treatment of symptomatic venous thromboembolism [91,92]. These studies were not comparable in terms of dosage and duration of LMWH. It was concluded that review of the data did not provide conclusive evidence of whether LMWH treatment was as effective as warfarin therapy in the prevention of recurrent symptomatic venous thromboembolism after an initial episode of deep vein thrombosis [92]. There was less bleeding with LMWH, although the doses used were relatively low [92].

In a recent study, patients who had cancer and venous thromboembolism were treated with therapeutic doses of LMWH (dalteparin) for 1 month followed by two thirds of the therapeutic dose for a further 5 months and compared with patients treated with initial LMWH followed by warfarin for a total of 6 months [93]. There was a significant decrease in the incidence of recurrent venous thromboembolism, with comparable bleeding and mortality rates. In another study, LMWH (tinzaparin) was given in therapeutic doses for 3 months and compared with initial LMWH followed by warfarin for 3 months in patients who had proximal deep vein thrombosis who were stratified for the presence of cancer [94]. The incidence of recurrent venous thromboembolism was comparable in the two groups in the overall study, but in the patients who had cancer, there was a significant decrease in the incidence of recurrent venous thromboembolism. Also, there was a significant decrease in bleeding complications in the overall study [94]. These results are supported by a smaller study that compared long-term LMWH (enoxaparin) with LMWH followed by warfarin for 3 months in patients who had venous thromboembolism and cancer. Results showed a trend to decreased recurrent venous thromboembolism and major bleeding [95]. These studies indicate that long-term use of LMWH is an alternative to VKA therapy, particularly in patients who have cancer and venous thromboembolism [93–95].

Ximelagatran, an oral direct thrombin inhibitor

Melagatran is a synthetic small molecule that is specific and a direct inhibitor of thrombin [96–101]. It must be given by injection to achieve its antithrombotic effect. Ximelagatran is an oral compound that is absorbed rapidly and converted to its active form, melagatran, with bioavailability of approximately 20%. Following ingestion of ximelagatran, peak plasma levels of melagatran occur in approximately 2 to 3 hours, with a half-life of 4 to 5 hours in most patients [96,97]. Melagatran has predictable pharmacokinetic and pharmacodynamic properties, with low binding affinity for plasma proteins and no known food interactions. Its pharmacokinetic profile is unaffected by body weight, age, sex, or ethnic origin [96–99]. The drug metabolism is independent of the hepatic P450 enzyme system and has no interaction with drugs metabolized through that route [100]. Because excretion is mainly renal, dose reduction or a longer dosing interval may be required in patients who have severe renal impairment [101]. Ximelagatran has a relatively wide therapeutic window, and the predictable pharmacokinetic profile of this drug allows administration in fixed doses without coagulation monitoring or dose adjustments.

Ximelagatran for initial and long-term treatment of thrombotic disorders

In preclinical studies, melagatran was shown to inhibit thrombus formation in venous and arterial models and to inhibit clot-bound thrombin [102–105]. In phase II and phase III clinical trials, ximelagatran with or without subcutaneous melagatran was shown to be efficacious and safe for the prevention of venous thromboembolism following total hip or total knee replacement surgery [106–108]. These trials established dosing profiles for the long-term treatment of venous thromboembolism, the prevention of stroke in patients who have atrial fibrillation, and the prevention of recurrent myocardial infarction after an initial episode.

Treatment of acute venous thromboembolism

In a dose-finding study (THRIVE [Thrombin Inhibitor in Venous Thromboembolism] I), ximelagatran in four different doses was compared with LMWH (dalteparin, 200 U/kg subcutaneously once daily) followed by adjusted-dose VKA with a target INR of 2.0 to 3.0 [109]. Marder scores, measured on repeat bilateral venography at 2 weeks of treatment, showed similar favorable results with all doses of ximelagatran and with dalteparin/warfarin. There was no dose-response relationship with regard to thrombus regression or bleeding over the four doses studied.

In the THRIVE treatment study, a double-blind, double-dummy, multinational randomized clinical trial compared fixed-dose oral ximelagatran (36 mg twice daily) with enoxaparin (1 mg/kg twice daily subcutaneously) for a minimum of 5 days, with VKA adjusted to a target INR of 2.0 to 3.0 for 6 months in patients who had acute symptomatic deep vein thrombosis with or without pulmonary embolism (37% of patients had confirmed pulmonary embolism at baseline) [110]. At 6 months, the cumulative risk of venous thromboembolism was comparable in the two groups, indicating that ximelagatran was noninferior to adjusted-dose VKA for the prevention of recurrent venous thromboembolism. The risk of major bleeding was similar. In this study, 9.6% of the patients in the ximelagatran group had an alanine transaminase (ALT) level more than three times the upper limit of normal.

Long-term treatment of venous thromboembolism

In the THRIVE III study, patients with venous thromboembolism who had received standard anticoagulation therapy with VKA for 6 months were randomized in a double-blind fashion to fixed-dose oral ximelagatran (25 mg twice daily) or placebo for 18 months without any coagulation monitoring [111]. The incidence of symptomatic recurrent venous thromboembolism at 18 months was 2.8% in the patients assigned to ximelagatran and 12.6% in patients assigned to placebo ($P < 0.001$) Rates of all-cause mortality and of major and minor bleeding were similar in the two groups. Elevation of the ALT levels above three times the upper limit of normal was found in 6% of patients in the ximelagatran group.

Ximelagatran for stroke prevention in patients with atrial fibrillation

In the SPORTIF (Stroke Prevention Using Oral Thrombin Inhibitor in Atrial Fibrillation) trials, patients with nonvalvular atrial fibrillation received oral ximelagatran or adjusted dose VKA (target INR 2.0–3.0) for the prevention of stroke. In the SPORTIF II study, patients with nonvalvular atrial fibrillation received oral ximelagatran (20, 40, or 60 mg twice daily) or adjusted-dose warfarin for 12 weeks [112]. Thromboembolic and bleeding events were uncommon and similar in the two groups; minor bleeding increased slightly with dose escalation of ximelagatran. For subsequent studies, a dose of 36 mg twice daily was chosen.

In the SPORTIF III trial, 3410 patients who had atrial fibrillation and one or more stroke risk factors were randomized to adjusted-dose VKA (with a target INR of 2.0 to 3.0) or to ximelagatran (36 mg twice daily) in an open-labeled fashion for a mean duration follow-up of 17.4 months [113]. The primary endpoint was stroke or systemic embolism. The primary event rate by intention to treat was 2.3% per year with VKA and 1.6% per year with ximelagatran, a relative risk reduction of 29% (95% confidence interval: 6.5–52). The rates of disabling or fatal stroke, mortality, and major bleeding were similar between in two groups. Combined major and minor bleeding was lower in the ximelagatran group compared with VKA (25.8% versus 29.8% per year, $P = 0.007$). ALT levels three times above the upper limit of normal were seen in 6% of patients in the ximelagatran group. Further SPORTIF trials are ongoing.

Ximelagatran for prevention of cardiovascular events after acute coronary syndromes

In the ESTEEM study (efficacy and safety of the oral thrombin inhibitor ximelagatran in combination with aspirin in patients with recent myocardial damage), 1883 patients who had recent ST segment elevated or non–ST segment elevated myocardial infarction were studied in a randomized, double-blind, dose-guiding study [114]. Eligible patients were randomized to receive oral ximelagatran in four doses twice daily or placebo for 6 months, along with aspirin (160 mg/day). The primary efficacy outcome was a composite of all-cause mortality, nonfatal myocardial infarction, or severe recurrent ischemia. Ximelagatran reduced the incidence of the primary endpoint from 16.3% to 12.7%, an absolute risk reduction of 24% ($P = 0.036$). Efficacy was similar in all four ximelagatran groups. Major bleeding rates did not differ in the five groups, but there was a dose-related increase in the combination of major and minor bleeding. Levels of ALT three times the upper limit of normal were seen in 5% of patients in the lowest dose group and in 12.2% to 13% in the three higher doses of ximelagatran.

In all of the studies on the long-term use of ximelagatran, between 6% and 13% of patients developed levels of ALT more than three times the upper limit of normal. These elevations usually are seen between 2 and 6 months of treatment;

most return to normal levels within 60 to 90 days and, in many cases, when the drug has been continued. Approximately 1% of patients in the control groups developed similar elevations of ALT, usually much earlier on in the treatment phase. The significance of these ALT elevations is uncertain but appears to be benign. When this drug becomes available for long-term use, it is likely that periodic ALT monitoring will be necessary for several months.

Summary

The VKAs (warfarin and related compounds) have been in clinical use for more than 50 years. The use of these agents has been shown to be efficacious and safe in a wide variety of clinical thrombotic disorders (including venous thromboembolism, stroke prevention in nonvalvular atrial fibrillation, prevention of systemic emboli in patients who have myocardial infarction, valvular heart disease, prosthetic heart valves, and peripheral vascular disease) and for the prevention of venous thromboembolism in a wide variety of patients. These drugs have a narrow therapeutic window with respect to INR, with inadequate therapy being associated with an increased thrombotic risk and overanticoagulation being associated with bleeding complications. Although much has been learned about the use of these agents (with safety being improved with the use of anticoagulant management clinics and point-of-care testing), the use of these agents is still problematic. Long-term LMWH provides an alternative to long-term treatment of patients who have venous thromboembolism but requires daily subcutaneous injection and is costly. For these reasons, there has been a search for newer oral antithrombotic agents, the most advanced of which are the thrombin and factor Xa inhibitors. Ximelagatran is an oral antithrombin that has been studied in a number of clinical settings and recently approved by the regulatory agencies for prophylaxis in orthopedic surgery in France and Germany. It is anticipated that this agent will be on the market in North America within the next 2 years. Agents such as this will markedly decrease the burden for physicians and patients with respect to long-term anticoagulation therapy.

References

[1] Wallin R, Martin LF. Vitamin K-dependent carboxylation and vitamin K metabolism in liver: effects of warfarin. J Clin Invest 1985;76:1879–84.

[2] Vermeer C. Gamma-carboxylglutamate-containing proteins and the vitamin K-dependent carboxylase. Biochem J 1990;266:625–36.

[3] Furie B, Furie BC. Molecular basis of vitamin K-dependent gamma carboxylation. Blood 1990;75:1753–62.

[4] Furie B, Bouchard BA, Furie BC. Vitamin K-dependent biosynthesis of gamma-carboxyglutamic acid. Blood 1999;93:1798–808.

[5] Choonara IA, Malia RG, Haynes BP, et al. The relationship between inhibition of vitamin K1 2,3-epoxide reductase and reduction of clotting factor activity with warfarin. Br J Clin Pharmacol 1988;25:1–7.

[6] Malhotra OP. Dicoumarol-induced 9-gamma-carboxyglutamic acid pro-thrombin: isolation and comparison with the 6-, 7-, 8-, and 10-gamma-carboxyglutamic acid isomers. Biochem Cell Biol 1990;68:705–15.
[7] Malhotra OP. Dicoumarol-induced prothrombins containing 6, 7, and 8 gamma-carboxyglutamic acid residues: isolation and characterization. Biochem Cell Biol 1989;67:411–21.
[8] Pineo GF, Gallus AS, Hirsh J. Unexpected vitamin K deficiency in hospitalized patients. Can Med Assoc J 1973;109:880–3.
[9] Lipsky JJ. Antibiotic-associated hypoprothrombinaemia. J Antimicrobrial Chemotherapy 1998; 21:281–300.
[10] Chakraverty R, Davidson S, Peggs K, et al. The incidence and cause of coagulopathies in an intensive care population. Br J Haemotol 1996;93:460–3.
[11] Udall JA. Human sources and absorption of vitamin K in relation to anticoagulation stability. JAMA 1965;194:127–9
[12] Frick PG, Riedler G, Brogli H. Dose response and minimal daily requirement for vitamin K in man. J Appl Physiol 1967;23:387–9.
[13] Exner DV, Brien WF, Murphy MJ. Superwarfarin ingestion. Can Med Assoc J 1992;146:34–5.
[14] Lipton RA, Klass EM. Human ingestion of a 'superwarfarin' rodenticide resulting in a prolonged anticoagulant effect. JAMA 1984;252:3004–5.
[15] O'Reilly RA, Pool JG, Aggeler PM. Hereditary resistance to coumarin anticoagulant drugs in man and rat. Ann N Y Acad Sci 1968;151:913–31.
[16] Alving BM, Strickler MP, Knight RD, et al. Hereditary warfarin resistance: investigation of a rare phenomenon. Arch Intern Med 1985;145:499–501.
[17] Freedman MD. Oral anticoagulants: pharmacodynamics, clinical indication and adverse effects. J Clin Pharmacol 1992;32:196–209.
[18] Hirsh J, Dalen JE, Anderson D, et al. Oral anticoagulants; mechanism of action, clinical effectiveness, and optimal therapeutic range. Chest 2000;119:8S–2S.
[19] Breckenridge A, Orme M, Wesseling H, et al. Pharmacokinetics and pharmacodynamics of the enantiomers of warfarin in man. Clin Pharmacol Ther 1974;15:424–30.
[20] Kelly JG, O'Malley K. Clinical pharmacokinetics of oral anticoagulants. Clin Pharmacokinet 1979;4:1–15.
[21] Sutcliffe FA, MacNicoll AD, Gibson GG. Aspects of anticoagulant action: a review of the pharmacology, metabolism and toxicology of warfarin and congeners. Rev Drug Metab Drug Interact 1987;5:225–72.
[22] Aithal GP, Day CP, Kesteven PJ, et al. Association of polymorphisms in the cytochrome P450 CYP2C9 with warfarin dose requirement and risk of bleeding complications. Lancet 1999;353:717–9.
[23] Miners JO, Birkett DJ. Cytochrome P4502C9: an enzyme of major importance in human drug metabolism. Br J Clin Pharmacol 1998;45:525–38.
[24] Shikata E, Leiri I, Ishiguro S, et al. Association of pharmacokinetic (CYP2C9) and pharmacodynamic (factors II, VII, IX, and X; proteins S and C; and γ-glutamyl carboxylase) gene variants with warfarin sensitivity. Blood 2004;103:2630–5.
[25] Oldenburg J, Quenzel EM, Harbrecht U, et al. Missense mutations at ALA-10 in the factor IX propeptide: an insignificant variant in normal life but a decisive cause of bleeding during oral anticoagulant therapy. Br J Haematol 1997;98:240–4.
[26] Broze GJ. Protein Z-dependent regulation of coagulation. Thromb Haemost 2001;86:8–13.
[27] Clouse LH, Comp PC. The regulation of hemostasis: the protein C system. N Engl J Med 1986; 314:1298–304.
[28] Brandjes DP, Heijboer H, Buller HR, et al. Acenocoumarol and heparin compared with acenoucoumarol alone in the initial treatment of proximal-vein thrombosis. N Engl J Med 1992;327:1485–9.
[29] Vigano S, Mannucci PM, Solinas S, et al. Decrease in protein C antigen and formation of an abnormal protein soon after starting oral anticoagulant therapy. Br J Haematol 1984;57: 213–20.

[30] O'Reilly RA, Aggeler PM. Studies on coumarin anticoagulant drugs: initiation of warfarin therapy without a loading dose. Circulation 1968;368:169–77.
[31] Wessler S, Gitel SN. Warfarin: from bedside to bench. N Engl J Med 1984;311:645–52.
[32] Hellemans J, Vorlat M, Verstraete M. Survival time of prothrombin and factors VII, IX, X after complete synthesis blocking doses of coumarin derivatives. Br J Haematol 1963;9:506–12.
[33] Patel P, Weitz J, Brooker LA, et al. Decreased thrombin activity of fibrin clots prepared in cord plasma compared with adult plasma. Pediatr Res 1996;39:826–30.
[34] Zivelin A, Rao LV, Rapaport SI. Mechanism of the anticoagulant effect of warfarin as evaluated in rabbits by selective depression of individual procoagulant vitamin K-dependent clotting factors. J Clin Invest 1993;92:2131–40.
[35] Khan T, Wynne H, Wood P, et al. Dietary vitamin K influences intra-individual variability in anticoagulant response to warfarin. Br J Haematol 2004;124:348–54.
[36] O'Reilly RA, Rytand DA. "Resistance" to warfarin due to unrecognized vitamin K supplementation. N Engl J Med 1980;303:160–1.
[37] Ansell J, Hirsh J, Dalen J, et al. Managing oral anticoagulant therapy. Chest 2001;119:22S–38S.
[38] Wells PS, Holbrook AM, Crowther R, Hirsh J. Warfarin and its drug/food interactions: a critical appraisal of the literature. Ann Intern Med 1994;121:676–83.
[39] Hylek EM, Heiman H, Skates SJ, et al. Acetaminophen and other risk factors for excessive warfarin anticoagulation. JAMA 1998;279:657–62.
[40] Turpie AG, Gent M, Laupacis A, et al. A comparison of aspirin with placebo in patients treated with warfarin after heart-valve replacement. N Engl J Med 1993;329:524–9.
[41] Poller L, Taberner DA. Dosage and control of oral anticoagulants: an international collaborative survey. Br J Haematol 1982;51:479–85.
[42] Hull R, Hirsh J, Jay R, et al. Different intensities of oral anticoagulant therapy in the treatment of proximal-vein thrombosis. N Engl J Med 1982;307:1676–81.
[43] Crowther MA, Ginsberg J, Kearon C, et al. A randomized trial comparing 5-mg and 10-mg warfarin loading doses. Arch Intern Med 1999;159:46–8.
[44] O'Donnell M, Hirsh J. Establishing an optimum therapeutic range for coumarins. filling in the gaps. Arch Intern Med 2004;164:588–90.
[45] Perret-Guillaume C, Wahl DG. Low-dose warfarin in atrial fibrillation leads to more thromboembolic events without reducing major bleeding when compared to adjusted-dose. A meta-analysis. Thromb Haemost 2004;91:394–402.
[46] Ridker PM, Goldhaber SZ, Danielson E, et al. Long-term, low-intensity warfarin therapy for the prevention of recurrent venous thromboembolism. N Engl J Med 2003;348:1425–34.
[47] Kearon C, Ginsberg JS, Kovacs MJ, et al. Comparison of low-intensity warfarin therapy with conventional-intensity warfarin therapy for long-term prevention of recurrent venous thromboembolism. N Engl J Med 2003;349:631–9.
[48] Couban S, Goodyear M, Burnell M, et al. A randomized double-blind placebo-controlled study of low dose warfarin for the prevention of symptomatic central venous catheter-associated thrombosis in patients with cancer [abstract]. Blood 2002;100:703a.
[49] Heaton DC, Han DY, Inder A. Minidose (1 mg) warfarin as prophylaxis for central vein catheter thrombosis. Intern Med J 2002;32:84–8.
[50] Masci G, Magagnoli M, Zucali PA, et al. Minidose warfarin prophylaxis for catheter-associated thrombosis in cancer patients: can it be safely associated with fluorouracil-based chemotherapy? J Clin Oncol 2003;21:736–9.
[51] Hyers T, Agnelli G, Hull R, et al. Antithrombotic therapy for venous thromboembolic disease. Chest 2001;119:176S–93S.
[52] Khamashta MA, Cuadrado MJ, Mujic F, et al. The management of thrombosis in the antiphospholipid-antibody syndrome. N Engl J Med 1995;332:993–7.
[53] Rosove MH, Brewer PM. Antiphospholipid thrombosis: clinical course after the first thrombotic event in 70 patients. Ann Intern Med 1992;117:303–8.
[54] Ruiz-Irastorza G, Khamashta MA, Hunt BJ, et al. Bleeding and recurrent thrombosis in definite antiphospholipid syndrome: analysis of a series of 66 patients treated with oral anticoagulation to a target international normalized ratio of 3.5. Arch Intern Med 2002;162:1164–9.

[55] Crowther MA, Ginsberg JS, Julian J, et al. A comparison of two intensities of warfarin for the prevention of recurrent thrombosis in patients with the antiphospholipid antibody syndrome. N Engl J Med 2003;349(12):1133–8.
[56] Landefeld CS, Rosenblatt MW, Goldman L. Bleeding in outpatients treated with warfarin: relation to the prothrombin time and important remediable lesions. Am J Med 1989;87:153–9.
[57] Cannegieter SC, Rosendaal FR, Wintzen AR, et al. Optimal oral anticoagulant therapy in patients with mechanical heart valves. N Engl J Med 1995;333(1):11–7.
[58] Levine MN, Raskob G, Landefeld S, et al. Hemorrhagic complications of anticoagulant treatment. Chest 2001;119:108S–21S.
[59] Torn M, van der Meer FJM, Rosendaal FR. Lowering the intensity of oral anticoagulant therapy. Effects on the risk of hemorrhage and thromboembolism. Arch Intern Med 2004; 164:668–73.
[60] Launbjerg J, Egeblad H, Heaf J, et al. Bleeding complications to oral anticoagulant therapy: multivariate analysis of 1010 treatment of overanticoagulated patients. Chest 1995;108:987–90.
[61] Hylek EM, Regan S, Go AS. Clinical predictors of prolonged delay in return of the international normalized ratio to within the therapeutic range after excessive anticoagulation with warfarin. Ann Intern Med 2001;135:393–400.
[62] Ansell JE, Hughes R. Evolving models of warfarin management: anticoagulation clinics, patient self-monitoring and patient self-management. Am Heart J 1996;132:1095–100.
[63] Ansell JE, Buttaro ML, Voltis-Thomas O, et al. Consensus guidelines for coordinated outpatient oral anticoagulation therapy management. Ann Pharmcother 1997;31:604–15.
[64] Poller L, Shiach CR, MacCalluk PK, et al. Multicentre randomized study of computerized anticoagulant dosage. European Concerted Action on Anticoagulation. Lancet 1998;352(9139): 1505–9.
[65] Leaning KE, Ansel JE. Advances in the monitoring of oral anticoagulation. J Thromb Thrombolysis 1996;3:377–83.
[66] White RH, McCurdy SA, von Marensdorff H, et al. Home prothrombin time monitoring after initiation of warfarin therapy. Ann Intern Med 1989;111:730–7.
[67] Bernardo A. Experience with patient self-management of oral anticoagulation. J Thromb Thrombolysis 1996;2:321–5.
[68] Gadisseur APA, Kaptein AA, Breuknink-Engbers WGM, et al. Patients' self-management of oral anticoagulant care vs. management by specialized anticoagulation clinics: positive effects on qualify of life. J Thromb Haemost 2003;2:584–91.
[69] Henderson MC, White RH. Anticoagulation in the elderly. Curr Opin Pulm Med 2001;7: 365–70.
[70] White RH, Beyth RJ, Zhou H, et al. Major bleeding after hospitalization for deep-vein thrombosis. Am J Med 1999;107:414–24.
[71] Fihn SD, McDonell M, Martin D, et al. Risk factors for complications of chronic anticoagulation: a multicentre study. Warfarin Optimized Outpatient Follow-up Study Group. Ann Intern Med 1993;118:511–20.
[72] Beyth BJ, Quinn LM, Landefeld CS. Prospective evaluation of an index for predicting risk of major bleeding in outpatients treated with warfarin. Am J Med 1998;105:91–9.
[73] Kuijer PM, Hutten BA, Prins MH, et al. Prediction of the risk of bleeding during anticoagulant treatment for venous thromboembolism. Arch Intern Med 1999;159:457–60.
[74] Crowther MA, Julian J, Douketis JD, et al. Treatment of warfarin-associated coagulopathy with oral vitamin K: a randomized clinical trial. Lancet 2000;3356:1551–3.
[75] Pengo V, Banzato A, Garelli E, et al. Reversal of excessive effect of regular anticoagulation: low oral dose of phytonadione (vitamin K1) compared with warfarin discontinuation. Blood Coagul Fibrinolysis 1993;4:739–41.
[76] Wilson SE, Watson HG, Crowther MA. Low-dose oral vitamin K therapy for the management of asymptomatic patients with elevated international normalized ratios: a brief review. Can Med Assoc J 2004;170(5):821–4.
[77] Johnsen SP, Sorensen HT, Mellemkjoer L, et al. Hospitalisation for upper gastrointestinal bleeding associated with use of oral anticoagulants. Thromb Haemost 2001;86:563–8.

[78] Grimaudo V, Gueissaz F, Hauert J, et al. Necrosis of skin induced by coumarin in a patient deficient in protein S. BMJ 1989;298:233–4.
[79] Becker CG. Oral anticoagulant therapy of skin necrosis: speculation on pathogenesis. Adv Exp Med Biol 1987;214:217–22.
[80] Broekmans AW, Bertina RM, Loeliger EA, et al. Protein C and the development of skin necrosis during anticoagulant therapy. Thromb Haemost 1983;49:251.
[81] Monagle P, Andrew M, Halton J, et al. Homozygous protein C deficiency: description of a new mutation and successful treatment with low molecular weight heparin. Thromb Haemost 1998;79:756–61.
[82] Samama M, Horellou MH, Soria J, et al. Successful progressive anticoagulation in a severe protein C deficiency and previous skin necrosis at the initiation of oral anticoagulant treatment. Thromb Haemost 1984;51:132–3.
[83] Kearon C, Hirsh J. Management of anticoagulation before and after elective surgery. N Engl J Med 1997;336(21):1506–11.
[84] Stein PD, Alpert JS, Bussey HI, et al. Antithrombotic therapy in patients with mechanical and biological prosthetic heart valves. Chest 2001;119:220S–7S.
[85] Dunn AS, Turpie AGG. Perioperative management of patients receiving oral anticoagulants. Arch Intern Med 2003;163:901–8.
[86] Douketis JD, Johnson JA, Turpie AG. Low-molecular-weight heparin as bridging anticoagulation during interruption of warfarin. Arch Intern Med 2004;164:1319–26.
[87] Tinmouth A, Kovacs MJ, Cruikshank M, et al. Out-patient peri-operative and peri-procedure treatment with dalteparin for chronically anticoagulated patients at high risk for thromboembolic complications [abstract]. Thromb Haemost 1999;(Suppl Aug):662.
[88] Spandorfer JM, Lynch S, Weitz HH, et al. Use of enoxaparin for the chronically anticoagulated patient before and after procedures. Am J Cardiol 1999;84:478–80.
[89] Jafri SM. Periprocedural thromboprophylaxis in patients receiving chronic anticoagulation therapy. Am Heart J 2004;147(1):1–25.
[90] Spyropoulos AC, Frost FJ, Hurley JS, et al. Costs and clinical outcomes associated with low-molecular weight heparin vs unfractionated heparin for perioperative bridging in patients receiving long-term oral anticoagulant therapy. Chest 2004;125:1642–50.
[91] Kakkar VV, Gebska M, Kadziola Z, et al. Low-molecular-weight heparin in the acute and long-term treatment of deep vein thrombosis. Thromb Haemost 2003;89:674–80.
[92] van der Heijden JF, Hutten BA, Buller HR, et al. Vitamin K antagonists or low-molecular-weight heparin for the long term treatment of symptomatic venous thromboembolism. Cochrane Database Syst Rev 2000;1:1–28.
[93] Lee A, Levine M, Baker R, et al, for the CLOT Investigators. Low-molecular-weight heparin versus a coumarin for the prevention of recurrent venous thromboembolism in patients with cancer. N Engl J Med 2003;349:146–53.
[94] Hull RD, Pineo GF, Mah AF, et al. A randomized trial evaluating long-term low-molecular-weight heparin therapy for three months vs. intravenous heparin followed by warfarin sodium in patients with current cancer [abstract]. Thromb Haemost 2003;1(Suppl July):137a.
[95] Meyer G, Marjanovic Z, Valcke J, et al. Comparison of low-molecular-weight heparin and warfarin for the secondary prevention of venous thromboembolism in patients with cancer: a randomized controlled study. Arch Intern Med 2002;162:1729–35.
[96] Eriksson UG, Bredberg U, Gislen K, et al. Pharmacokinetics and pharmacodynamics of ximelagatran, a novel oral direct thrombin inhibitor, in young healthy male subjects. Eur J Clin Pharmacol 2003;59:35–43.
[97] Eriksson UG, Mandema J, Karlsson MO, et al. Pharmacokinetics of melagatran and the effect on ex vivo coagulation time in orthopaedic surgery patients receiving subcutaneous melagatran and oral ximelagatran: a population model analysis. Clin Pharmacokinet 2003;42:687–701.
[98] Wåhlander K, Lapidus L, Olsson CG, et al. Pharmacokinetics, pharmacodynamics and clinical effects of the oral direct thrombin inhibitor ximelagatran in acute treatment of patients with pulmonary embolism and deep vein thrombosis. Thromb Res 2002;107:93–9.

[99] Johansson LC, Frison L, Logren U, et al. Influence of age on the pharmacokinetics and pharmacodynamics of ximelagatran, an oral direct thrombin inhibitor. Clin Pharmacokinet 2003;42:381–92.
[100] Bredberg E, Andersson TB, Frison L, et al. Ximelagatran, an oral direct thrombin inhibitor, has a low potential for cytochrome P450-mediated drug-drug interactions. Clin Pharmacokinet 2003;42:765–77.
[101] Eriksson UG, Johansson S, Attman P-O, et al. Influence of severe renal impairment on the pharmacokinetics and pharmacodynamics of oral ximelagatran and subcutaneous melagatran. Clin Pharmacokinet 2003;42:743–53.
[102] Boström SL, Hansson G, Sarich TC, et al. The inhibitory effect of melagatran, the active form of the oral direct thrombin inhibitor ximelagatran, compared with enoxaparin and r-hirudin on ex vivo thrombin generation in human plasma. Thromb Res 2004;113:85–91.
[103] Klement P, Carlsson S, Rak J, et al. The benefit-to-risk profile of melagatran is superior to that of hirudin in a rabbit arterial thrombosis prevention and bleeding model. J Thromb Haemost 2003;1:587–94.
[104] Sarich TC, Osende JI, Eriksson UG, et al. Acute antithrombotic effects of ximelagatran, an oral direct thrombin inhibitor, and r-hirudin in a human ex vivo model of arterial thrombosis. J Thromb Haemost 2003;1:999–1004.
[105] Sarich TC, Wolzt M, Eriksson UG, et al. Effects of ximelagatran, an oral direct thrombin inhibitor, r-hirudin and enoxaparin on thrombin generation and platelet activation in healthy male subjects. J Am Coll Cardiol 2003;41:557–64.
[106] Heit JA, Colwell CW, Francis CW, et al. AstraZeneca Arthroplasty Study Group: comparison of the oral direct thrombin inhibitor ximelagatran with enoxaparin as prophylaxis against venous thromboembolism after total knee replacement: a phase 2 dose-finding study. Arch Intern Med 2001;161:2215–21.
[107] Eriksson BI, Bergqvist D, Kalebo P, et al. Melagatran for Thrombin Inhibition in Orthopaedic surgery. Ximelagatran and melagatran compared with dalteparin for prevention of venous thromboembolism after total hip or knee replacement: the METHRO II randomised trial. Lancet 2002;360:1441–7.
[108] Francis CW, Davidson BL, Berkowitz SD, et al. Ximelagatran versus warfarin for the prevention of venous thromboembolism after total knee arthroplasty. A randomized, double-blind trial. Ann Intern Med 2002;137:648–55.
[109] Eriksson H, Wahlander K, Gustafsson D, et al. THRIVE Investigators: a randomized, controlled, dose-guiding study of the oral direct thrombin inhibitor ximelagatran compared with standard therapy for the treatment of acute deep vein thrombosis. THRIVE I. J Thromb Haemost 2003;1:41–7.
[110] Huisman MV, on behalf of the THRIVE Treatment Study Investigators. Efficacy and safety of the oral direct thrombin inhibitor ximelagatran compared with current standard therapy for acute symptomatic deep vein thrombosis, with or without pulmonary embolism: a randomized, double-blind, multinational study. J Thromb Haemost 2003;1(Suppl):OC003.
[111] Schulman S, Wahlander K, Lundstrom T, et al. Secondary prevention of venous thromboembolism with the oral direct thrombin inhibitor ximelagatran. N Engl J Med 2003;349(18): 1713–21.
[112] Petersen P, Grind M, Adler J, SPORTIF II Investigators. Ximelagatran versus warfarin for stroke prevention in patients with nonvalvular atrial fibrillation. SPORTIF II: a dose-guiding, tolerability, and safety study. J Am Coll Cardiol 2003;41:1445–51.
[113] Executive Steering Committee on behalf of the SPORTIF III Investigators. Stroke prevention with the oral direct thrombin inhibitor ximelagatran compared with warfarin in patients with non-valvular atrial fibrillation (SPORTIF III): randomized controlled trial. Lancet 2003;362: 1691–8.
[114] Wallentin L, Wilcox RG, Weaver WG, et al. Oral ximelagatran for secondary prophylaxis after myocardial infarction: the ESTEEM randomised controlled trial. Lancet 2003;362:789–97.

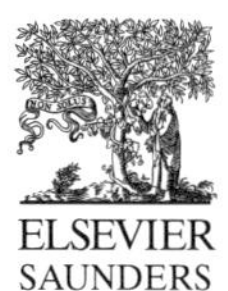
ELSEVIER
SAUNDERS

Hematol Oncol Clin N Am
19 (2005) 87–117

HEMATOLOGY/
ONCOLOGY
CLINICS OF
NORTH AMERICA

Antiplatelet Agents: Current Drugs and Future Trends

Harry L. Messmore, Jr, MD[a,b,*], Walter P. Jeske, PhD[c], William Wehrmacher, MD[d], Erwin Coyne, PhD[a], Sohrab Mobarhan, MD[e], Leslie Cho, MD[f], Fred S. Leya, MD[f], John F. Moran, MD[f]

[a]*Hines Veteran's Affairs Hospital, Hines, IL 60141, USA*
[b]*Loyola University Stritch School of Medicine, Cancer Center, Loyola University Medical Center, 2160 South First Avenue, Maywood, IL 60153, USA*
[c]*Loyola University Stritch School of Medicine, Cardiovascular Institute, Loyola University Medical Center, 2160 South First Avenue, Maywood, IL 60153, USA*
[d]*Loyola University Stritch School of Medicine, Department of Physiology, Loyola University Medical Center, 2160 South First Avenue, Maywood, IL 60153, USA*
[e]*Loyola University Stritch School of Medicine, Department of Gastroenterology, Loyola University Medical Center, 2160 South First Avenue, Maywood, IL 60153, USA*
[f]*Loyola University Stritch School of Medicine, Division of Cardiology, Loyola University Medical Center, 2160 South First Avenue, Maywood, IL 60153, USA*

The clinical use of antiplatelet drugs has developed over the past 40 years, beginning with the discovery that platelets underwent adhesion and aggregation under the influence of ADP released from red blood cells [1,2]. Investigations of the biochemical pathways involved were greatly stimulated by the discovery that aspirin could prolong the bleeding time [3,4]. Over the next 10 years, the importance of prostaglandins in platelet function and the actions of thrombin, collagen, ADP, and serotonin on platelets were discovered. The discovery of the cyclic (c)AMP pathway within platelets soon led to experiments with drugs that impaired the enzyme phosphodiesterase in platelets. Thus, dipyridamole became an "antiplatelet drug" [5]. Because of the suggestion by Craven in 1954 that aspirin could protect against coronary artery thrombosis and death, it was rational to consider that the effect of aspirin on platelets was the explanation for

* Corresponding author. Hines Veteran's Affairs Hospital, Hines, IL 60141.
E-mail address: hlmehd64@aol.com (H.L. Messmore, Jr).

doi:10.1016/j.hoc.2004.09.004 **hemonc.theclinics.com**

Craven's findings in an observational study [6]. It was assumed at that time and remains so at present that dysfunctional platelets are not the cause of atherothrombotic disease. Consequently, the use of aspirin and dipyridamole could have only modest benefit in the absence of effective prevention and treatment of atherosclerosis.

Current research is focused on the pathogenesis and risk factors for atherosclerosis. Early intervention to prevent atherothrombosis and the treatment of platelets with inhibitory drugs when atherothrombosis is present constitutes the current strategy to prevent disability and death. There are uncommon disorders in which platelets in increased numbers are responsible for vascular occlusion. These are myeloproliferative disorders in which high levels of platelets and possibly other factors result in platelet thromboemboli and vascular occlusion [7]. Heparin-induced thrombocytopenia–thrombosis is a unique disorder in which immune-mediated platelet aggregation is associated with platelet-rich arterial thrombi that occlude arteries and arterioles. Endothelial injury and leukocytes also are involved in the pathogenesis [8]. Venous thrombosis also occurs in heparin-induced thrombocytopenia–thrombosis. Antiplatelet drugs have not been found to be useful for the treatment of heparin-induced thrombocytopenia–thrombosis despite the fact that platelet aggregation is a prominent part of the process. A recent report suggests, however, that some antiplatelet drugs have been useful [9].

The clinical use of antiplatelet drugs has advanced steadily for the past 30 years as knowledge of the physiology of platelets and the pathogenesis of thromboembolic disorders, particularly those of the arterial circulation, has expanded. The driving force for the clinical use of some antiplatelet drugs has been the increased prevalence of cardiovascular disease in the western countries of the world and in the recognition of the therapeutic value of antiplatelet drugs. There are now nine clinically useful dedicated antiplatelet drugs approved for use

Table 1
Summary of recommended antiplatelet drug therapy

Clinical indication	Antiplatelet drug
Stable coronary artery disease (with or without angina)	Aspirin
Acute coronary syndrome	
Non-Q-wave MI	Aspirin, heparin or LMWH, clopidogrel, GP IIb/IIIa inhibitor
Q-wave MI with PCI	Aspirin, heparin or LMWH, clopidogrel, GpIIb/IIIa inhibitor
Q-wave MI with thrombolysis	Aspirin, heparin or LMWH (post lytic therapy)
PCI	Aspirin, clopidogrel, heparin, GpIIb/IIIa inhibitor
Post CABG	Aspirin
Mechanical heart valve	Heparin, aspirin, or dipyridamole
TIA and stroke	Aspirin, dipyridamole-aspirin, clopidogrel
Peripheral arterial disease	Clopidogrel, cilostazol
Nonvalvular atrial fibrillation	Aspirin (low-risk patients)

Abbreviations: CABG, coronary artery bypass grafting; Gp, platelet glycoprotein; LMWH, low molecular weight heparin; MI, myocardial infarction; PCI, percutaneous coronary intervention; TIA, transient ischemic attack.

in the United States. In addition, there are anticoagulant drugs such as heparin, low molecular weight heparins, antithrombin, and anti-Xa drugs that reduce the activation of platelets by way of the modulation of thrombin generation and its action as a platelet agonist (Table 1). When used selectively and in combination, these drugs have a reasonably safe yet effective suppressant action on platelet activity. There remains a need for improvement in both effectiveness and safety, which is being met by vigorous research efforts in the fields of physiology and basic and clinical pharmacology and in clinical trials.

Physiology

The platelet circulates in the blood in an inactive state, having been released into the blood from the bone marrow as an anucleate fragment of the cytoplasm of a disintegrating megakaryocyte. In the absence of interaction with foreign surfaces and agonists, a platelet circulates for approximately 10 days. It travels in the outer lane of a column of moving red blood cells and leukocytes. It is thus conveniently adjacent to the endothelial surface where it performs its hemostatic function by adhering to sites of disruption or denudation of the vascular lining. The specific processes traditionally have been described as shape change, adhesion, spreading, activation (release reaction), and aggregation. Over the past half-century, detailed studies have revealed the microscopic anatomy, the biochemical features of the surface membrane, the activation pathways to enzyme activity, and the release of platelet contents, along with the powers of contraction (clot retraction).

Shape change and subsequent reactions

The concentration of platelets in the blood is 150,000/μL to 400,000/μL. The platelet at rest is disk-shaped, is approximately 3 μm in diameter, and has a volume of 7 μm^3. When platelets contact exposed subendothelium (collagen and von Willebrand factor [vWF]), they change shape rapidly from discoid to round and spread with filopodia and lamellipodia formation (stellate form). As this process takes place, biochemical pathways are "activated" and various surface and internal reactions result in the release of ADP, the generation of thromboxane A_2 (TXA_2) and prostaglandins G and H, and the release of multiple proteins stored in the α-granules. Integrins such as platelet glycoprotein (Gp)Ib/IX-V complex that binds to vWF and GpIIb/IIIa (αIIbβ3), which in turn binds to the γ chain of fibrinogen, link the platelets to each other. Calcium ions are necessary for this process. As the activation process proceeds, the actin–myosin complexes within each platelet shorten and draw the platelet mass together (clot retraction). TXA_2 generation induces further platelet aggregation and induces blood vessel contraction and vasoconstriction, slowing the flow of blood and increasing the shear forces. Platelet function is regulated in vivo by the presence of nitric oxide. It has been shown that inhibition of nitric oxide production in humans results in rapid platelet activation that can be reversed by the administration of exogenous nitric oxide [10]. Many details of the processes that have been briefly reviewed here can be found in several excellent references [11–14].

Pathogenesis of thrombosis

Any damage to the endothelium by a multiplicity of causes can result in the formation of a thrombus at that site. This thrombus commonly is the result of the atherosclerotic process in which the deposition of cholesterol in the subendothelium results in plaque formation. Where the flow of blood becomes severely restricted and the endothelium becomes dysfunctional or disrupted in the region of atherosclerotic vascular disease (commonly, plaque formation), platelets begin to become part of the physical process of vascular occlusion (atherothrombosis) by concomitantly releasing substances that interact with and recruit leukocytes and additional platelets [15–17].

Recently, more attention has been given to atherosclerosis superimposed by thrombosis, and this attention already has generated an atherothrombosis society. For adequate contemporary application of platelet physiology and pathology, this concept requires thorough exploration that supplements the originally competing fundamental proposals made by Virchow [18], von Rokitansky [19], and Duguid [20], which are now combined to include low-grade injury resulting in inflammatory insudation (Virchow) and encrustation of mural thrombi (von Rokitansky and Duguid). The initial atherosclerotic lesion is characterized by adhesion and invasion of mononuclear leukocytes and progression to a fibrous plaque involving the accumulation of smooth muscle cells and lipids. Thrombotic complications result from contact between circulating blood and the highly thrombogenic material located in the lesion's lipid core. Current evidence supports the central role of an inflammatory process in the pathogenesis of the atherothrombosis and subsequent recruitment of thrombotic material that may support healing or lead to vascular occlusion and death.

Substances that cause vasoconstriction are simultaneously released (TXA_2). In the healing process of such vascular lesions, platelets may participate by releasing platelet-derived growth factor and other substances. Suppression of platelet functions may logically retard the process of vascular occlusion by preventing thrombosis on atherosclerotic vascular lesions. When endothelial, subendothelial, and smooth muscle injury occur during therapeutic angioplasty, antiplatelet therapy is mandatory [21]. The insertion of intravascular stenting materials likewise requires antiplatelet therapy for 9 to 12 months to prevent occlusion by platelet thrombi [22,23]. Because inflammation is potentially a part of any disease process in the vascular system, the possibility of thrombosis is enhanced. This process may occur as an interaction with leukocytes in the surrounding circulation, with leukocytes bound to endothelium or subendothelium, lipid-laden macrophages in the plaque, and endothelial cells damaged by cytokines generated by leukocytes [24]. Not only do the platelets become activated and release their contents, but they also express adhesion molecules that interact with adjacent leukocytes and endothelial cells [24].

The vascular lesions that are caused by autoimmunity such as lupus vasculitis and host-versus-graft disease might logically be treated with antiplatelet drugs, anticoagulants, or both, but this article does not address those problems. It has been reported that systemic lupus erythematosis is associated with accelerated atherosclerosis and treatment of such patients with antiplatelet drugs may be useful when they become symptomatic, but no new data exist to support this concept [25,26].

Platelets serve as a bridge between the hemostatic and inflammatory systems by virtue of their ability to release inflammatory mediators and the expression of various adhesion molecules on their surface after activation, leading to interactions with leukocytes and endothelial cells [27,28]. Platelets release a number of substances such as interleukin (IL)-1β, regulated on activation normal T cell expressed and secreted, platelet factor 4, macrophage inflammatory protein-1α, transforming growth factor β, platelet-derived growth factor, and 5-hydroxytryptamine (serotonin) that exhibit proinflammatory properties. Studies have shown that the deposition of regulated on activation normal T cell expressed and secreted and platelet factor 4 by platelets on the vessel wall leads to enhanced monocyte adhesion [29]. Contrary to long-standing belief, platelets have been shown to be capable of synthesizing a number of proteins including constitutive surface integrins (GpIb, GpIIb, GpIIIa), granule components (fibrinogen, vWF), and inflammatory substances (IL-1β, bcl-3) [30,31]. Ligand binding to GpIIb/IIIa appears to be an initiating factor leading to platelet production of inflammatory mediators [32,33].

After activation, platelets express two proteins on their surface that are linked to inflammation: P-selectin and CD40L. P-selectin becomes expressed on adherent platelets and provides a site for leukocyte tethering and rolling. Leukocyte binding to P-selectin is one of the signals required for leukocyte activation leading to the generation to inflammatory mediators and enhanced monocyte tissue factor expression [34]. Inhibition of leukocyte binding to P-selectin through the use of recombinant soluble P-selectin glycoprotein-1 has been shown to promote clot lysis [35,36].

Thus, it is apparent that strategies to prevent thrombosis from occurring on injured or diseased vascular endothelium may use many different single or combinations of antiplatelet drugs. A rationale for using these strategies is presented in a review by Rauch et al [37].

Antiplatelet drugs currently in use

Aspirin

Platelets are activated by a large number of substances. One of the strongest activators is TXA_2. TXA_2 is formed when arachidonic acid is acted on by

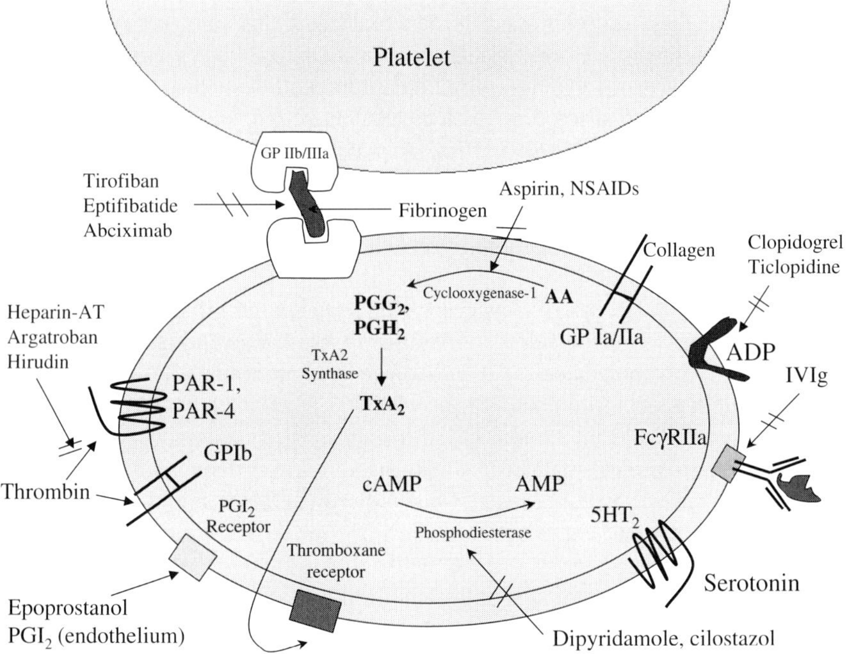

Fig. 1. Sites of action of currently approved antiplatelet drugs. Antiplatelet drugs are capable of inhibiting platelet activation by blocking cell surface receptors and inhibiting the generation of bioactive substances. Platelet aggregation is potently inhibited by blocking fibrinogen binding to glycoprotein IIb/IIIa. AA, arachidonic acid; AT, antithrombin; GP, glycoprotein; $5HT_2$, serotonin; IVIg, intravenous immunoglobulin; PAR, protease activated receptor; PG, prostaglandin; Tx, thromboxane.

cyclooxygenase 1 (COX-1). Aspirin and other nonsteroidal anti-inflammatory drugs (NSAIDs) inhibit COX-1, thereby preventing the generation of TXA_2 and other prostaglandin metabolites (Fig. 1) [38]. Aspirin exhibits several desirable properties as an antiplatelet drug; namely, it can be taken orally, its effects are irreversible, and monitoring of drug levels is not required [39]. It is important to recognize that aspirin does not completely inhibit platelet function because high concentrations of ADP, collagen, and thrombin can activate platelets through alternate pathways [40]. Although the effect of aspirin on COX-1 is irreversible (acetylation of the enzyme), the effect of some other nonspecific NSAIDs such as ibuprofen is reversible and, as such, these agents may produce a weaker antiplatelet effect and may, in fact, antagonize the antiplatelet effect of low-dose aspirin [41].

Because aspirin irreversibly inhibits COX-1 and the anucleate platelets are unable to synthesize new enzyme, a single daily dose of aspirin is sufficient to inhibit platelet function for the life of the platelet. The dose of aspirin required to inhibit platelet function is relatively low compared with that required to achieve an anti-inflammatory effect. The antithrombotic effect of aspirin saturates at doses of approximately 100 mg [40]. The incidence of adverse effects of aspirin, particularly in terms of local bleeding in the gastrointestinal tract, correlates with the frequency of dosing and the size of the dose. The major side effect associated with aspirin usage is hemorrhage. Upper gastrointestinal bleeding can be attributable to the antiplatelet effects of aspirin and to the inhibition of gastric mucosal cytoprotection. The incidence of major gastrointestinal bleeding is estimated to be 1 to 2 per 1000 patient years [41]. Thus, in patients who have stable angina, previous myocardial infarction (MI), and high-risk states such as unstable angina, the benefits of the antiplatelet effect far outweigh the potential for adverse effects [41].

Recently, considerable attention has focused on the possibility that a subpopulation of patients is resistant to the antiplatelet effects of aspirin [42]. The exact incidence of aspirin resistance is not clear because several tests have been used to characterize this condition. There is some evidence that increasing doses of aspirin in such patients overcomes this resistance.

Thienopyridines

ADP, a component of platelet dense granules, activates platelets by way of several distinct receptors on the platelet surface. ADP binding to $P2Y_1$ receptors results in intracellular calcium mobilization and platelet shape change, whereas the activation of $P2Y_{12}$ receptors leads to an inhibition of cAMP formation and the granule release response. Both receptors need to be activated to induce the aggregation response [43]. Metabolites of the thienopyridines ticlopidine and clopidogrel selectively inhibit ADP-induced platelet aggregation. The in vivo hepatic metabolism of clopidogrel by way of cytochrome P450-1A leads to the generation of an active metabolite that induces irreversible alteration of the $P2Y_{12}$ receptor [44]. Like aspirin, clopidogrel is administered orally in a once-daily dose. The onset of antiplatelet effect with clopidogrel is slow, although this can be overcome with the use of a loading dose [45]. The inhibition of platelet aggregation can be detected as early as 2 hours after administration of an oral loading dose. Repeated daily dosing results in steady-state levels of inhibition (~50%) after 4 to 7 days of therapy [45]. Platelet function returns to normal 7 days following the last dose. Intravenous ADP receptor antagonists such as AR-C69931MX are under development [46].

Platelet glycoprotein IIb/IIIa complex inhibitors

GpIIb/IIIa is the most abundant receptor on the platelet surface and serves as the primary receptor in the mediation of platelet aggregation. On unactivated platelets, GpIIb/IIIa is found in an inactive conformation, unable to bind fibrinogen with high affinity. When platelets are stimulated with any of a wide variety of agonists, a calcium-dependent conformational change occurs in GpIIb/IIIa, allowing it to bind to fibrinogen with higher affinity. Because fibrinogen is bivalent, its binding to GpIIb/IIIa leads to cross-linking of platelets [47]. The active site of GpIIb/IIIa recognizes the R(K)GD sequence in fibrinogen and a number of other adhesive ligands [48]. Although these drugs potently inhibit platelet aggregation, they have little-to-no effect on platelet activation/degranulation.

Because fibrinogen binding to GpIIb/IIIa is the final common pathway of platelet aggregation irrespective of the initiating stimulus, its blockade is of considerable clinical interest. A number of GpIIb/IIIa inhibitors have been developed, including abciximab (ReoPro), tirofiban (Aggrastat), and eptifibatide (Integrilin) [49]. The preceding agents are representative of the three major subclasses of GpIIb/IIIa antagonists. Abciximab is a humanized Fab fragment that also inhibits the vitronectin receptor ($\alpha v\beta 3$). The inhibition of GpIIb/IIIa and $\alpha v\beta 3$ is likely due to steric hindrance. Unlike aspirin and clopidogrel, the antiplatelet effect of currently available GpIIb/IIIa inhibitors is reversible, the effect being present only when the drug is bound to the receptor. The ultimate antiplatelet effect is directly related to the percentage of receptors bound. Too few bound receptors limits efficacy, whereas too many bound receptors compromises safety. It has been shown that an inhibition of at least 80% of receptors is required to completely inhibit platelet aggregation. Following cessation of dosing (typically, bolus followed by intravenous [IV] infusion), platelet function returns to near normal within 48 hours. In vitro studies have suggested that abciximab can attenuate adhesion-dependent platelet procoagulant activity [50].

Eptifibatide is a cyclic heptapeptide containing the KGD sequence. Tirofiban is a small molecular weight peptidomimetic that mimics the RGD sequence of fibrinogen and binds to GpIIb/IIIa with high affinity. Both small-molecule inhibitors are reversible antagonists. Because of their short half-lives and the potential for additional GpIIb/IIIa receptors to become expressed on the platelet surface after activation, GpIIb/IIIa antagonists are dosed intravenously on a weight basis as repeated boluses or as a bolus followed by a maintenance infusion.

Due to their pharmacokinetic properties, these agents are not suitable for indications in which long-term inhibition of platelet function is required. Several GpIIb/IIIa inhibitors for oral use have been developed as potential long-term antiplatelet agents. These agents are limited by their relatively low bioavailability and inability to maintain desirable levels of platelet inhibition [49].

Although hemorrhage remains the major concern with the use of these agents, transient, severe thrombocytopenia occurs within the first few hours of administration in a small fraction of patients. Although this complication occurs most frequently with abciximab, cases have been reported with the other two inhibitors. Because of the potential for enhanced bleeding, careful management of dosing of the drug and coadministration of antiplatelet and concomitant anticoagulants must be performed.

Phosphodiesterase inhibitors

An older member of this class of drugs currently in use as an antiplatelet agent is sustained-release dipyridamole. It typically has been used in conjunction with warfarin sodium as prophylaxis against embolization from mechanical heart valves. Recently, it was reformulated in combination with aspirin (Aggrenox) to reduce the risk of stroke in patients who have had transient ischemia of the brain or completed ischemic stroke due to thrombosis. Dipyridamole affects platelets through a complex mechanism of action that leads to an increase in intraplatelet cyclic nucleotides [51]. The increase in cAMP/cGMP in platelets by dipyridamole is due to an inhibition of the adenosine transporter and the inhibition of cGMP and cAMP phosphodiesterases. An increase in platelet cGMP leads to a potentiation of effect of nitric oxide. An increase in intracellular cAMP stimulates prostacyclin production. Dipyridamole reversibly inhibits platelet aggregation induced by platelet activating factor, collagen, and ADP.

Cilostazol (Pletal) is a selective and potent inhibitor of the phosphodiesterase 3 isozyme that leads to an inhibition of agonist and shear-induced platelet aggregation, release, and TXA_2 production [52]. Unlike aspirin, cilostazol inhibits primary and secondary platelet aggregation induced by ADP and epinephrine but does not decrease endothelial production of prostacyclin.

Indirect-acting antiplatelet drugs

Inhibitors of factor Xa and thrombin decrease the level of the agonist thrombin, diminishing the probability of platelet activation at sites of endothelial dysfunction (Fig. 2). In effect, this is no different than blocking the receptor for thrombin on platelets. Drugs in this category include heparin; low molecular weight heparin; the direct antithrombin drugs argatroban, bivalirudin, hirudin,

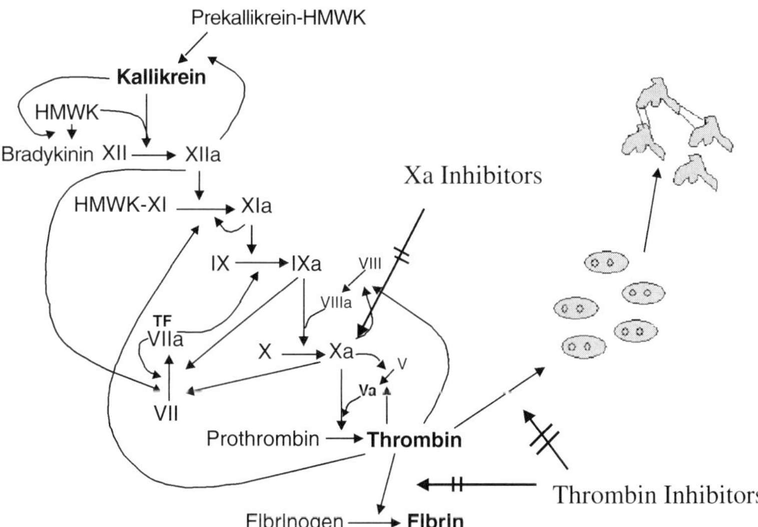

Fig. 2. Inhibition of thrombin or its generation by specific, direct enzyme inhibitors—heparin or low molecular weight heparins—not only prevents clot formation but also limits platelet activation. HMWK, high molecular weight kininogen; TF, tissue factor. Cartoon-platelets represent aggregated platelets.

and ximelagatran; and the direct anti-Xa drug fondaparinux. These drugs are effective and reasonably safe unless they are given in doses that nearly completely block the generation of thrombin or thrombin itself, in which case serious bleeding can occur. Heparin prolongs the bleeding time at higher doses by way of its antithrombin effect and also impairs the action of vWF on platelets [53–55]. Synthetic, selective factor Xa inhibitors do not completely inhibit thrombin generation and, as such, have minimal affect on tissue factor–induced platelet aggregation [56]. Recently, a synthetic hexadecasaccharide with anti-Xa and antithrombin activity was shown to produce a dose-dependent inhibition of platelet adhesion [57].

Clinical use of antiplatelet drugs

It is particularly important to note that in acute vascular events such as acute coronary syndrome, multiple antiplatelet agents are necessary to achieve optimal results with reasonable safety. In contrast, stable vascular disease such as post MI, post unstable angina, post angioplasty of any artery, post stroke, stable angina pectoris, and post coronary artery bypass grafting (CABG) are, as a rule, treated prophylactically with a single agent, usually low-dose aspirin. In patients who have stents in place, two antiplatelet agents may be needed for up to 12 months [23,58–61]. The foregoing is defined as secondary prevention.

Primary prevention is more problematic for the clinician because the risk/benefit ratio is not as favorable as in secondary prevention. This is due to the fact that the risk of hemorrhage, especially cerebral, which is less common than gastrointestinal but has a greater probability of disability and death, may outweigh any advantage in preventing nonfatal MIs. In primary prevention trials, death due to vascular events is not reduced by the use of antiplatelet drugs. Reviews of the data recently have been published [62–64].

The rationale for using multiple antiplatelet drugs in high-risk arterial thrombotic disease is based on the knowledge that no dose of aspirin completely blocks platelet function. ADP causes the release of α-granules from aspirin-treated platelets and thrombin also can aggregate such platelets when present in high concentrations. By inhibiting phosphodiesterases, dipyridamole inhibits platelets by increasing cAMP levels in the platelet, thus adding to the aspirin effect [62,65].

Acute coronary syndrome

Antiplatelet drugs have had a major impact on the treatment of ischemic heart disease. The first clue was the very favorable effect of aspirin on the outcome of unstable angina [66]. When this result was compared with that of intravenous heparin, it was found to be superior [67]. Presently, all patients who have acute coronary syndrome are given aspirin. From the results of the initial evaluation of such patients, decisions must be made regarding additional antithrombotic/anticoagulant drugs depending on a number of factors. If the patient has acute MI, then he or she may go to thrombolytic therapy or to percutaneous transluminal coronary angioplasty (PTCA). Heparin or low molecular weight heparin will be given depending on the plan, as may clopidogrel, a GpIIb/IIIa inhibitor, or both depending on the level of risk. In October 2002, the American College of Cardiology and the American Heart Association (ACC/AHA) developed guidelines designed to help with the management of these patients [68]. The clinician's first decision is to establish that the patient's symptoms of chest pain are highly suspicious for acute ischemia. The development of the Thrombosis in Myocardial Infarction risk score has helped to stratify high-risk patients and low-risk patients [69]. High-risk patients are those older than age 65 years with the presence of diabetes, hypertension, and an anginalike chest pain. Systolic blood pressure of less than 100 mmHg and a heart rate of greater than 100 beats/minute with a Killup class II to IV go a long way to establish acute ischemia. The Killup score speaks for the degree of left ventricular dysfunction. Important ECG changes include an acute injury current or a ST segment elevation or ST segment depression greater than 1 mm. New-onset complete left bundle branch block is significant. In the Thrombosis in Myocardial Infarction risk score article [69], a low body weight of less than 67 kg or 147 lb and time to treatment greater than 4 hours increased the risk score. In addition, prolonged chest pain at rest or worsening accelerated chest pain, especially with hemodynamic instability or hypotension, leads to a high-risk profile for acute ischemia. In addition, three or more coronary risk factors for coronary artery disease and the development of serum markers such as an elevated troponin are helpful in the diagnosis. These ischemic patients—examples of acute coronary syndrome—present commonly but with widely varying risks. Various subgroups have different outcomes. The ACC/AHA guidelines address these risks and attempt to match treatment plans with the varying subgroups of acute coronary syndrome. There are four important parts to the treatment: anti-ischemic, anticoagulant/antiplatelet, a decision for an invasive approach, and finally, discharge and post hospital care. The goal is to relieve symptoms and prevent or ameliorate damage of an acute MI (see Table 1).

Antiplatelet therapy in acute coronary syndrome—high-risk patients

A 325-mg aspirin is given, followed by 81 mg aspirin daily. Intravenous GpIIb/IIIa inhibitors have added benefit in these patients. Finally, large benefits have been seen when two antiplatelet agents are added together, such as clopidogrel and aspirin, provided the risks of bleeding are acceptable [70]. Finally, IV unfractionated heparin or low molecular weight heparin is ordered. For anticoagulation, heparin, aspirin, clopidogrel, and GpIIb/IIIa inhibitors are indicated for high-risk patients when percutaneous coronary intervention (PCI) is planned (Box 1).

If CABG is to be performed, then clopidogrel should be withheld. In the PCI–Clopidogrel in Unstable Angina to Prevent Recurrent Events (CURE) study [71], it was clear that somewhere between 32% and 45% of patients eventually would undergo CABG surgery. The risk of bleeding was 5 to 10 times higher in those patients who had been treated with clopidogrel and aspirin beforehand. For that

Box 1. Antiplatelet therapy in acute coronary syndrome—high-risk patients

Chest pain

- High suspicion for acute ischemia: abnormal ECG, non-Q-wave MI or ST segment elevation MI, acute injury current, hemodynamic instability, life-threatening arrhythmias; history of prior MI
- Prolonged chest pain at rest
- Worsening accelerated chest pain
- Cardiogenic shock

ECG

- ST elevation or depression >1 mm ST
- New complete left bundle branch block
- Dynamic or labile ECG changes

Hemodynamic instability

- Brady- or tachyarrhythmias with hypotension
- Dynamic ECG changes or active chest pain

Treatment pathways

- IV unfractionated heparin or low molecular weight heparin
- IV metoprolol
- IV nitroglycerine for chest pain control or hypertension
- Aspirin, 325 mg
- IV GpIIb/IIIa inhibitors
- Clopidogrel

reason, it is prudent to hold the clopidogrel before the diagnostic angiogram to learn whether CABG is a strong consideration. GpIIb/IIIa inhibitors have relatively shorter duration of action and, therefore, can be used in that preoperative setting. Finally, early treatment with 3-hydroxy-3-methylglutaryl coenzyme A reductase inhibitors ("statins") following acute MI will improve 1-year survival.

Antiplatelet drugs such as aspirin are used in patients who have acute MI who may receive thrombolytic therapy or, alternatively, PCI. If they are to receive thrombolytic therapy, then heparin or low molecular weight heparin may be added post therapy.

Antiplatelet therapy in acute coronary syndrome—intermediate-risk patients

An intermediate-risk group of patients who have chest pain can be defined as those with exertional angina prolonged to greater than 30 minutes, an acute change in the severity of their angina, or resting chest pain of greater than 20 minutes, especially with a history of prior coronary artery disease, MI, or CABG surgery (Box 2). The ECG is nondiagnostic. The treatment plan for this group is similar, with IV metoprolol, IV nitroglycerine, IV unfractionated heparin or low molecular weight heparin, and aspirin (325 mg acutely, followed by 81 mg of aspirin daily for chronic treatment). Clopidogrel can be used as an alternative to aspirin in those patients who are aspirin resistant or intolerant. Finally, a protocol to follow patients and to rule out myocardial damage is an important part of the plan.

Antiplatelet therapy in acute coronary syndrome—low-risk patients

Low-risk patients are those with typical or atypical symptoms not suggestive of unstable angina or an acute MI (Box 3). There is no evidence of an abnormal stress test or a previous revascularization procedure. The ECG is nondiag-

Box 2. Antiplatelet therapy in acute coronary syndrome—intermediate-risk patients

Chest pain

Symptoms suggestive of unstable angina: prolonged exertional angina (> 30 minutes), acute changes in severity or frequency of angina, resting chest pain > 20 minutes, prior coronary artery disease

ECG

Nondiagnostic of acute injury
Includes old complete left bundle branch block, Q waves, left ventricular hypertrophy with ST segment changes
No serious arrhythmias

Treatment plan

IV β-blocker
IV nitroglycerine
IV heparin or low molecular weight heparin
Rule out MI protocol
Aspirin 325 acutely, and 81 mg chronically
Clopidogrel as an alternative to aspirin

Box 3. Antiplatelet therapy in acute coronary syndrome—low-risk patients

Chest pain

Typical or atypical symptoms not suggestive of unstable angina or acute MI
No abnormal stress test or revascularization (CABG or percutaneous transluminal coronary angioplasty [PTCA]) within the last 6 months at least

ECG

Nondiagnostic for acute event (eg, normal, near normal, or unchanged from a prior ECG)

Laboratory

Normal myoglobin, troponin

Treatment

No IV heparin
No IV nitroglycerine

nostic and laboratory markers are normal. The treatment should include a 325 mg aspirin dose, followed by 81 mg/day if atherosclerotic coronary artery disease is the cause of the symptoms. Intravenous heparin and nitroglycerin are not necessary.

Chronic angina patients

These patients should be treated with low-dose aspirin (81 mg/d) and with maximally tolerated doses of β-blockers and angiotensin converting enzyme inhibitors. Sublingual nitroglycerine can be used for intermittent anginal episodes and for prophylaxis in those patients who have documented coronary artery disease. Statin treatment is important. Previously, the Adult Treatment Panel III [149] guidelines recommended lowering low-density lipoprotein cholesterol to less than 100 mg/dL, with total cholesterol less than 200 mg/dL, triglycerides less than 150 mg/dL, and high-density lipoprotein cholesterol over 40 mg/dL. Recent trials (PROVE-IT and REVERSAL) have suggested that the targeted low-density lipoprotein cholesterol level should now be as low as 70 mg/dL. Incapacitating chronic stable angina with poor exercise tolerance requires coronary angiography for the full assessment. At that point, revascularization therapies with angioplasties, stents, or CABG surgery can be considered.

Antiplatelet therapy in percutaneous coronary intervention

From the first percutaneous coronary angioplasty by Andreas Grüntzig in 1977, adjunctive antiplatelet therapy has played an integral part of PCI. All PCIs involve plaque fracture, medial disruption, and vessel dissection that serve as potent stimuli for platelet and coagulation system activation. Platelet deposition and mural thrombus formation occur after PCI depending on the level of vessel wall injury. The most important risk factor for ischemic complications after PCI is formation of a platelet thrombus at the site of vessel injury and at sites of subsequent rupture/thrombus of other plaques.

Aspirin

Aspirin has been used since the first PCI in 1977 and is now routinely used in all PCIs. Although aspirin is a cost-effective platelet inhibitor, it provides only a partial inhibition of platelet aggregation. Therefore, not many studies have been performed with aspirin alone in PCI. Barnathan et al [72] studied aspirin and dipyridamole in the prevention of acute coronary thrombosis complicating coronary angioplasty. Patients pretreated with aspirin and dipyridamole before admission and angioplasty had the lowest rates of thrombosis following coronary angioplasty. Aspirin given in combination with dipyridamole also was associated with a significant reduction in periprocedural Q-wave MI compared with placebo (1.6% versus 6.9%, $P = 0.011$) in patients undergoing PTCA [73]. In the era of coronary stenting, aspirin was used in combination with warfarin (Coumadin) but was associated with poor clinical outcomes and more procedural bleeding complications. The Stent Anticoagulation Restenosis Study (STARS) [21] established the superiority of aspirin and the ADP receptor antagonist ticlopidine over aspirin alone or aspirin plus warfarin in patients undergoing coronary artery stenting. Patients had a significant reduction in the primary end point of death, target vessel revascularization (TVR), target vessel thrombosis, or recurrent MI.

ADP receptor antagonists

Thienopyridines irreversibly inhibit platelet aggregation by selectively blocking the recently identified $P2Y_{12}$ platelet ADP receptors [44,70,74]. There have been few studies assessing the role of ADP receptor antagonists in patients undergoing balloon angioplasty. A study by Bertrand et al [75] randomized patients to ticlopidine (250 mg twice a day) or placebo beginning 2 days before and continuing for 6 months following PTCA to assess the effect of ticlopidine on acute vessel closure and angiographic restenosis. Although there was no difference in restenosis, there was a significant reduction in acute vessel closure between the two groups (5.1% versus 16.2%, $P < 0.01$).

There have been four randomized trials comparing anticoagulation to antiplatelet therapy in the setting of coronary artery stenting. The Intracoronary Stenting and Antithrombotic Regimen (ISAR) trial [76] and STARS [21] demonstrated a significant reduction in death, MI, or TVR with antiplatelet therapy. In the ISAR trial, the primary end point of cardiac death, MI, or TVR occurred in 1.6% of the antiplatelet group versus 6.2% of the anticoagulation group ($P = 0.01$). In the larger STARS trial, 1653 patients were randomized to aspirin alone, aspirin with warfarin, or aspirin with ticlopidine. The primary end point of death, MI, or TVR occurred in 3.6% in the aspirin monotherapy group, 2.7% in the aspirin with warfarin group, and 0.5% in the aspirin and ticlopidine group ($P = 0.001$). The Multicenter Aspirin and Ticlopidine Trial after Intracoronary Stenting study [77] found a trend toward reduction in death, MI, and target lesion revascularization with ticlopidine plus aspirin compared with warfarin (5.6% versus 11.0%, $P = 0.07$). In these studies and in the Full Anticoagulation versus Aspirin and Ticlopidine study [78] that specifically addressed bleeding complications, ticlopidine plus aspirin significantly reduced bleeding complications compared with warfarin.

Thienopyridines prolong the bleeding time; however, the most serious side effects with ticlopidine have been neutropenia and thrombotic thrombocytopenic purpura. The incidence of neutropenia was 2.4% in one study and the incidence of thrombotic thrombocytopenic purpura is estimated to be 1 case in every 2000 to 4000 patients exposed [79]. The incidence of neutropenia with clopidogrel was 0.1% in the Clopidogrel versus Aspirin in Patients at Risk of Ischemic Events (CAPRIE) trial [80], which was similar to aspirin, and there have been rare case reports of clopidogrel-associated thrombotic thrombocytopenic purpura, although it is not clear whether clopidogrel was really the cause. Due to the serious hematologic side effects of ticlopidine, clopidogrel has now become the preferred thienopyridine.

To date, there have been 10 studies comparing ticlopidine versus clopidogrel. Data from three large randomized trials [81–83] and numerous registry data [84–89] have shown that clopidogrel in combination with aspirin has a reduction in major cardiac events similar to ticlopidine plus aspirin and appeared to be safer. For example, the Clopidogrel Aspirin Stent International Cooperative Study compared clopidogrel with ticlopidine. The primary end point (adverse drug events) occurred in 9.1% of patients in the ticlopidine group and in 4.6% of patients in the clopidogrel group (relative risk, 0.40; 95% confidence interval: 0.31 to 8.1; $P = 0.005$), showing improved tolerability with clopidogrel. Overall, rates of major cardiac events (cardiac death, MI, target lesion revascularization) were low and comparable between treatment groups and not statistically significant. A large meta-analysis of these trials [90] showed that clopidogrel was associated with significant reduction in the incidence of major adverse cardiac events (odds ratio 0.50, 0.41–0.62, $P = 0.001$) including mortality (odds ratio 0.43, 0.28–0.66, $P = 0.001$). Thus, the data support substitution of ticlopidine with clopidogrel.

Recently, there has been much discussion regarding the timing of pretreatment and the length of post-treatment with ADP receptor antagonists before coronary stenting. Steinhubl et al [91] observed that patients treated with ticlopidine greater than 3 days before the procedure had the lowest rates of postprocedure MI. A beneficial effect of pretreatment with clopidogrel also has been described [92,93]. In the PCI-CURE study [71], 1313 patients were randomized to clopidogrel and 1345 to placebo. All patients received standard drug therapy including aspirin, heparin, β-blockers, angiotensin converting enzyme inhibitors, lipid-lowering agents, and GpIIb/IIIa inhibitors. In addition to aspirin, patients were pretreated with study drug clopidogrel for a median of 6 days before their PCI. Most patients were given open-label thienopyridine for 4 weeks following PCI. The study drug was subsequently reinitiated for up to 1 year (8 months on average). Clopidogrel pretreatment subsequently reduced the incidence of the primary composite end point of death, nonfatal MI, or urgent TVR at 30 days compared with placebo (4.5% versus 6.4%; relative risk, 0.70; $P = 0.03$). The incidence of MI before the PCI also was significantly reduced by clopidogrel (15.3% versus 12.1%, $P = 0.008$). Patients who received clopidogrel after PCI for up to 12 months (an average of 8 months) had a lower rate of cardiac death, MI, or urgent TVR (18.3% versus 21.7%; relative risk, 0.83; $P = 0.03$). Also, overall (including events before and after PCI), there was a 31% reduction cardiovascular death or MI ($P = 0.002$). In terms of safety, there was no difference in major bleeding in the short-term (at 30 days) or long-term (at follow-up) with clopidogrel use; however, minor bleeding was greater with long-term clopidogrel use ($P = 0.03$). The results of the PCI-CURE study also support the use of prolonged outpatient clopidogrel use in patients undergoing PCI from the usual 1 month to longer treatment. The results of the CURE [150] and PCI-CURE trials have prompted the revision of the ACC/AHA guidelines on the treatment of unstable angina/ST segment elevation MI. In patients in whom PCI is planned, clopidogrel should be started and continued for at least 1 month and up to 9 months in patients who are not at high risk for bleeding. The recently completed Clopidogrel for Reduction of Events During Extended Observation trial showed benefit from prolonged use of clopidogrel and aspirin versus aspirin alone for reducing late ischemic events in patients undergoing PCI.

Prolonged dual antiplatelet therapies with aspirin and thienopyridines have been used in patients undergoing brachytherapy for in-stent restenosis due to late ischemic events. For patients who receive balloon angioplasty in the setting of brachytherapy, life-long aspirin plus 6-month clopidogrel treatment is commonly used, whereas stented patients receive life-long aspirin followed by 9 months to 1 year of clopidogrel treatment. With the emergence of drug-eluting stents, the role for prolonged dual antiplatelet therapy will only increase. The new drug-eluting stents require 3 to 6 months of clopidogrel treatment plus aspirin.

Platelet glycoprotein IIb/IIIa inhibitors in percutaneous coronary intervention

The GpIIb/IIIa receptor is the final common pathway leading to platelet aggregation (Table 2). GpIIb/IIIa inhibitors do not have effects on platelet activation as does aspirin and thienopyridines. There are three GpIIb/IIIa inhibitors

Table 2
Platelet glycoprotein IIb/IIIa inhibitors and percutaneous coronary intervention: the trials

GpIIb/IIIa inhibitor	PCI	NSTEMI ACS	Acute MI
Abciximab	EPIC	CAPTURE	RAPPORT
	EPILOG		ADMIRAL
	EPISTENT		CADILLAC
	TARGET		
Eptifibatide	IMPACT II		
	ESPRIT		
Tirofiban	RESTORE		
	TARGET		

Abbreviations: ACS, acute coronary syndrome; ADMIRAL, Abciximab before Direct angioplasty and stenting in Myocardial Infarction; CADILLAC, Controlled Abciximab and Device Investigation to Lower Late Angioplasty Complications; CAPTURE, Chimeric 7E3 AntiPlatelet Therapy in Unstable angina REfractory to standard treatment; EPIC, Evaluation of Platelet IIb/IIIa Inhibition for Prevention of Ischemic Complications; EPILOG, Evaluation of PTCA to Improve Long-Term Outcome with Abciximab GPIIb/IIIa Blockade; EPISTENT, Evaluation of Platelet IIb/IIIa Inhibitor for Stenting; ESPRIT, Enhanced Suppression of the Platelet Receptor Glycoprotein IIb/IIIa using Integrilin Therapy; IMPACT II, Integrilin to Minimize Platelet Aggregation and Coronary Thrombosis II; NSTEMI ACS, non–ST segment elevation myocardial infarction; RAPPORT, ReoPro And Primary PTCA Organization and Randomized Trial; RESTORE, Randomized Efficacy Study of Tirofiban for Outcomes and Restenosis; TARGET, Tirofiban and Abciximab for Revascularization Give Equivalent Outcomes Trial.

available. Abciximab is the Fab fragment of a murine monoclonal antibody to the GpIIb/IIIa receptor that has been humanized to reduce immunogenicity. Eptifibatide is a synthetic peptide compound and tirofiban is a nonpeptide mimetic. Lamifiban, a synthetic peptide, currently is unavailable. Abciximab has a biologic half-life of 8 to 12 hours, whereas eptifibatide and tirofiban have shorter biologic half-lives of approximately 2 hours. Eptifibatide, tirofiban, and lamifiban are eliminated by the kidneys and require adjustment in patients who have renal insufficiency. Because these agents inhibit platelet aggregation at different sites of action, the use of triple therapy with aspirin, thienopyridine, and GpIIb/IIIa inhibitor is the most potent antiplatelet therapy. A study by Klinkhardt et al [94] showed the augmentation of the antiaggregatory effects of GpIIb/IIIa inhibitors by aspirin and clopidogrel. The present article does not discuss GPIIb/IIIa inhibitor trials in the setting of acute coronary syndrome or acute MI.

Evaluation of c7E3 for the Prevention of Ischemic Complications was the first clinical trial that demonstrated the benefit of GpIIb/IIIa inhibition in high-risk patients undergoing PCI [95]. Abciximab bolus and infusion significantly lowered major ischemic events at 30 days, especially nonfatal MI and urgent TVR (12.8% rate of death, MI, and urgent TVR with placebo; 11.5% for abciximab bolus; 8.3% for abciximab bolus and infusion; $P = 0.008$). This benefit was maintained at 6 months [96] and at 3 years [80,97]. Abciximab use with 10,000 to 12,000 U of heparin, however, was associated with higher bleeding complications. The Evaluation of PTCA to Improve Long-Term Outcome with Abciximab GpIIb/IIIa Blockade trial studied abciximab in patients undergoing urgent or elective PCI and the role of weight-adjusted heparin dosing to reduce bleeding complications [98]. At 30 days, abciximab use significantly reduced death, MI, or urgent TVR event rates regardless of the heparin dosing (11.7% in placebo, 5.4% for abciximab bolus and infusion with standard heparin dosing, 5.2% for abciximab bolus and infusion with weight-adjusted heparin dosing; $P<0.001$). Although major bleeding rates were similar in the placebo group, weight-adjusted heparin dosing group with abciximab, and standard heparin dosing group with abciximab, more minor bleeding was seen in the abciximab plus standard heparin dosing group. At 6 months, the incidence of death, MI, or TVR was reduced in the abciximab group. In the Evaluation of Platelet IIb/IIIa Inhibitor for Stenting trial [99], abciximab was tested in patients undergoing elective PCI. Patients were randomized to stent with abciximab, PTCA with abciximab, or stent with placebo. The incidence of death, nonfatal MI, or urgent TVR was significantly reduced in the stent with abciximab group at 30 days (10.8% in stent with placebo group, 6.9% in PTCA with abciximab group, 5.3% in stent with abciximab group; $P = 0.007$). Continued benefit was seen at 6 months and 1 year in the abciximab group. There also appears to be a benefit on mortality that emerges with longer-term follow-up [100]. The benefit is especially notable in diabetic patients [101].

Small-molecule GpIIb/IIIa inhibitors also have been studied in the setting of PCI. The Integrilin to Minimize Platelet Aggregation and Coronary Thrombosis II study evaluated eptifibatide in patients undergoing elective, urgent, or emergent PCI. Patients were randomized to eptifibatide (135 μg/kg) bolus followed by an infusion of 0.5 μg/kg/min for 20 to 24 hours, eptifibatide (135 μg/kg) bolus followed by infusion of 0.75 μg/kg/min for 20 to 24 hours, or placebo [102]. The primary end point of death, MI, or urgent TVR at 30 days was not significantly different between the groups (9.2% in the eptifibatide 0.5 μg/kg/min infusion group, 9.9% in the eptifibatide 0.75 μg/kg infusion group, 11.4% in the placebo group; $P = 0.22$). The Enhanced Suppression of the Platelet Receptor Glycoprotein IIb/IIIa Using Integrilin Therapy trial [103] studied whether patients undergoing elective PCI would benefit from eptifibatide versus placebo using a different eptifibatide dosing of 180 μg/kg double bolus with 2.0 μg/kg/minute for 18 to 24 hours infusion. The study end point of death, MI, urgent TVR, or bailout GpIIb/IIIa inhibitor use at 48 hours was significantly reduced with eptifibatide (6.6% versus 10.5%, $P = 0.0015$). At 30 days, the composite secondary end point of death, MI, or urgent TVR also was reduced with eptifibatide (6.8% versus 10.5%, $P = 0.0034$). This benefit was sustained at 6 months (7.5% versus 11.5%, $P = 0.002$) and also at 1 year [104].

The Randomized Efficacy Study of Tirofiban for Outcomes and Restenosis trial evaluated the role of tirofiban in 2139 patients undergoing balloon angioplasty or directional atherectomy within 72 hours after presenting with unstable angina or acute MI [105]. Patients were given a tirofiban bolus of 10 μg/kg followed by a 36-hour infusion of 0.15 μg/kg/minute or placebo. The primary end point of death, MI, or urgent TVR was not significantly different between the groups (12.2% in the placebo group, 10.3% in the tirofiban group; $P = 0.16$).

Recently, the Tirofiban and Abciximab for Revascularization Give Equivalent Outcomes trial [106] compared abciximab and tirofiban in patients undergoing coronary stenting. This study was the first large randomized study to test two different types of GpIIb/IIIa inhibitors. Abciximab was found to be superior to tirofiban in preventing the composite end point of death, MI, or urgent TVR at 30 days (6.0% versus 7.6%, $P = 0.038$).

Antiplatelet therapies have played an important role since the first PCI in 1977. The understanding of antiplatelet therapies in PCI has been enlarged by the many trials in the last decade. Oral and intravenous antiplatelet therapies have become critical adjuncts to maximize the benefits of percutaneous coronary revascularization.

Antiplatelet drugs for cerebrovascular disease

Cerebrovascular disease may result in focal ischemia, focal cerebral infarction, or focal hemorrhage. Embolization from the heart or carotid vessels and from the venous circulation by way of a patent foramen ovale may produce ischemia with or without accompanying hemorrhage in the ischemic area. Antiplatelet agents have been found to be useful in some of these clinical circumstances. Aspirin, clopidogrel, and aspirin/dipyridamole in combination have been evaluated in clinical trials of primary and secondary prevention and in therapeutic trials. Summations of these trials have been published by Albers and colleagues [107,108] and by del Zoppo [109]. In general, it may be stated that in patients who have had a recent transient ischemic attack, aspirin is effective in preventing subsequent stroke, MI, and death. Aspirin alone is not sufficient when transient ischemic attacks are caused by embolization from carotid stenosis of 70% to 90%. After carotid endarterectomy, however, aspirin is useful. Aspirin/dipyridamole in combination is effective in preventing recurrence following completed stroke (secondary prevention), as is aspirin alone or clopidogrel in aspirin-resistant patients.

Peripheral occlusive arterial disease

The two antiplatelet agents that appear to be most useful in peripheral vascular disease to prevent ischemic necrosis are clopidogrel and cilostazol. When aspirin and clopidogrel were compared in the CAPRIE trial, clopidogrel was superior [80]. Cilostazol is a phosphodiesterase inhibitor that is effective for peripheral vascular disease but has adverse effects on congestive heart failure and should not be used in patients in or at risk of overt failure [110].

Intracardiac sources of arterial emboli

Atrial fibrillation

In atrial fibrillation associated with valvular disease, antiplatelet drugs may be useful when added to oral anticoagulant therapy after that treatment alone fails.

Aspirin alone or substitutes for aspirin may be useful in younger (<65 years) patients who have isolated atrial fibrillation (nonvalvular without cardiomyopathy or congestive heart failure) [111,112].

Patent foramen ovale

Embolization to the brain from peripheral venous sources may occur in the presence of patent foramen ovale. In such cases, antiplatelet drugs are not known to be clinically useful. Such patients are treated with anticoagulants with or without surgical correction of the patent foramen ovale. Following patent foramen ovale repair and in the absence of peripheral venous thromboembolism, antiplatelet therapy with aspirin or clopidogrel for a limited postoperative period may be advisable [112].

Congestive heart failure

Congestive heart failure is associated with coronary artery disease for which patients take aspirin for secondary prevention of thrombosis. Thus, any antithrombotic agent added to that may have added benefit but also added risk of hemorrhage. A study in progress (Warfarin Aspirin Reduced Ejection Fraction) is comparing the relative effectiveness of aspirin and warfarin in preventing death or stroke and recurrent hospitalizations.

Adverse effects of aspirin

The risk of gastrointestinal hemorrhage, particularly from aspirin doses higher than 325 mg/d is well known. It also is known that the lowest effective dose also is associated with a risk of gastrointestinal bleeding. The local effect of aspirin in the mucosa of the stomach is likely to be more prevalent with the higher doses, but patients who have mucosal lesions or vascular malformations may bleed at any dose.

There also is a risk of cerebral hemorrhage associated with aspirin therapy, which is more difficult to treat. This complication occurs more frequently in patients with prior stroke or with hypertension. Thus, a detailed history and physical examination are essential before antiplatelet therapy is started.

It recently was reported that *Helicobacter pylori* infection doubles the risk of gastrointestinal hemorrhage in patients taking aspirin or other NSAIDs [113,114]. It is not known whether diagnostic tests for the detection of *H pylori* followed by endoscopic evaluation or directed therapy with antibiotics or acid-suppressing drugs will reduce the rate of NSAID-induced bleeding complications. Certainly, a history of *H pylori* infection should be considered a risk factor for bleeding. The importance of this information on the use of aspirin for cardiovascular disease remains to be determined.

Bleeding complications

Antiplatelet drugs seldom cause bleeding when used as single agents in recommended dosages except in surgical or invasive procedures. The gastrointestinal bleeding due to aspirin is dose- and gastric disease–related as mentioned previously in the discussion on *H pylori* infection, gastric and duodenal ulcers, and gastritis. Bleeding of that type requires endoscopic evaluation and treatment by a gastroenterologist, if possible. The effect of aspirin and the thienopyridines clopidogrel and ticlopidine lasts for the life of the platelet. If the bleeding is severe and potentially life threatening, then platelet transfusions should be given even when the platelet count is normal. It recently was reported that recombinant factor VIIa (NovoSeven) may be useful in the case of bleeding induced by antiplatelet drugs. It acts by the enhancement of thrombin generation at the site of bleeding, which could activate and aggregate platelets even though an antiplatelet drug is present [115,116].

Thrombocytopenia may occur during antiplatelet therapy due to the drug causing immediate destruction, as was seen in the early onset of platelet destruction reported with abciximab [117]. Late-onset immune destruction sometimes is observed in abciximab-treated patients [118,119]. Platelet transfusions are recommended when there is life-threatening hemorrhage or extremely low platelet counts. Other supportive measures also may be needed. This type of platelet destruction does not respond to corticosteroids.

Resistance to antiplatelet drugs

Resistance to antiplatelet drugs has been limited to aspirin and clopidogrel. Failure of the drug to have the desired clinical effect is the prime reason to suspect that resistance exists, but first it is necessary to make sure that there are no errors in drug labeling and compliance. Assuming that those are not the problems and failure of absorption is improbable, true resistance to the drug may exist. Abnormalities in the COX-1 molecule may limit acetylation by aspirin. Abnormal metabolic pathways may limit the biotransformation of clopidogrel to its active metabolite. Unusually rapid generation of thrombin at the thrombotic site may constitute a "relative resistance." There is some evidence to suggest that some individuals require higher doses than those being given for arterial thrombotic disease. Such a finding may be related to metabolic control because a weaker aspirin response was observed in type 2 diabetes mellitus patients compared with nondiabetic individuals [120,121].

Coadministration of reversible NSAIDs that block COX-1 and COX-2 may interfere with the irreversible effect of aspirin on cyclooxygenase. Ibuprofen has been shown to interfere with the effect of aspirin on platelets. Pure COX-2 inhibitors do not compete with aspirin for interaction with cyclooxygenase.

Aspirin resistance can be tested by demonstrating that the expected impairment of platelet function is not present when the patient has taken the drug. For aspirin resistance, the two most reliable tests are platelet aggregation testing, with arachidonic acid as the agonist, or measurement of thromboxane B_2 levels in the urine. The bleeding time is too insensitive to be used for this purpose. Resistance to clopidogrel can be demonstrated by showing normal response to ADP by patients' platelets ex vivo in the aggregometer [122–124].

Future antiplatelet agents

There area a number of additional targets that may lead to effective antiplatelet therapy (Fig. 3). Among those developing the most interest are thromboxane receptor antagonists/thromboxane synthase inhibitors and Gplb inhibitors. Thromboxane is a powerful platelet agonist that is formed from arachidonic acid by way of COX-1. A number of thromboxane receptor antagonists have been identified [125,126]. In addition, a number of these compounds are dual-function inhibitors, inhibiting the receptor and the enzyme thromboxane synthase [127–129]. These compounds offer an advantage over aspirin because prostacyclin synthesis is not compromised. As expected, these agents potently inhibit arachidonic acid and U-46619 (thromboxane receptor agonist)–induced

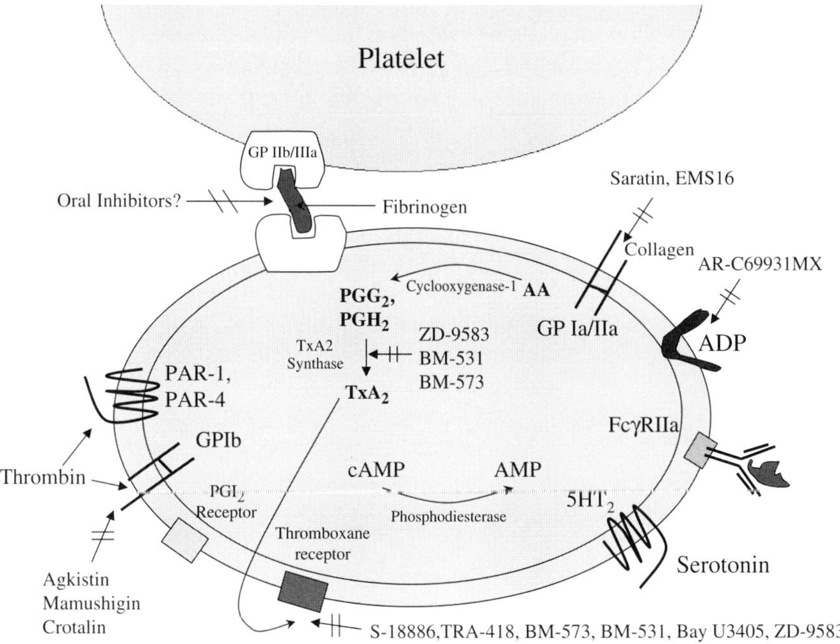

Fig. 3. Sites of action of experimental antiplatelet agents. New drugs that block platelet adhesion by inhibiting Gplb or the collagen receptor currently are being developed. A number of compounds capable of inhibiting thromboxane generation or blocking the thromboxane receptor also are being developed. AA, arachidonic acid; $5HT_2$, serotonin; PAR, protease activator receptor; PG, prostaglandin.

platelet aggregation, with higher concentrations required to inhibit aggregation induced by other agonists. Several in vitro studies have shown that thromboxane receptor antagonists are more effective than aspirin at inhibiting platelet adhesion to subendothelial matrix [127,130]. Several of the identified thromboxane receptor antagonists exhibit significant oral bioavailability [131,132].

Although the GpIIb/IIIa receptor antagonists are effective at preventing platelet thrombus formation, they have little effect on platelet adhesion to the vessel wall [133]. GpIb, therefore, is another potentially attractive target for antiplatelet therapy because vWF binding to this receptor plays a key role in the initial platelet adhesion response, particularly at sites of high shear stress [134]. A number of proteins isolated from snake venoms [135–138] and other antibodies that inhibit vWF binding to GpIb [139] are being studied as potential antiplatelet agents. In vitro, such agents inhibit ristocetin-induced platelet agglutination. In addition, various inhibitors have been shown to inhibit thrombus formation in models of arterial thrombosis [136]. Aurin tricarboxylic acid, which binds to high molecular weight multimers of vWF, prevents vWF from binding to GpIb. In vitro studies have shown that aurin tricarboxylic acid prevents shear-induced platelet adhesion to rabbit aorta [140]. The GpIb receptor also is important to platelet function in light of findings that thrombin binding to this receptor induces platelet aggregation and clot retraction without inducing high-affinity GpIIb/IIIa receptor expression on the platelet surface [141].

Platelets contain a number of receptors for collagen, allowing platelets to adhere to sites of vascular damage [142]. This platelet adhesion also may be mediated by vWF binding to exposed subendothelial collagen. Collagen also is a potent agonist for platelet activation. The main platelet receptors for collagen are $\alpha_2\beta_1$ and GpVI. Several natural inhibitors of the platelet–collagen interaction have been identified in snake venoms and the saliva of blood-sucking animals [142–144]. Such proteins target $\alpha_2\beta_1$, GpVI, or the vWF binding site on collagen. In addition, peptide inhibitors to block the platelet–collagen interaction are being developed [145]. Limited studies performed to date have suggested that inhibition of the platelet–collagen interaction can inhibit thrombogenesis and may be associated with a lower bleeding potential [146–148].

References

[1] Born GVR. Aggregation of blood platelets by adenosine diphosphate and its reversal. Nature 1962;194:927–9.

[2] Gaarder A, Jonssen J, Laland S, et al. Adenosine diphosphate in red cells as a factor in the adhesiveness of human blood platelets. Nature 1961;192:531–2.

[3] Beaumont JL, Caen JP, Bernard J. Influence de l'acid acetyl salicyliqe dan les maladies hemorrhagiques. Sang 1956;27:43–8.

[4] Quick AJ. Analgesia in hemophilia. Anesth Analg 1963;42:475–6.

[5] Fitzgerald GA. Dipyridamole. N Engl J Med 1987;316:1247–57.

[6] Craven LL. Experiences with aspirin (acetylsalicylic acid) in the nonspecific prophylaxis of coronary thrombosis. Miss Val Med J 1953;75:38–40.

[7] Wu KK. Platelet hyperaggregability and thrombosis in patients with thrombocythemia. Ann Intern Med 1978;88:7–11.
[8] Walenga JM, Jeske W, Messmore H. Mechanisms of venous and arterial thrombosis in heparin-induced thrombocytopenia. J Thromb Thrombolysis 2000;10:S13–9.
[9] Walenga JM, Jeske WP, Wallis DE, et al. Clinical experience with combined treatment of thrombin inhibitors and GPIIb/IIa inhibitors in patients with HIT. Semin Thromb Hemost 1999;25(Suppl 1):77–81.
[10] Schafer A, Wiesmann F, Neubauer S, et al. Rapid regulation of platelet activation in vivo by nitric oxide. Circulation 2004;109:1819–22.
[11] Badimon L, Badimon JJ, Fuster V. Pathophysiology of arterial thrombosis. In: Gresele P, Page C, Vermylen J, editors. Platelets in thrombotic and non-thrombotic disorders. Pathophysiology, pharamcology and therapeutics. Cambridge, UK: Cambridge University Press; 2002. p. 727–37.
[12] Brass LF, Manning DR, Cichowski K, et al. Signaling through G-proteins in platelets to the integrins and beyond. Thromb Haemost 1997;78:581–9.
[13] Hynes RO. Integrins, versatility, modulation and signaling in cell adhesion. Cell 1992;69: 11–25.
[14] White JG. An overview of platelet structural physiology. Scand Microbiol 1988;1:1677–700.
[15] Guyton JR, Klemps KF. Development of the lipid-rich core in human atherosclerosis. Arterioscler Thromb Vasc Biol 1996;16:4–11.
[16] Virmani R, Kolodgie FD, Burke AP, et al. Lessons from sudden coronary death. A comprehensive morphological classification scheme for atherosclerotic lesions. Arterioscler Thromb Vasc Biol 2000;20:1262–75.
[17] Kolodgie FD, Gold HK, Burke AP, et al. Intraplaque hemorrhage and progression of atheroma. N Engl J Med 2003;349:2316–25.
[18] Virchow R. Plogose u thrombose in gefaesssystem gessamelte abhandlungen zur wissenschaftlichen medizin. Frankfurt, Germany: Meidinger Sohn; 1856.
[19] von Rokitansky C. A manual of pathological anatomy. London, UK: The Sydenham Society; 1852.
[20] Duguid JB. Thrombosis as a factor in pathogenesis or coronary atherosclerosis. J Pathol Bacteriol 1946;58:207–12.
[21] Leon MB, Baim DS, Popma JJ, et al. A clinical trial comparing three antithrombotic drug regimens after coronary artery stenting. Stent Anticoagulation Restenosis Study Investigators. N Eng J Med 1998;339:1665–71.
[22] Steinbuhl SR, Berger PB, Mann JT. Early and sustained dual oral antiplatelet therapy following percutaneous coronary intervention: a randomized controlled trial. JAMA 2002;288:2411–20.
[23] Lange RA, Hillis LD. Antiplatelet therapy for ischemic heart disease. N Engl J Med 2004; 350:277–80.
[24] Heistad DD. Unstable coronary artery plaques. N Engl J Med 2003;349:2285–7.
[25] Roman M, Shankar BA, Davis A, et al. Prevalence and correlates of accelerated atherosclerosis is systemic lupus erythematosis. N Engl J Med 2003;349:2399–406.
[26] Hahn B. Systemic lupus erythematosis and accelerated atherosclerosis. N Engl J Med 2003; 349:2379–80.
[27] McIntyre TM, Prescott SM, Weyrich AS, et al. Cell-cell interactions: leukocyte-endothelial interactions. Curr Opin Hematol 2003;10:150–8.
[28] Elstad MR, McIntyre TM, Prescott SM, et al. The interaction of leukocytes with platelets in blood coagulation. Curr Opin Hematol 1995;2:47–54.
[29] von Hundelshausen P, Weber KS, Huo Y, et al. RANTES deposition by platelets triggers monocyte arrest on inflamed and atherosclerotic endothelium. Circulation 2001;103:1772–7.
[30] Lindemann S, Tolley ND, Dixon DA, et al. Activated platelets mediate inflammatory signaling by regulated interleukin 1beta synthesis. J Cell Biol 2001;154:485–90.
[31] Weyrich AS, Dixon DA, Pabla R, et al. Signal-dependent translation of a regulatory protein, Bcl-3, in activated human platelets. Proc Natl Acad Sci USA 1998;95:5556–61.
[32] Lindemann S, Tolley ND, Eyre JR, et al. Integrins regulate the intracellular distribution of

eukaryotic initiation factor 4E in platelets: a checkpoint for translational control. J Biol Chem 2001;276:33947–51.
[33] Pabla R, Weyrich AS, Dixon DA, et al. Integrin-dependent control of translation: engagement of integrin alphaIIbbeta3 regulates synthesis of proteins in activated human platelets. J Cell Biol 1999;144(1):175–84.
[34] Celi A, Pelligrini G, Lorenzet R, et al. P-selectin induces the expression of tissue factor on monocytes. Proc Natl Acad Sci USA 1994;91:8767–71.
[35] Myers D, Wrobleski S, Londy F, et al. New and effective treatment of experimentally induced venous thrombosis with anti-inflammatory rPSGL-Ig. Thromb Haemost 2002;87:374–82.
[36] Kumar A, Villani MP, Patel UK, et al. Recombinant soluble form of PSGL-1 accelerates thrombolysis and prevents reocclusion in a porcine model. Circulation 1999;99:1363–9.
[37] Rauch U, Osende JI, Fuster V, et al. Thrombus formation on atherosclerotic plaques: pathogenesis and clinical consequences. Ann Intern Med 2001;134:224–38.
[38] Roth GJ, Majerus PW. The mechanism of the effect of aspirin on human platelets. I. Acetylation of a particulate fraction protein. J Clin Invest 1975;56:624–32.
[39] Patrono C. Aspirin as an antiplatelet drug. N Engl J Med 1994;330:1287–94.
[40] Awtry EH, Loscalzo J. Aspirin. In: Michelson AD, editor. Platelets. Amsterdam: Academic Press; 2002. p. 745–68.
[41] Patrono C, Bachmann F, Baigent C, et al. Expert consensus document on the use of antiplatelet agents. Eur Heart J 2004;25:166–81.
[42] Christiaens L, Macchi L. [Resistance to aspirin: up to date 2003.] Arch Mal Coeur Vaiss 2004; 97(4):320–6.
[43] Rao AK. Inherited defects in platelet signaling mechanisms. J Thromb Haemost 2003;1(4): 671–81.
[44] Hollopeter G, Jantzen HM, Vincent D, et al. Identification of the platelet ADP receptor targeted by antithrombotic drugs. Nature 2001;409:202–7.
[45] Curtin R, Cox D, Fitzgerald D. Clopidogrel and ticlopidine. In: Michelson AD, editor. Platelets. Amsterdam: Academic Press; 2002. p. 787–801.
[46] Storey F. The P2Y12 receptor as a therapeutic target in cardiovascular disease. Platelets 2001; 12:197–209.
[47] Coller BS, Peerschke EI, Scudder LE, et al. A murine monoclonal antibody that completely blocks the binding of fibrinogen to platelets produces a thrombasthenic-like state in normal platelets and binds to glycoproteins IIb and/or IIIa. J Clin Invest 1983;72:325–38.
[48] Plow EF, Pierschbacher MD, Ruoslahti E, et al. The effect of Arg-Gly-Asp containing peptides on fibrinogen and von Willebrand factor binding to platelets. Proc Natl Acad Sci USA 1985; 82:8057–61.
[49] Agah R, Plow EF, Topol EJ. GPIIb-IIIa Antagonists. In: Michelson AD, editor. Platelets. Amsterdam: Academic Press; 2002. p. 769–85.
[50] Ilveskero S, Lassila R. Abciximab inhibits procoagulant activity but not the release reaction upon collagen- or clot-adherent platelets. J Thromb Haemost 2003;1:805–13.
[51] Eisert WG. Dipyridamole. In: Michelson AD, editor. Platelets. Amsterdam: Academic Press; 2002. p. 803–15.
[52] Ikeda Y, Sudo T, Kimura Y. Cilostazol. In: Michelson AD, editor. Platelets. Amsterdam: Academic Press; 2002. p. 817–23.
[53] Sobel M, McNeill PM, Carlson PL. Heparin inhibition of von Willebrand factor–dependent platelet function in vitro and in vivo. J Clin Invest 1991;87:1787–93.
[54] Messmore H, Griffin B, Fareed J, et al. In vitro studies of the interaction of heparin, low molecular weight heparin and heparinoids with platelets. Ann N Y Acad Sci 1989;556:217–32.
[55] Messmore H, Griffin B, Koza M, et al. Interactions of heparinoids with platelets. Comparison with heparin and low molecular weight heparin. Semin Thromb Hemost 1991;17(Suppl 1): 57–9.
[56] Ieko M, Tarumi T, Takeda M, et al. Synthetic selective inhibitors of coagulation factor Xa strongly inhibit thrombin generation without affecting initial thrombin forming time necessary for platelet activation in hemostasis. J Thromb Haemost 2004;2:612–8.

[57] Bal dit Sollier C, Kang C, Berge N, et al. Activity of a synthetic hexadecasaccharide (SanOrg123781A) in a pig model of arterial thrombosis. J Thromb Haemost 2004;2(6):925–30.
[58] Mukherjee DP, Fang J, Chetcuti S, et al. Impact of combination evidence-based medical therapy on mortality in patients with acute coronary syndrome. Circulation 2004;109:745–9.
[59] The Clopidogrel in Unstable Angina to Prevent Recurrent Events Trial Investigators. Effects of clopidogrel in addition to aspirin in patients with acute coronary syndromes without S-T segment elevation. N Engl J Med 2001;345:494–502.
[60] Helft G, Osende JI, Worthley SG, et al. Acute antithrombotic effects of a front-loaded regimen of clopidogrel in patients with atherosclerosis on aspirin. Arterioscler Thromb Vasc Biol 2000; 20(11):2316–21.
[61] Gibbons RJ, Abrams J, Chatterjee K, et al. ACC/AHA 2002 guideline update for the management of patients with chronic stable angina—summary article: a report of the American College of Cardiology/American Heart Association Task Force on Practice Guidelines (Committee on the Management of Patients with Chronic Stable Angina). Circulation 2003;107: 149–58.
[62] Nappi J, Talbert R. Dual antiplatelet therapy for prevention of recurrent ischemic events. Am J Health Syst Pharm 2002;59:1723–34.
[63] Eidelman R, Hebert P, Weisman S, et al. An update on aspirin in the primary prevention of cardiovascular disease. Arch Intern Med 2003;163:2006–10.
[64] The Steering Committee of the Physician's Health Study Research Group. Findings from the aspirin component of the ongoing Physician's Health Study. N Eng J Med 1988;318:262–4.
[65] White HD, Willerson JT. We must use the knowledge we have to treat patients with acute coronary syndrome. Circulation 2004;109:698–700.
[66] Lewis HD, Davis JW, Arcibald DG, et al. Protective effects of aspirin against acute myocardial infarction and death in men with unstable angina. Results of a Veterans Administration Cooperative Study. N Engl J Med 1983;309(7):396–403.
[67] Theroux P, Ouimet H, McCans J, et al. Aspirin, heparin, or both to treat acute unstable angina. N Engl J Med 1988;319(17):1105–11.
[68] Braunwald E, Antman EM, Beasley JW. ACC/AHA guidelines update for the management of patients with unstable angina and non-ST segment myocardial infarction—2000: summary article. Circulation 2002;106:1893–900.
[69] Morrow DA, Antman EM, Charlesworth A, et al. TIMI risk score for ST-elevation myocardial infarction: a combined bedside, clinical score for risk assessment at presentation. Circulation 2000;102:2031–7.
[70] Cadroy Y, Bossavy JP, Thalamas C. Early potent antithrombotic effect with combined aspirin and a loading dose of clopidogrel on experimental arterial thrombogenesis in humans. Circulation 2000;101:2833–8.
[71] Mehta SR, Yusaf S, Peters RJ, et al. Effects of pretreatment with clopidogrel and aspirin followed by long-term therapy in patients undergoing percutaneous coronary intervention: the PCI-CURE study. Lancet 2001;358:527–33.
[72] Barnathan ES, Schwartz JM, Taylor L, et al. Aspirin and dipyridamole in the prevention of acute coronary thrombosis complicating coronary angioplasty. Circulation 1987;76:125–34.
[73] Schwartz L, Bourassa MG, Lesperance J, et al. Aspirin and dipyridamole in the prevention of restenosis after percutaneous transluminal coronary angioplasty. N Engl J Med 1988;318: 1714–9.
[74] Herbert JM, Dol F, Bernat A, et al. The antiaggregating and antithrombotic activity of clopidogrel is potentiated by aspirin in several experimental models in the rabbit. Thromb Haemost 1998;80:512–8.
[75] Bertrand ME, Allain H, Lablanche JM. Results of a randomized trial of ticlopidine versus placebo for the prevention of acute closure and restenosis after coronary angioplasty. Circulation 1990;82(Suppl III):90.
[76] Schomig A, Neumann FJ, Kastrati A, et al. A randomized comparison of antiplatelet and anticoagulant therapy after the placement or coronary artery stents. N Engl J Med 1996;334: 1084–9.

[77] Urban P, Macaya C, Rupprecht HJ, et al. Randomized evaluation of anticoagulation versus antiplatelet therapy after coronary stent implantation in high-risk patients: the multicenter aspirin and ticlopidine trial after coronary stenting (MATTIS). Circulation 1998;98:2126–32.
[78] Bertrand ME, Legrand V, Boland J, et al. Randomized multicenter comparison of conventional anticoagulation versus antiplatelet therapy in unplanned and elective coronary stenting The full anticoagulation versus aspirin and ticlopidine (FANTASTIC) study. Circulation 1998;98: 1597–603.
[79] Steinbuhl SR, Tan WA, Foody JM. Incidence and clinical course of thrombotic thrombocytopenic purpura due to ticlopidine following coronary stenting EPISTENT Investigators Evaluation of Platelet IIb/IIIa Inhibitor for Stenting. JAMA 1999;281:806–10.
[80] CAPRIE Steering Committee. A randomised, blinded trial of clopidogrel versus aspirin in patients at risk of ischemic events (CAPRIE). Lancet 1996;348:1329–39.
[81] Bertrand ME, Rupprecht HJ, Urban P, et al. Double-blind study of the safety of clopidogrel with and without a loading dose in combination with aspirin compared with ticlopidine in combination with aspirin after coronary stenting: the clopidogrel aspirin stent international cooperative study (CLASSICS). Circulation 2000;102:624–9.
[82] Taniuchi M, Kuraz HI, Smith SC, et al. Ticlid or plavix post-stent (TOPPS): Randomization to 2-week treatment [abstract]. Circulation 1999;100(Suppl I):379.
[83] Muller C, Buttner HJ, Petersen J, et al. A randomized comparison of clopidogrel and aspirin versus ticlopidine and aspirin after placement of coronary-artery stents. Circulation 2000;101: 590–3.
[84] Berger PB, Bell MR, Rihal CS, et al. Clopidogrel versus ticlopidine after intracoronary stent placement. J Am Coll Cardiol 1999;34:1891–4.
[85] Moussa I, Oetgen M, Roubin G, et al. Effectiveness of clopidogrel and aspirin versus ticlopidine and aspirin in preventing stent thrombosis after coronary stent implantation. Circulation 1999;99:2364–6.
[86] L'Allier PL, Aronow HD, Yadav J, et al. Is clopidogrel a safe and effective adjunctive anti-platelet therapy for coronary artery stenting? [abstract]. J Am Coll Cardiol 2000;35(Suppl A):66A.
[87] Mishkel GJ, Aguirre FV, Ligon RW, et al. Clopidogrel as adjuctive antiplatelet therapy during coronary stenting. J Am Coll Cardiol 1999;34:1884–90.
[88] Plucinski DA, Scheltema K, Krusmark J, et al. A comparison of clopidogrel to ticlopidine therapy for the prevention of major adverse cardiac events at thirty days and six months following coronary stent implantation [abstract]. J Am Coll Cardiol 2000;35:67A.
[89] Calver AL, Blows LJ, Harmer S, et al. Clopidogrel for prevention of major cardiac events after coronary stent implantation: 30-day and 6-month results in patients with smaller stents. Am Heart J 2000;140:483–91.
[90] Bhatt DL, Bertrand ME, Berger PB, et al. Meta-analysis of randomized and registry comparisons of ticlopidine and clopidogrel after stenting. J Am Coll Cardiol 2002;39:9–14.
[91] Steinhubl SR, Lauer MS, Mukherjee DP, et al. The duration of pretreatment with ticlopidine prior to stenting is associated with the risk of procedure-related non-Q-wave myocardial infarctions. J Am Coll Cardiol 1998;32:1366–70.
[92] Assili AR, Salloum J, Sdringola S, et al. Effects of clopidogrel pretreatment before percutaneous coronary intervention in patients treated with glycoprotein IIb/IIIa inhibitors (abciximab or tirofiban). Am J Cardiol 2001;88:884–6.
[93] Chew DP, Bhatt DL, Robbins MA, et al. Effect of clopidogrel added to aspirin before percutaneous coronary intervention on the risk associated with C-reactive protein. Am J Cardiol 2001;88:672–4.
[94] Klinkhardt U, Kirchmaier CM, Westrup D, et al. Ex vivo–in vitro interaction between aspirin, clopidogrel, and the glycoprotein IIb/IIIa inhibitors abciximab and SR 121566A. Clin Pharmacol Ther 2000;67(3):305–13.
[95] The EPIC Investigators. Use of a monoclonal antibody directed against the platelet glycoprotein IIb/IIIa receptor in high-risk coronary angioplasty. N Engl J Med 1994;330:956–61.
[96] Topol EJ, Callif RM, Weisman HF, et al. Randomised trial of coronary intervention with

antibody against platelet IIb/IIIa integrin for reduction of clinical restenosis: results at six months. Lancet 1994;343:881–6.
[97] Topol EJ, Ferguson JJ, Weisman HF, et al. Long-term protection from myocardial ischemic events in a randomized trial of brief integrin beta3 blockade with percutaneous coronary intervention EPIC Investigator Group Evaluation of Platelet IIb/IIIa Inhibition for Prevention of Ischemic Complication. JAMA 1997;278:479–84.
[98] The EPILOG Investigators. Platelet glycoprotein IIb/IIIa receptor blockade and low-dose heparin during percutaneous coronary revascularization. N Engl J Med 1997;336:1689–96.
[99] The EPISTENT Investigators. Randomised placebo-controlled and balloon-angioplasty-controlled trial to assess safety of coronary stenting with use of platelet glycoprotein-IIb/IIIa blockade. Lancet 1998;352:87–92.
[100] Topol EJ, Mark DB, Lincoff AM, et al. Outcomes at 1 year and economic implications of platelet glycoprotein IIb/IIIa blockade in patients undergoing coronary stenting: results from a multicentre randomised trial. EPISTENT Investigators. Evaluation of Platelet IIb/IIIa Inhibitor for Stenting. Lancet 1999;354:2019–24.
[101] Bhatt DL, Marso SP, Lincoff AM, et al. Abciximab reduces mortality in diabetics following percutaneous coronary intervention. J Am Coll Cardiol 2000;35:922–8.
[102] The IMPACT II Investigators. Randomised placebo-controlled trial of effect of eptifibatide on complications of percutaneous coronary intervention: IMPACT-II. Integrilin to Minimise Platelet Aggregation and Coronary Thrombosis-II. Lancet 1997;349:1422–8.
[103] The ESPRIT Investgators. Novel dosing regimen of eptifibatide in planned coronary stent implantation (ESPRIT): a randomised, placebo-controlled trial. Lancet 2000;356:2037–44.
[104] O'Shea JC, Hafley GE, Greenberg S, et al. Platelet glycoprotein IIb/IIIa integrin blockade with eptifibatide in coronary stent intervention: the ESPRIT trial: a randomised controlled trial. JAMA 2001;285:2468–73.
[105] The RESTORE Investigators. Effects of platelet glycoprotein IIb/IIIa blockade with tirofiban on adverse cardiac events in patients with unstable angina or acute myocardial infarction undegoing coronary angioplasty. Randomized Efficacy Study of Tirofiban for Outcomes and REstenosis. Circulation 1997;96:1445–53.
[106] Topol EJ, Moliterno DJ, Herrmann HC, et al. Comparison of two platelet glycoprotein IIb/IIIa inhibitors, tirofiban and abciximab, for the prevention of ischemic events with percutaneous coronary revascularization. N Engl J Med 2001;344:1888–94.
[107] Albers G, Easton JD, Sacco RL, et al. Antithrombotic and thrombolytic therapy in ischemic stroke. Chest 2001;119(Suppl 1):300S–20S.
[108] Albers G. Role of ticlopidine for prevention of stoke. Stroke 1992;23:912–6.
[109] del Zoppo GJ. Antithrombotic intervention in cerebrovascular disease. In: Loscalzo J, Schafer A, editors. Thrombosis and hemorrhage. 3rd edition. Philadelphia: Lippincott, Williams and Wilkins; 2003. p. 1021–9.
[110] Dawson DL, Culter BS, Meissner MH, et al. Cilostazol has beneficial effects in treatment of intermittent claudication: results from a multicenter, randomized prospective double-blind trial. Circulation 1998;98(7):678–86.
[111] Albers G, Dalen J, Laupacis A, et al. Antithrombotic therapy in atrial fibrillation. Chest 2001; 119:194S–206S.
[112] van Walraven C, Hart RG, Wells GA, et al. Clinical prediction rule to identify patients with atrial fibrillation and a low risk for stroke while taking aspirin. Arch Intern Med 2003;163: 936–43.
[113] Papatheodoidis GV, Papadelli D, Cholongitas E, et al. Effect of *Helicobactor pylori* infections on the risk of upper gastrointestinal bleeding in users of nonsteroidal anti-inflammatory drugs. Am J Med 2004;116:601–5.
[114] Hawkey CJ, Tulassay Z, Szczepanski L. Randomised control trial of *Helicobactor pylori* eradication in patients on non-steroidal anti-inflammatory drugs: HELP NSAIDs study. Helicobacter Eradication for Lesion Protection. Lancet 1998;352:1016–21.
[115] Lisman T, De Groot PG. Mechanism of action of recombinant factor VIIa. J Thromb Haemost 2003;1(6):1138–9.

[116] Hu Q, Brady JO. Recombinant activated factor VII for treatment of enoxaparin-induced bleeding. Mayo Clin Proc 2004;79:827.
[117] Berkowitz SD, Sane DC, Sigman KN, et al. Occurence and clinical significance of thrombocytopenia of a population of high-risk percutaneous coronary revascularization. J Am Coll Cardiol 1998;32:311–9.
[118] Curtis BR, Divgi A, Garrity M, et al. Delayed thrombocytopenia after treatment with abciximab: a distinct clinical entity associated with the immune response to the drug. J Thromb Haemost 2004;2:985–92.
[119] Curtis BR, Swyers J, Divgi A, et al. Thrombocytopenia after second exposure to abciximab is caused by antibodies that recognize abciximab-coated platelets. Blood 2002;99:2054–9.
[120] Watala C, Golanski J, Pluta J, et al. Reduced sensitivity of platelets from type 2 diabetic patients to acetylsalicylic acid (aspirin)—its relation to metabolic control. Thromb Res 2004; 113:101–13.
[121] Di Minno G, Violi F. Aspirin resistance and diabetic angiopathy: back to the future. Thromb Res 2004;113:97–9.
[122] Garcia-Rodriguez LA, Vara C, Patrono C. Differential effects of aspirin and non-aspirin nonsteroidal antiinflammatory drugs in the primary prevention of myocardial infarction in women. Epidemiology 2000;11:382–7.
[123] Patrono C, Coller BS, Dalen J, et al. Platelet-active drugs: the relationships among dose, effectiveness and side-effects. Chest 2001;119:39S–63S.
[124] Weber AA, Zimmermann KC, Meyer-Kirchrath J, et al. Cyclooxygenase 2 in human platelets. A possible factor is aspirin resistance. Lancet 1999;353:900.
[125] Yamada N, Miyamoto M, Isogaya M, et al. TRA-418, a novel compound having both thromboxane A(2) receptor antagonistic and prostaglandin I(2) receptor agonistic activities: its antiplatelet effects in human and animal platelets. J Thromb Haemost 2003;1(8):1813–9.
[126] Villalobos MA, De La Cruz JP, Escalante R, et al. Effects of camonagrel, a selective inhibitor of platelet thromboxane synthase, on platelet-subendothelium interaction. Pharmacology 2003; 69(1):44–50.
[127] De La Cruz JP, Villalobos MA, Escalante R, et al. Effects of the selective inhibition of platelet thromboxane synthesis on the platelet-subendothelial interaction. Br J Pharmacol 2002;137(7): 1082–8.
[128] Rolin S, Dogne JM, Michaux C, et al. Activity of a novel dual thromboxane A(2) receptor antagonist and thromboxane synthase inhibitor (BM-573) on platelet function and isolated smooth muscles. Prostaglandins Leukot Essent Fatty Acids 2001;65(2):67–72.
[129] Muck S, Weber AA, Schror K. Effects of terbogrel on platelet function and prostaglandin endoperoxide transfer. Eur J Pharmacol 1998;344(1):45–8.
[130] Escolar G, Albors M, Garrido M, et al. Inhibition of platelet-vessel wall interactions by thromboxane receptor antagonism in a human in vitro system: potentiation of antiplatelet effects of aspirin. Eur J Clin Invest 1998;28(7):562–8.
[131] Osende JI, Shimbo D, Fuster V, et al. Antithrombotic effects of S 18886, a novel orally active thromboxane A2 receptor antagonist. J Thromb Haemost 2004;2(3):492–8.
[132] Brownlie RP, Brownrigg NJ, Butcher HM, et al. ZD9583, an orally effective thromboxane A2 synthase inhibitor and receptor antagonist with a sustained duration of action in rat and dog. J Pharm Pharmacol 1997;49(2):187–94.
[133] Melis E, Bonnefoy A, Daenens K, et al. αIIbβ3 antagonism vs. antiadhesive treatment to prevent platelet interactions with vascular subendothelium. J Thromb Haemost 2004;2:993–1002.
[134] Vanhoorelbeke K, Ulrichts H, Schoolmeester A, et al. Inhibition of platelet adhesion to collagen as a new target for antithrombotic drugs. Curr Drug Targets Cardiovasc Haematol Dis 2003;3: 125–40.
[135] Lee WH, Zhang Y. Molecular cloning and characterization of a platelet glycoprotein Ib-binding protein from the venom of *Trimeresurus stejnegeri*. Toxicon 2003;41(7):885–92.
[136] Yeh CH, Chang MC, Peng HC, et al. Pharmacological characterization and antithrombotic effect of agkistin, a platelet glycoprotein Ib antagonist. Br J Pharmacol 2001;132(4): 843–50.

[137] Sakurai Y, Fujimura Y, Kokubo T, et al. The cDNA cloning and molecular characterization of a snake venom platelet glycoprotein Ib-binding protein, mamushigan, from *Agkistrodon halys bomhoffii* venom. Thromb Haemost 1998;79(6):1199–207.

[138] Chang MC, Lin HK, Peng HC, et al. Antithrombotic effect of crotalin, a platelet membrane glycoprotein Ib antagonist from venom of *Crotalus atrox*. Blood 1998;91(5):1582–9.

[139] Kageyama S, Yamamoto H, Nakazawa H, et al. Pharmacokinetics and pharmacodynamics of AJW200, a humanized monoclonal antibody to von Willebrand factor, in monkeys. Arterioscler Thromb Vasc Biol 2002;22(1):187–92.

[140] Owens MR, Holme S. Aurin tricarboxylic acid inhibits adhesion of platelets to subendothelium. Thromb Res 1996;81(2):177–85.

[141] Dubois C, Steiner B, Kieffer N, et al. Thrombin binding to GPIbα induces platelet aggregation and fibrin clot retraction supported by resting αIIbβ3 interaction with polymerized fibrin. Thromb Haemost 2003;89:853–65.

[142] Clemetson KJ. Platelet collagen receptors: a new target for inhibition? Haemostasis 1999;29: 16–26.

[143] Smith TP, Alshafie TA, Cruz CP, et al. Saratin, an inhibitor of collagen-platelet interaction, decreases venous anastomotic intimal hyperplasia in a canine dialysis access model. Vasc Endovasc Surg 2003;37(4):259–69.

[144] Horii K, Okuda D, Morita T, et al. Structural characterization of EMS16, an antagonist of collagen receptor (GPIa/IIa) from the venom of *Echis multisquamatus*. Biochemistry 2003; 42(43):12497–502.

[145] Chiang TM. Development of peptide inhibitors to block type I and type III collagen-platelet interaction. Curr Med Chem Cardiovasc Hematol 2003;1(2):171–5.

[146] Siljander PR, Munnix IC, Smethurst PA, et al. Platelet receptor interplay regulates collagen-induced thrombus formation in flowing human blood. Blood 2004;103(4):1333–41.

[147] Goto S, Ikeda Y, Saldivar E, et al. Distinct mechanisms of platelet aggregation as a consequence of different shearing flow conditions. J Clin Invest 1998;101:479–86.

[148] Andre P, Hainaud P, Bal dit Sollier C, et al. Relative involvement of GPIb/IX–vWF axis and GPIIb/IIIa in thrombus growth at high shear rates in the guinea pig. Arterioscler Thromb Vasc Biol 1997;17:919–24.

[149] Grundy SM, Cleeman JI, Merz CNB, et al. Implications of recent clinical trials for the national cholesterol education program adult treatment panel III guidelines. Arteriosclerosis, Thrombosis, and Vascular Biology 2004;24(e149):1–2.

[150] Mehta SR, Yusuf S, on behalf of the CURE Investigators. The Clopidogrel in Unstable angina to Prevent Recurrent Events (CURE) trial programe: rationale, design, and baseline characteristics including a meta-analysis of the effects of thienopyridines in vascular disease. Eur Heart J 2000;21:2033–41.

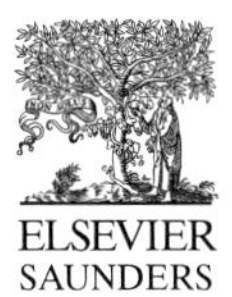

ELSEVIER
SAUNDERS

Hematol Oncol Clin N Am
19 (2005) 119–145

HEMATOLOGY/
ONCOLOGY
CLINICS OF
NORTH AMERICA

The Direct Thrombin Inhibitors: Their Role and Use for Rational Anticoagulation

Eugene P. Frenkel, MD*, Yu-Min Shen, MD,
Barbara B. Haley, MD

Harold C. Simmons Comprehensive Cancer Center, University of Texas Southwestern Medical School, 2201 Inwood Road, Dallas, TX 75235-8852, USA

Anticoagulant therapy entered the clinical arena following the isolation of a sulfated glycosaminoglycan from canine liver, termed *heparin*, by Howell in 1923 [1] and was employed in the treatment of thromboembolism in 1939 [2]. Shortly thereafter, bishydroxycoumarin was defined as a vitamin K antagonist, and its potential for oral therapy of thromboembolic disease was recognized. This recognition led to the development of other structurally related antagonists for clinical use [3–5]. The efficacy of these agents led to their use in the prophylaxis of thromboembolic disease in the surgical and nonsurgical setting [6]. Despite this long-standing approach, it has long been evident that these agents commonly fail in thromboembolic therapy, have a variety of side effects, have complex and multiple drug–drug interactions, and are inadequate in prophylaxis. These problems and issues have led to an intense pursuit of more effective, less toxic, and better-targeted agents.

Role of thrombin in thrombogenesis

The significant clinical burden of thrombotic disease has led to an explosion of interest in the development of agents with the potential of effectively interfering with thrombogenesis. Virtually every site in the coagulation schema has seen a focus of interest.

This research was funded in part by the Nasher Cancer Research Fund.

* Corresponding author.
E-mail address: eugene.frenkel@utsouthwestern.edu (E.P. Frenkel).

0889-8588/05/$ – see front matter
doi:10.1016/j.hoc.2004.09.002

It is thrombin, however, that is the most important focal point in thrombogenesis. Appropriately, thrombin has been termed the *master enzyme* of coagulation [7]. It is the last enzyme in the coagulation cascade and its ultimate product. It is a serine protease that originates from the circulating zymogen precursor protein, prothrombin [8,9].

A cogent summary of the complex steps in the activation of prothrombin to thrombin has been well delineated and expanded by the Furies [5,10] and by the extensive, brilliant studies by Kenneth Mann and coworkers [8,11–20]. These sequential steps and interactions are depicted in Fig. 1.

In brief, the conversion of prothrombin to thrombin results from the enzymatic action of factor Xa and the cofactor Va in a complex formed on membrane surfaces. This complex, situated on a membrane (either platelet or endothelial) in the presence of calcium, has been termed the *prothrombinase complex* because its action is to "alter" or "activate" the substrate prothrombin. The prothrombinase complex has an unusual affinity for phospholipid (vesicles) membranes. Factor Va of this complex binds to specific sites on the platelet surface, and the binding provides a structural receptor (complex) on the platelets for binding of factor Xa.

Two major pathways for prothrombin activation exist at the molecular level, and this sequence is displayed in Fig. 2.

Prothrombin can be activated by factor Xa, producing prothrombin fragment 1•2 and some $\propto$ thrombin, but the latter is produced at a very slow rate. Stepwise cleavage at Arg 271 (step 1) produces the prethrombin fragment 1•2, which

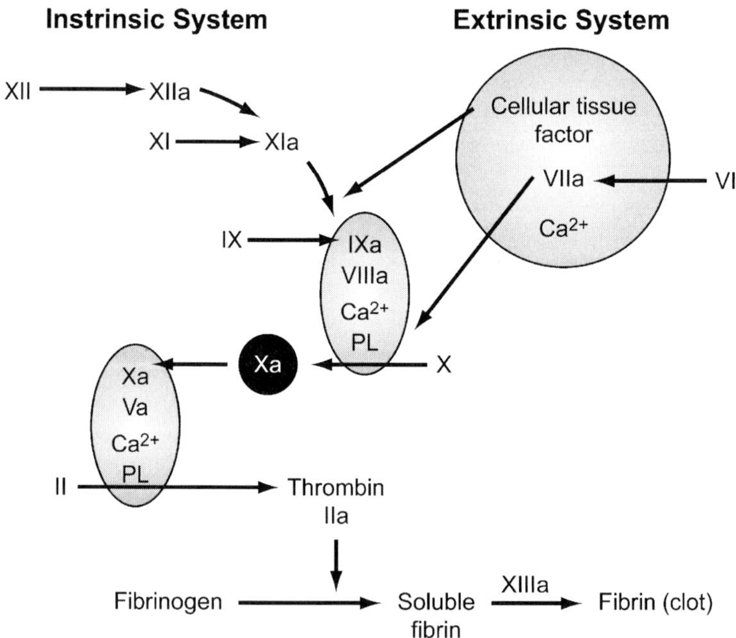

Fig. 1. The coagulation schema.

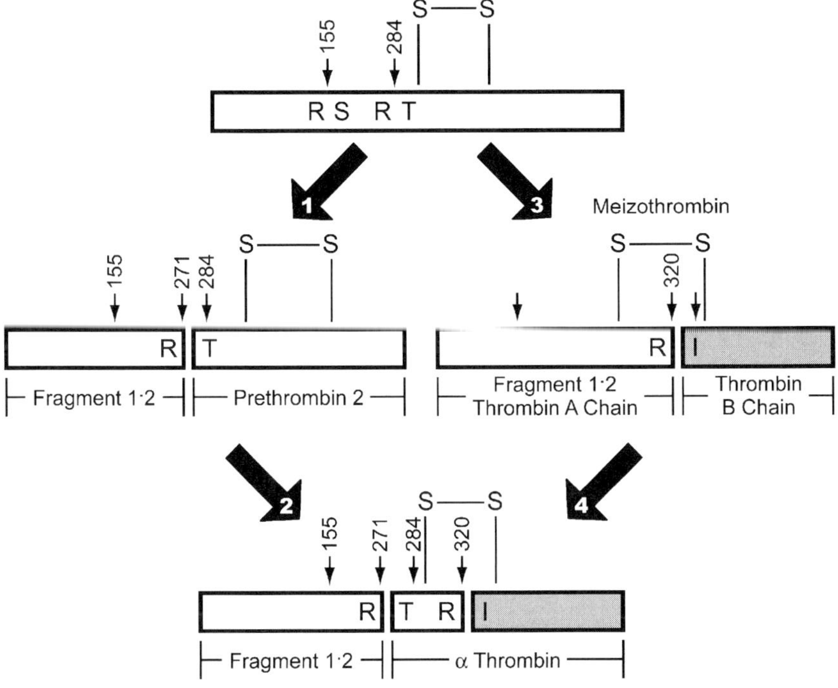

Fig. 2. The activation sequence of prothrombin.

contains the Gla domain and kringles 1 and 2, and prothrombin 2. Cleavage of prethrombin 2 at Arg 320 (step 2) gives rise to prothrombin fragment 1•2 and ∝ thrombin [8,13,16,19].

When prothrombin is activated by the prothrombinase complex, the reaction proceeds with an order of bond cleavage that is reversed compared with that for factor Xa. The initial cleavage is at Arg 320, producing an obligate intermediate meizothrombin, an active enzyme but one that actually lacks clotting or platelet-activating activity. It is cleaved at Arg 271, resulting in thrombin and prothrombin fragment 1•2. It merits emphasis that production of factor Xa (which also may serve as an initial activation mechanism for factor V to Va, thereby triggering the prothromboninase complex formation) serves as a slow and relatively minor independent prothrombin activation mechanism. Indeed, assembly of the prothrombinase complex results in about 300,000 times greater prothrombin activation [8,10,11].

Recent studies have examined clotting in a sequential manner [17,20] and have shown that at the "initiation phase" of coagulation activation of thrombin, substrates occur at concentrations of less than 2 nmol thrombin (0.2%). Most thrombin (96%) is formed well after initial "triggered" clotting occurs [20]. The reason for this late overabundance of thrombin generation after (some) clot is present is still unknown, but this sequence appears very important in the issues of thrombogenesis.

The final product of this sequence is thrombin, perhaps the most versatile enzyme in humans. The usual focus of its function is that of clot production by virtue of its attachment to a thrombin-binding domain on fibrinogen. This results in the release of fibrinopeptides A and B in the primary initiation of fibrin generation. This pivotal action of thrombin, however, is only one of its important functions. The many and varied hemostatic effects of thrombin at virtually every step in the coagulation sequence are presented in Box 1.

Clearly, the enzymatic role of thrombin in the hemostatic process is important and impressive. Thrombin, however, also has many biologic effects that are far more complex than merely hemostatic ones [7,9–11]. As shown in Box 2, these "nonhemostatic" actions involve the stimulation of chemotaxis of white blood cells and cytokine generation and release by them. It has complex effects on the endothelial cells, with the release of a variety of biologic mediators. Finally, it also has a role in fibroblast proliferation and mitogenesis. Although not clearly defined, evidence of a role in cancer cell adhesion has been postulated.

Recent observations have shown that the thrombin receptor, which is a member of the 7-transmembrane domain family, is found in platelets, endothelial

Box 1. Hemostatic effects of thrombin

Clot formation

- Cleaves fibrinogen → fibrin
- Cleaves factor XIII → factor XIIIa

Amplification of clot

- Cleaves factor V → factor Va
- Cleaves factor VIII → factor VIIIa
- Feedback enhancement of further prothrombin activation

Platelet activation

- Stimulates platelet aggregation
- Stimulates platelet release of storage granules
- Increases thromboxane A_2 formation (which further activates platelets)

Physiologic coagulation "inhibitors"

- Activates protein C to PCa: thrombomodulin

Box 2. Nonhemostatic effects of thrombin

Effects on white blood cells

Stimulates chemotaxis
Triggers cytokine generation

Effects on endothelial cells

Effects synthesis and release of prostacyclin, nitrous oxide, tissue plasminogen activator, endothelin, tissue factor

Effects on other tissue sites

Fibroblast: proliferation
Smooth muscle: mitogenesis

Other potential effects

Cancer cells: affects adhesion, metastasis, cellular proliferation

and smooth muscle cells, and fibroblasts. Indeed, the receptor appears critical in the mediation of many of the cellular effects of thrombin [9,21–24].

Absolutely critical and of physiologic importance is the mechanism or mechanisms for the control of an overabundance of thrombin generation after the reaction is "triggered." Two reaction systems are responsible for alternating the expression of the activity of the prothrombinase complex in generating thrombin. These safeguards limit "relentless massive thrombosis":

1. The antithrombin–(heparin) system that inhibits the proteases, factor Xa, and $\propto$ thrombin
2. The thrombomodulin–protein C system in which thrombin escaping from the site of the reaction binds to thrombomodulin on the vascular cell surface and activates protein C. Activated protein C recognizes factor Va as a substrate and cleaves the light and the heavy chains, resulting in an incompetent form that is incapable of producing the binding sites needed for the production of the prothrombinase complex and thereby blocking subsequent attachments to the membrane binding site [8].

Another important issue relative to thrombin is that it has at least four distinct binding sites that function relative to substrates, inhibitors, cofactors, and Na^+. The Na^+ binding site appears to help determine whether thrombin acts as a procoagulant by recognizing fibrinogen as a subtrate (in the presence of sodium ions) or acts as an anticoagulant by recognizing protein C as a substrate (in the absence of sodium ions) [20]. The other three sites are exosite I, exosite II, and the active site that recognizes a variety of different molecules and provides for the diverse functions of thrombin [25].

All of the physiologic effects of thrombin directly relate and completely depend on its catalytic activity. Substrate specificity, however, is determined by several accessory binding domains that exist in clusters.

Differences between indirect and direct thrombin inhibitors

The critical importance of thrombin in thrombogenesis and thrombotic states has made it the focus of clinical and pharmacologic attempts at intervention. Two types of inhibitors of thrombin generation have become part of the clinical armemtarium for the prevention and therapy of thrombotic events. Until recently, only indirect inhibitors were available; now, excellent direct thrombin inhibitors have entered clinical practice, and the spectrum of these exciting agents is expanding rapidly.

The most critical and important issue relative to attempts to alter thrombin-related thrombosis formation is the fact that during clot formation, thrombin (in its near-native state) exists bound to fibrin. This fibrin-bound thrombin remains enzymatically active and is critically protected from inactivation by classic circulating inhibitors (such as heparin). Thrombus thus serves as a reservoir of active thrombin that stimulates thrombus growth by locally activating platelets [26–28], converting proximal fibrinogen to fibrin [29], and further continued activation of factors V and X [26,28].

In addition, after an indirect inhibitor of thrombin such as heparin is stopped, there can be a reactivation of the coagulation system as the fibrin-bound thrombin reactivates factor X within the thrombus, triggering further thrombin generation.

It also merits emphasis that thrombin generation at sites of arterial injury appears to have a very broad and extensive coagulation cascade stimulus because it has been well documented that specific inhibitors of thrombin are far more effective than heparin at blocking injury-induced arterial thrombosis in baboons [30,31] and in humans [32,33].

Finally, the important and dramatic role of continued thrombin generation is aptly defined in the syndrome of heparin-induced thrombocytopenia (HIT), whereby despite stopping heparin, increased thrombin generation can be seen for as long as 21 days after its cessation, with resultant risk of new thrombosis [34].

Current status of clinically used indirect thrombin inhibitors

Currently, two drugs (heparin and warfarin) are part of the common armamentarium for the management of thrombotic circumstances. Recently, a new agent, fondaparinux, a synthetic heparin pentasaccharide that inhibits factor Xa binding to antithrombin, has entered the clinical arena (this topic is discussed extensively elsewhere in this issue). Fondaparinux has excellent bioavailability by the subcutaneous route, with a rapid onset of action and a prolonged half-life (14–20 hours). It is unfortunate that its function critically depends on endogenous antithrombin levels [35–37]. In addition to this critical requirement and its obvious indirect inhibition of thrombin, it requires normal renal function because there is no metabolism before its renal execution. It is difficult to monitor because the activated partial thromboplastin time (aPTT) cannot be used. Finally, no antidote exists should excessive bleeding occur [37].

Heparin is the classic indirect thrombin inhibitor. It is well acknowledged that it has only modest efficacy as an agent to limit thrombin generation and thrombogenesis. The limitations of efficacy and some of the underlying mechanisms for such limitations have been well delineated (Table 1) [26,38,39]. The variable response to a given initial dose of heparin poses a common confounding clinical problem. Because heparin has nonspecific binding to circulating proteins (especially acute-phase type) and to products released from activated platelets and endothelial cells, it will always present a problem in focused dose/response predictability. Physiologically, however, its major deficit, as noted earlier, is its mobility to inactivate fibrin-bound thrombin or inactivate factor Xa of the prothrombinase complex.

In addition to these significant limitations in efficacy, a variety of side effects complicate heparin therapy [35]. These side effects are related problems that are extensively delineated in the article found elsewhere in this issue.

The second common clinical therapeutic approach to affect thrombin generation has focused on activating or supplementing naturally occurring thrombin

Table 1
Limitations of heparin efficacy

Limitation	Mechanism
Variable anticoagulant response	Heparin binds to various acute-phase proteins and proteins released from activated platelets or endothelial cells
Dose-dependent clearance	Heparin binding sites on endothelium and macrophages must be saturated before heparin appears in the circulation
Reduced activity in the presence of platelets	Platelet factor 4 released from activated platelets neutralizes heparin
Unable to inactivate fibrin-bound thrombin	Heparin binds to fibrin and exosite 2 on thrombin, thereby heightening the thrombin-fibrin interaction and rendering exosite 2 on thrombin inaccessible to antithrombin-bound heparin
Unable to inactivate factor Xa within the prothrombinase complex	Factor Xa bound to the platelet surface is relatively resistant to inactivation by the heparin/antithrombin complex

Data from Weitz J, Hirsh J. New antithrombotic drugs. In: Colman RW, et al, editors. Hemostasis and thrombosis: basic principles and clinical practice, vol. 91. 4th edition. Philadelphia: Lippencott Williams & Wilkins; 2002. p. 1531.

inhibitors (ie, antithrombin or heparin cofactor II). The most classic anticoagulant used to reduce the generation of thrombin has been the coumarin (warfarin) derivatives. These function by reducing the concentrations of prothrombin and the other vitamin K–dependent clotting factors (factors VII, IX, and X and the physiologic anticoagulants protein C and S). Warfarin acts by blocking the regeneration of reduced vitamin K, which in essence, induces a functional vitamin K deficiency. Reduced vitamin K serves as a critical cofactor for the microsomal carboxylation of glutemic acid residues (residues 9–12), a step critical for the activation and function of these vitamin K–dependent coagulation factors.

Certainly, the major asset of this class of drugs is their oral availability; however, the complex mechanism of action and the extensive serious problems of absorption, drug–drug interactions, and biologic variation represent serious therapeutic limitations to their use [40–42]. Because warfarin does not have an effect on the activity of the fully carboxylated coagulation factors, the efficacy and function relate to the actual clearance of the individual circulating factor. In addition, there is no selectivity relative to suppression of any of these moieties.

Rationale and function of direct thrombin inhibitors

Approaches to inhibition of thrombin generation

Historically, the recognition of naturally occurring inhibitors (what was subsequently learned to be thrombin) of coagulation came from the study of blood-sucking animals. During evolutionary development, hematophagia developed in several species of animals, particularly leeches and bugs [43–46]. Such a form of nutrition for the blood-sucking parasites required their development of substances to counteract blood clotting in the host (ie, their dinner) [44,45,47,48]. Certainly, the best-studied hematophagus animal was the medicinal leech, *Hirudo medicinalis*. The isolation of the active moiety hirudin was performed in the late 1800s, and it was the first parenteral anticoagulant to be used. Indeed, in 1909, it was used to treat eclampsia [49]. In 1926, it was used in hemodialysis in patients [50]. Problems of availability and purification, however, led to its disuse when heparin became available.

Molecular cloning and recombinant technology that exploited point mutations and N-terminal modifications has led to the development and availability of recombinant forms of hirudin, one of which (lepiridin [Refludan]) has become an available clinically applicable direct thrombin inhibitor [51–54].

The serious deficits of heparin, particularly in the new understanding of the hemostatic and biologic aspects related to the management of arterial thrombotic disease [55–57], has led to an explosion of pharmaceutical interest in the development of agents capable of altering thrombin generation. This interest has included exploration of inhibitors from a variety of hemophagocytic leaches and bugs.

Box 3. The rationale for using thrombin as the therapeutic target in thrombogenesis

1. Thrombin has a central role in thrombogenesis.
2. It amplifies its own generation.
3. It activates factors V, VIII, and XI, providing positive feedback to enhance (further) thrombin formation.
4. It activates platelets: it is a potent agonist.
5. It converts fibrinogen to clottable fibrin.
6. It activates factor XIII cross-linking of fibrin to form a stable clot.
7. It enhances resistance of thrombin to fibrinolysis.

The "why" of direct thrombin inhibition

Clearly, thrombin has a premier and central role in thrombogenesis, thereby making it the ideal "target site" for therapeutic manipulation (Box 3). Because it amplifies its own generation and activates factors V, VIII, and XI, thereby providing positive feedback to enhance further thrombin formation, it is pivotal in any attempt to alter thrombogenesis. Its many other correlate functions (see Box 3) that include serving as a potent platelet agonist and an activator of the conversion of fibrinogen to clottable fibrin, and the subsequent activation of factor XIII for the cross-linking of the fibrin to form a stable clot serve to emphasize its central value as the appropriate target site for therapeutic interdiction.

The functional bases for the role of direct thrombin inhibitors are quite clear. As delineated in Box 4, these include the ability of such agents to inhibit fibrin-bound thrombin, which is pivotal to delimit thrombus growth, and their ability to bind thrombin at its active site, thereby inhibiting the downstream events discussed previously. Finally, they inhibit the activation of platelet factor 4, thereby further serving to delimit thrombogenesis. Because platelet factor 4 is a heparin-binding protein, this sequelae of thrombin activation further reflects on the

Box 4. The functional bases for role of direct thrombin inhibitors

1. Inhibit fibrin-bound thrombin, thereby delimiting thrombus growth
2. Bind thrombin at its active site, thereby inhibiting downstream events
3. Inhibit platelet factor 4 activation (an agonist that also inactivates heparin)
4. Provide more predictable anticoagulant responses because they are not bound to plasma proteins and have no drug–drug interactions

potential problems that exist with heparin and other indirect thrombin inhibitors. Two added valuable assets have been identified for practical therapeutics: (1) the agents identified do not bind to plasma proteins, which can result in altered, complex, and unpredictable physiologic delivery; and (2) to date, no known drug–drug interactions exist with these inhibitors.

Status and use of currently available direct thrombin inhibitors

Presently, four direct inhibitors of thrombin generation are available for clinical use:

1. Hirudin (Refludan): approved for the treatment of HIT
2. Bivalirudin (Hirulog): approved for use in angioplasty
3. Argatroban: approved for the treatment of HIT
4. Melagatran and its oral prodrug ximilagatran (Exanta): currently in the Food and Drug Administration approval process

Although these all are direct thrombin inhibitors, they differ somewhat in their specific binding site or sites on thrombin and have different modes of delivery, metabolism, and excretion. Some are reversible inhibitors, and these have better efficacy to safety ratios from the data in animal studies. These issues served as the basis for their approval for clinical use.

Recombinant hirudin: lepirudin (Refludan)

Recombinant hirudin, lepirudin (Refludan [nDNA]), entered the clinical sequelae of HIT, and its evident therapeutic efficacy in randomized prospective trials led to approval for use in the European community in 1997, by the US Food and Drug Administration in 1998, and in Canada in 1999 [51–54]. Lepirudin has been examined in prospective trials of HIT and HIT with associated thromboembolic complications (HIT-T) and shown to be effective and safe [50,51], thereby establishing its initial clinical role.

Hirudin functions by noncovalent binding to the active catalytic site of thrombin, thereby inducing a blockade of its variegated hemostatic and nonhemostatic functions [54]. Although recombinant hirudins have lack of sulfation on the tyrosine, they have proper conformation and disulfide bridging for correct inhibition of thrombin [51,54].

Lepirudin, as recombinant hirudin, is derived from yeast cells. It is a bivalent thrombin inhibitor (Fig. 3) that simultaneously binds to the active (catalytic site of thrombin) and to the accessory (fibrinogen) binding site. The NH_2–terminal region amino acids bind to the thrombin site cleft while the core of the hirudin molecule closes off the active site pocket. The carboxy-terminal tail interacts with the fibrinogen–anion binding site, thereby blocking thrombin-catalyzed cleavage. The inhibition constant for thrombin is in the picomolar range

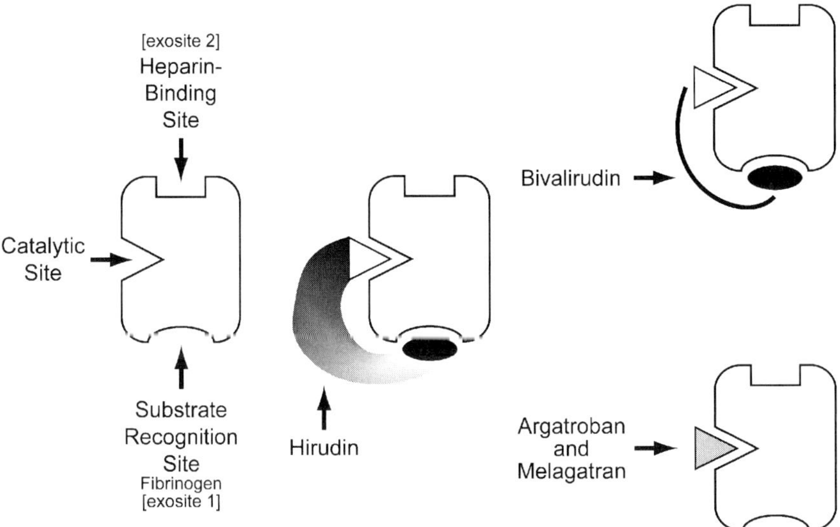

Fig. 3. The sites of action of the direct thrombin inhibitors. Hirudin (lepirudin) has fixed binding to the catalytic site and the fibrinogen recognition site (exosite 1). Lesser binding is seen with bivalirudin at exosite 1. None occurs with argatroban or melagatran.

(K_1 = 20 fmol), and lepirudin forms a noncovalent, irreversible 1:1 complex with thrombin, thereby inhibiting all of the biologic activities of thrombin.

Plasma pharmacokinetics of lepirudin have been extensively studied [53,54]. Intravenous administration results in a two-compartment model, with an initial $T_{1/2}$ of 8 to 12 minutes and a terminal elimination of 0.8 to 1.7 hours. In general, the half-life can be considered approximately 1 hour. Given subcutaneously, peak concentration is reached at 3 to 4 hours. Interestingly, it is not transported into the central nervous system or into breast milk [53,54]. The pharmacokinetic profile does not change with repeated doses; however, approximately 50% of patients treated for more than 5 days develop antibodies to lepirudin [58,59]. Still unclear is an unusual observation that in 2% of the patients who develop these antibodies, there appears to be an enhancement of function so that the dose must be reduced, often by 50% to 60%. One proposed mechanism for this paradox is that the antibodies form immunoglobulin complexes that then result in reduced renal clearance of lepirudin [58,59].

Lepirudin clearance is by the kidneys. In fact, a significant fraction (30%–60%) of the administered dose appears in the urine intact [44,46,51] and the clearance approximates the creatinine clearance [46]. An interesting observation is that during prolonged surgical procedures (ie, 3–5 hours or more), the half-life is prolonged, presumably due to decreased blood flow during anesthesia; the resultant consideration is that dose reduction (30%–50%) is needed during the procedure.

The commonly recommended dose schedules are shown in Box 5, including the approach in a patient with decreased renal function.

The issue of monitoring therapeutic levels is complex, and in truth, the best method is not yet firmly established. The thrombin time is not linear and is too sensitive for clinical use. By contrast, the prothrombin time is too insensitive. The aPTT can be used in the low–hirudin-level range at which the standard curve is linear. The serious problem comes at the higher (potentially toxic range) levels because these cannot be determined with the aPTT. The best monitoring method, the Ecarin Clotting Time, was developed in Europe [60–62]. It was developed as a rapid "point of service" assay, applicable to the operating room, emergency suite, or the ICU. It is based on the evidence that a snake venom enzyme (a metalloprotease of *Echis carinatus*) specifically cleaves prothrombin at the Arg 320/isoleucine bond, thereby generating meizothrombin. Interestingly, lepirudin inhibits meizothrombin with the same kinetics as the active site of thrombin, thus providing a direct clot monitoring method [60–62] applicable to rapid analysis such as in an operating room. It is unfortunate that Ecarin Clotting Time monitoring capability is not widely available and most clinicians have depended on the aPTT without adequate awareness of its problems in the higher therapeutic range.

Aside from the problems attendant to decreased renal function, the major adverse risk of lepirudin is that of bleeding. Because lepirudin is irreversibly bound to thrombin, no antidote for bleeding exists. Cerebral hemorrhage has been a noteworthy problem, and its incidence has slowed and even delayed enthusiastic encompassment of its therapeutic potential. In a multi-institutional trial of the clinical group GUSTO (Global Use of Strategies to Open Occluded Coronary Arteries) that randomized lepirudin or heparin in 2564 patients with an acute

Box 5. Lepirudin (Refludan) treatment schedules

Dosage

Obtain baseline aPTT*
Initial: Bolus-intravenous: 0.4 mg/kg/h (over 15–20 seconds)
Then: 0.15 mg/kg/h by continuous infusion

* Do not start if aPTT ratio of 2.5 or greater

Adjust dose downward in renal failure

Decrease by 50% for creatinine 1.6 to 2.0
Decrease by 70% to 75% for creatinine 2.1 to 3.0
Decrease by 80% to 85% for creatinine 3.0 to 6.0
(Therapeutic blood levels: 0.5–1.5 mg/mL)

coronary syndrome, the overall incidence of hemorrhagic stroke was 1.3% in the lepirudin-treated patients and 0.7% in the heparin-treated patients [63]. Subsequent studies using lower doses of lepirudin have shown a better safety margin; however, when bleeding complications occur, they have been difficult to manage. A well-recognized risk status has been identified: elevations of lepirudin levels to fivefold the therapeutic level are directly associated with life-threatening bleeding. Therapy for bleeding has included hemofiltration onto cellulose and trials of recombinant factor VIIa (r-VIIa).

Lepirudin, as the first direct thrombin that emerged from the pharmaceutical development activities, demonstrated efficacy in the management of HIT and quickly established a clinical presence [54,64]. Subsequent studies expanded the role of lepirudin in coronary artery disease with and in the absence of defined infarction [54,64] and in venous thromboembolism, particularly in surgical prophylaxis and therapy [65–67]. Clinical efficacy was quickly evident. Its irreversible thrombin binding and cost led to exploration of other agents that were direct thrombin inhibitors. Nevertheless, hirudin was the historical, biologic, and clinical agent that provided the fundamental platform for the developments in this arena.

Bivalirudin (Hirulog)

A variety of synthetic peptides based on the hirudin structure have been developed. A dodecapeptide, initially derived from the carboxyl-terminal region made up of residues 53 to 64, was developed that was an exosite-targeted peptide. By virtue of its binding to exosite 1 (the fibrinogen-binding site) it was, as expected, shown to inhibit fibrinogen binding and fibrin generation but failed to interrupt thrombin-mediated platelet-dependent thrombus propagation, which critically requires inhibition of the catalytic site. It was then combined by way of a four-glycene residue (Gly) 4 bridge with a tetrapeptide with active center specificity (D-Phe-Pro-Arg-Pro), resulting in a bifunctional antithrombin peptide, bivalirudin. This peptide is "bivalent" because there is binding to exosite 1 (ie, fibrinogen site) and the catalytic site, thereby decreasing platelet-dependent thrombosis.

Unlike hirudin, bivalirudin produces only transient inhibition of the active site of thrombin because after bonding to thrombin, the Arg-Pro band on the amino-terminal extension is cleared, thereby converting bivalirudin into a low-affinity inhibitor [67].

It has a variety of very desirable features compared with lepirudin. Most important is that the binding to thrombin is reversible, making it safer than lepirudin. In addition, it has a very short half-life. Only a small fraction of bivalirudin is excreted by the kidneys. Hepatic metabolism and proteolysis contribute to its clearance [64,68,69]. Currently, bivalirudin is approved as an alternate to heparin in patients undergoing angioplasty [64,68] and in the treatment of patients with unstable angina [69].

Argatroban

Argatroban was discovered and developed by Professor S. Okamoto in Tokyo in the 1970s. It is a small molecule (approximately 526 d) synthetically derived from L-arginine and is a complex mixture of R and S isomers. Early on, the Japanese recognized argatroban to be a unique direct inhibitor of thrombin generation with reversible features. In Japan in the 1980s, it was first used to treat peripheral arterial occlusive disease, and its approval in Japan now extends to that indication and to acute ischemic cerebral thrombosis, anticoagulation (largely hemodialysis) of antithrombin-deficient patients, and HIT-T [70,71]. It is now approved in the United States for use in HIT and HIT-T and for use in percutaneous coronary artery interventions.

It merits emphasis that this unique developmental activity by Okamoto and his team is an excellent example of the new vision in the approach to issues of thrombosis. They began this new arena by designing protease-inhibitors through the mimicry of substrates [47]. By imitating the amino acid sequence around the thrombin-scissile bond in fibrinogen, they examined and produced a protein that was able to enter by means of a covalent or noncovalent bond with the active site of thrombin.

Argatroban is uniquely of value by virtue of its direct "blockade" of the active catalytic site of thrombin (see Fig. 3); this blockade is competitive and reversible. Argatroban inhibits soluble and clot-bound thrombin. In essence, it inhibits thrombin-catalyzed or thrombin-induced reactions that include fibrin formation, activation of factors V, VIII, and XIII and protein C, and interferes with platelet aggregation [70,72,73]. It is highly selective for thrombin, with an excellent inhibitory constant (K_I of 0.04 μmol). It is fortunate that argatroban has no effect on other severe proteases and that heparin-induced antibodies do not react with it [71,73–75].

The pharmacokinetics and pharmacodynamics of argatroban have been extensively examined [70–76]. It has a rapid onset of action, with clear measured response within 30 minutes, and a linear relationship between the dose and plasma concentration is evident. Although bolus administration will shorten the steady-state plasma concentration, the typical therapy approach is by continuous infusion (at 2 mcg/kg/min), whereby steady-state levels are usually achieved by 1 to 3 hours following initiation of therapy. Plasma protein binding occurs at approximately 54% (with 20% to albumin and 34% to an α1-acid glycoprotein). Its major route of elimination is in the feces by way of biliary secretion. Its metabolism is in the liver by hydroxylation and aromatization by the cytochrome P450 microsomal system. It is of interest that four metabolites result from the metabolism and they appear to have independent, although weak, anticoagulant effects. As expected from this, liver impairment influences the kinetics of argatroban, with significant prolongation of the half-life, thereby requiring dose reduction. By contrast, age, gender, and renal dysfunction do not affect its kinetics [76].

Monitoring of therapy with argatroban can be done easily with the aPTT. It has a clear and reliable linear effect. Because argatroban causes an increase in the international normalized ratio (INR), special attention to this effect is needed for patients who are concurrently treated with warfarin [76,77]. Thus, a predictable effect of argatroban ($\leq$2 mcg/kg/min) on the INR during warfarin cotherapy has been documented [77]. An inverse prediction equation for such cotherapy has been developed that can be used to predict monotherapy [76,77]. Thus, for an INR of 4 during argatroban therapy at 2 μg/kg/min with warfarin cotherapy, the predicted warfarin monotherapy INR would equal 2.5 [77]. To avoid the abrupt risk of recurrent thrombosis on cessation of argatroban during cotherapy, it has been suggested that a repeat INR be done at approximately 4 hours when the effect of argatroban is negligible [77]. Sheth et al [77] also showed that at high infusion rates for argatroban (ie, 3 or 4 μg/kg/min), the estimates for warfarin monotherapy were more imprecise.

The recommended dosage schedule for argatroban therapy is displayed in Box 6.

The efficacy of argatroban for the treatment of patients with thrombosis was clearly established in a multicenter prospective open-label study of HIT and HIT-T [75,78]. The initial pivotal studies compared the results of argatroban therapy against historical controls because no other approved therapy for HIT/HIT-T was available in the United States. The primary efficacy endpoint was composite all-cause death, all-cause amputation, or new thrombosis, which was significantly reduced in the argatroban-treated HIT group (25.6% versus 38.8% in the controls [$P = 0.014$]) and HIT-T group (43.8% versus 56.5% in the controls [$P = 0.13$]) [78].

Other studies have examined argatroban's efficacy as an alternative to heparin in patients with a previous history of HIT or HIT-T who were to undergo percutaneous coronary intervention or related procedures. Clear evidence and safety of efficacy for such an approach has been shown [75,79]. In addition, argatroban has been evaluated as an adjunct to thrombolytic therapy in the treatment of myocardial infarction. In a double-blind study, argatroban was shown to be as beneficial as heparin as an adjunct to streptokinase or tissue

Box 6. Argatroban treatment schedule

Pretreatment

A baseline aPTT should be obtained.

Dose schedule

Initial dose: 2 μg/kg/min by continuous intravenous infusion

Monitor aPTT at 2 hours, then adjust dose to maintain aPTT at 1.5 to 3 times baseline (do not exceed a dose of 10 μg/kg/min or aPTT of 100 seconds)

plasminogen activator therapy, although bleeding as an adverse event was slightly more common [80].

The safety profile for therapy with argatroban is good. As expected, the major side effect is that of bleeding. The relatively short half-life and the reversible binding help provide a safety margin. It is unfortunate, however, that no specific antidote exists. The use of r-VIIa is believed to be a reasonable therapeutic approach. It is of interest that antibodies have not been identified with repeated infusions, and dosage requirements did not change with re-exposure [81].

Melagatran and ximelagatran (Exanta)

One of the most exciting and interesting direct thrombin inhibitor developments is that of melagatran and its oral prodrug ximelagatran (Exanta) [82]. The formulation and delineation of clinical efficacy of the prodrug form has been shown to have excellent oral bioavailability and has provided the construct for a truly new era of prophylaxis and therapy of thromboembolic disease.

Melagatran, the physiologically active direct thrombin inhibitor, fits directly into the catalytic site of thrombin (see Fig. 3). It is a low molecular weight (429.5 d) dipeptide analog designed to mimic fibrinopeptide A [83]. It is univalent, thereby binding only to the active site (see Fig. 3). As such, it is an active site–directed thrombin inhibitor that inhibits thrombin activity and thrombin generation. A significant asset is that the binding is reversible. It has very high potency for thrombin inhibition, with a low inhibition constant for thrombin (0.002 μmol/L). In addition, it inhibits thrombin-induced platelet aggregation at very low concentrations. Unlike many other direct thrombins, it has very low plasma protein binding (<15%). It has been shown to be highly effective at the inhibition of both arterial and venous thromboembolism in several animal models [81–83]. Also, it has shown virtually no inhibition of the fibrinolytic enzyme system.

The pharmacokinetics and pharmacodynamics have been extensively studied and characterized [84–86]. After intravenous or subcutaneous administration, a steady state is achieved in approximately 30 minutes, with a half-life of 2 to 4 hours. This short half-life obviates the need for prolonged discontinuation before a surgical procedure. Drug excretion is by way of the kidneys so that either drug monitoring or dose adjustment (downward) is appropriate for those patients with a serum creatinine above 1.8. By contrast, dose adjustment is not needed for obesity or altered liver function. As expected with a low molecular weight agent, it traverses the placenta.

It is now clear that a major advantage of this family of direct thrombin inhibitors is the lack of need for serial monitoring of the status of coagulation parameters. Nevertheless, the aPTT is an effective means of monitoring, with the goal of steady-state target of 1.5 to 2.5 times normal [87]. By contrast, the INR cannot be used to monitor activity. Careful studies have shown that the sensitivity of 17 separate available INR type assays to measure the anticoagulant effect of melagatran varied too widely to allow any of these to be identified as a valid monitoring method [87,88].

It is quite clear that melagatran has an excellent therapeutic window with easily achievable plasma concentrations that produce a beneficial antithrombin effect in the absence of a significant increase in the risk of bleeding. As clinical studies emerged, it became evident that the approach to the uncommon but worrisome event of bleeding was the cessation of the drug. With its very short half-life (2 to 4 hours), cessation generally is all that is needed. For urgent-emergent rescue, r-VIIa has been considered to be the reasonable approach.

The clinical efficacy of melagatran was clearly shown in a series of patients with phlebographically verified deep vein thrombosis who had significant regression of the size of the thrombus [84,88].

It was the prompt development of an oral formulation of a prodrug (H376/95) of melagatran, however, that has led to the introduction of an exciting new era in the prophylaxis and therapy of thromboembolic states. The drug ximelagatran has documented efficacy in the inhibition of thrombin generation [89,90] and platelet activation [90].

Excellent oral bioavailability of ximelagatran has been demonstrated in several species including humans [91–95]. Variations in the oral formulation (ie, whole tablets, crushed tablets, or dissolved tablets) have been explored, and the pharmacokinetics of melagatran were not significantly altered depending on the mode of delivery [95]. The time to mean peak concentration was 2.3 hours for the whole tablet and approximately 0.5 hours earlier for the crushed or dissolved tablet, presumably due to more rapid absorption. The mean half-life was 2.8 hours for each regardless of the mode of delivery [95]. Extensive studies of the pharmacokinetics and pharmacodynamics of ximelagatran confirmed rapid and complete metabolism into melagatran, with a mean value for melagatran clearance of approximately 20% predictable pharmacodynamics [16] and with rapid onset of anticoagulation [91–94].

The wide therapeutic index achieved with the consistent activation of melagatran by the oral administration of ximelagatran makes monitoring of the coagulation cascade unnecessary, except in patients with renal impairment [96,97]. With renal impairment, the resultant plasma concentrations of melagatran are higher than in patients with normal renal function, and a linear correlation has been shown between renal function and melagatran clearance [96]. Melagatran accounted for 13.9% of the oral dose of ximelagatran excreted in the urine of normal individuals compared with 8% in patients with renal impairment. In addition, melagatran was found to have a 32% higher relative bioavailability after oral ximelagatran in the renal failure patients, which in comparison to the normals, was double the elimination half-life [96]. Because the aPTT was nonlinear with severe renal dysfunction, the clinical recommendations for therapy in renal failure include increasing the interval between doses or decreasing the oral dose [96–98].

The serious and complex problems of drug–drug interactions that complicate and confound the oral indirect thrombin inhibitor warfarin (Coumadin) have led to extensive studies on potential variables that might affect ximelagatran. To date, no physiologic circumstances or drug–drug interactions have been identified. Thus, obesity does not affect the dose requirement of ximelagatran [99]. Extensive studies have shown that no age-dependent differences in the absorption or biotransformation of ximelagatran have been found [100]. Similarly, the pharmacokinetic and pharmacodynamic properties of ximelagatran are independent of ethnic origin [101], and the potential of drug–drug interactions has been examined for amcodorone, atorvastatin, or digoxin [102], acetylsalicylic acid [103], and alcohol [104], which have shown to have no effect. Even more interesting has been the data showing little or no effect on cytochrome P450-mediated drug–drug interactions [105]. Finally, an important clinical correlate—significant liver impairment—has now been shown to not affect the pharmacokinetics or pharmacodynamics of ximelagatran [106].

Appropriately, the clinical model used to define an appropriate dose and to institute evaluation of efficacy was that of prophylaxis against venous thromboembolism after joint replacement. The rationale focused on the significant risk of thromboembolic disease that exists in association with total knee or hip replacement surgery. Thus, venous thromboembolism is so commonly seen in patients with total knee replacement that in the absence of prophylaxis, almost 60% will have venographic evidence of deep vein thrombosis at the time of hospital discharge [107–109]. Prophylaxis with warfarin (Coumadin), although convenient because of its oral formulation, has been satisfactory but significantly less effective than with low molecular weight heparin [110]. The prevalence of proximal (ie, at or proximal to the popliteal site) deep vein thrombosis, however, is still approximately 30% despite low molecular weight heparin [110]. Because such sites of thrombosis are of particular importance as a cause for symptomatic venous thromboembolism or pulmonary emboli, it is evident that better means of prophylaxis are needed.

Multicenter studies [111] identified efficacy of ximelagatran at least equivalent to low molecular weight heparin for surgical venous thromboembolism prophylaxis. An excellent multi-institutional randomized, parallel dose-ranging study of 600 patients undergoing total knee replacement examined ximelagatran, twice daily, at a variety of fixed doses, and then compared these doses to exoxaparin given at a 30 mg dose twice daily [112]. The rate of overall venous thromboembolism, defined by unilateral ascending venography in the operated extremity, was 22.7% for enoxaparin and the rate of proximal deep vein thrombosis or pulmonary embolism was 3.1%. By comparison, the overall incidence at 8 mg twice daily of ximelagatran was 27%, 19.8% at 12 mg twice daily, 28.7% at 18 mg twice daily, and 15.8% at 24 mg twice daily. The rates for symptomatic deep vein thrombosis or pulmonary embolism were comparable to low molecular weight heparin and were 3.2% at 24 mg twice daily, a commonly accepted dose. There was no major bleeding. Thus, these investigators showed that fixed-dose unmonitored ximelagatran at 24 mg twice daily begun 12 to 24 hours after surgery was an effective oral prophylaxis against thromboembolism in the surgical setting [112].

Another multi-institutional randomized, double-blind, parallel phase III trial compared ximelagatran (at a fixed dose of 24 mg twice a day beginning on the morning after surgery) with warfarin (using a target INR of 2.5 [range 1.8–3.0] starting on the evening of the day of surgery). The study had 680 patients who had undergone total knee arthroplasty [113]. The incidence of venous thromboembolism was 19.2% in the ximelagatran group and 25.7% in the warfarin group. In the ximelagatran group, major bleeding was seen in 1.7% and minor bleeding was seen in 7.8%. For warfarin, the major bleeding rate was 0.9% and the minor bleeding rate was 6.4%. Appropriately, the investigators concluded that fixed-dose ximelagatran, at 24 mg twice a day beginning on the morning after surgery was effective and safe and did not require either coagulation monitoring or dose adjustment [113].

The evidence of equivalency of efficacy reported by Francis et al [114] led to an investigation of a higher dose of ximelagatran to see whether dose escalation would prove to be superior to warfarin. A multi-institutional randomized, double-blind trial that evaluated oral ximelagatran at two dose levels (24 or 36 mg twice daily) starting the morning after surgery was again compared with warfarin begun the evening of surgery. The study involved 1851 patients and was performed by a consortium named EXULT A (Exanta Used to Lessen Thrombosis A); thus, it was clearly associated with Astra-Zeneca, the pharmaceutical company associated with ximelagatran (Exanta).

The study was well done and provided important data [115]. Oral ximelagatran at a dose of 36 mg twice daily was clearly superior to warfarin. The primary endpoints were venous thromboembolism and death from all causes following total knee replacement. The ximelagatran group experienced primary endpoint issues in 20.3%; the warfarin group in 27.6% ($P = 0.003$). The bleeding incidence was essentially the same in each group (0.8% and 0.7%, respectively). Similarly, the composite secondary endpoints of proximal deep vein thrombosis, pulmonary embolism, and death were 2.7% in the oral ximelagatran group and 4.1% ($P = 0.17$) in the warfarin group [115].

The authors' Swedish colleagues performed an interesting correlative study that explored the issue of secondary prevention of venous thromboembolism following initial therapy [114]. The focused proposition of these investigators who make up the THRIVE (Thrombin Inhibitor in Venous Thromboembolism) group (also supported by Astra-Zeneca) is that the appropriate true duration of anticoagulant prophylaxis following venous thromboembolism is not known, but treatment for 6 months is a commonly used approach. They examined, in a double-blind, randomly assigned, multi-institutional study of 1233 patients, the role of secondary prevention with ximelagatran for 18 months beyond the initial 6 months of standard anticoagulant therapy for venous thromboembolism. The ximelagatran dose was 24 mg twice a day without monitoring of the coagulation status. Their baseline evaluation included bilateral ultrasonography of the legs and perfusion lung scans. The primary endpoint was symptomatic recurrent venous thromboembolism. There were 612 patients in the ximelagatran group and 12 had confirmed recurrence; there were 611 patients in the placebo group and 71 had confirmed recurrence (hazard ratio 0.16; $P = 0.001$). Death from all causes occurred in 6 patients in the ximelagatran group and in 7 patients in the placebo group. Bleeding occurred in 134 patients in the ximelagatran group and in 111 patients in the placebo group (hazard ratio 1.19; $P = 0.17$) [114].

This study, as has been true of several others using ximelagatran on a prolonged basis, identified increases in alanine transaminase levels (to more than three times the upper limit of normal) in 6.4% of the melagatran group and in only 1.2% in the placebo-treated patients ($P < 0.001$). Of interest is that these elevated enzyme levels generally were seen in the first 4 months of therapy and decreased with a similar time course whether the use of the drug was continued (median time to normalization 84 days) or discontinued (median time to normalization 129 days). Similar enzyme changes [34] have been seen in other studies of ximelagatran that had longer duration of therapy [116]. Nevertheless, this study demonstrated the feasibility, safety, and wisdom of secondary prevention of venous thromboembolism with ximelagatran.

Another pivotal study with ximelagatran has been a consortium effort of the SPORTIF (Stroke Prevention Using an Oral Thrombin Inhibitor in Atrial Fibrillation) team, again a group essentially developed and supported by AstraZeneca. Regardless of the source of support, the group has provided excellent multi-institutional randomized evidence that fixed-dose oral ximelagatran was at least as effective as dose-adjusted warfarin in stroke prevention in high-risk patients with nonvalvular atrial fibrillation [116,117].

This group studied 3410 patients with atrial fibrillation with one or more risk factors for stroke who were randomized to open label warfarin (dose-adjusted with INR 2.0–3.0) or to oral ximelagatran at an unmonitored fixed dose of 36 mg twice daily [117]. At 4941 patient years of therapy, 96 patients had primary events defined as stroke or systemic embolism; of these, 56 were in the warfarin group and 40 were in the ximelagatran group. The primary event rate by intention to treat was 2.3% per year for warfarin and 1.6% per year for ximelagatran, providing an absolute risk reduction of 0.7% and a relative risk reduction of 2.9% [117]. These investigators provided excellent evidence that in patients who are at high risk for stroke or systemic embolization fixed dose, unmonitored ximelagatran is at least as effective as adjusted-dose warfarin for prevention of these events [116,117].

Adverse events are always an issue in the anticoagulation prevention trials. Hemorrhagic stroke occurred in 9 patients (0.4% per year) in the warfarin group and in 4 patients in the ximelagatran group (0.2% per year). Major hemorrhage (other than stroke) occurred in 41 patients in the warfarin group (1.8% per year) and in 29 ximelagatran-treated patients (1.3% per year). It is noteworthy that 44% of the patients who bled on warfarin had INRs greater than 3.0 [117].

An issue of adverse effects related to ximelagatran induced elevations of the hepatic-related enzyme alanine transaminase. As seen in other studies, these elevations (commonly defined as greater than threefold normal) were seen in 6.3% of patients and usually occurred during the second to sixth month of treatment. As seen in all of the other trials, the values returned to normal either spontaneously or after cessation of therapy [117]. The mechanism of the alanine transaminase elevation has been examined carefully in each of the clinical trials and, to date, there is no clear explanation [115–117]. In this light, it appears prudent to monitor liver function for the first 6 to 12 months of therapy. This issue is interesting in light of the lack of need to monitor the coagulation status.

It is clear from these well-coordinated, large randomized trials that ximelagatran is an excellent oral agent for the prevention of thromboembolism in a wide variety of clinical circumstances in which warfarin or low molecular weight heparin classically have been used. Ximelagatran has a safety profile at least equivalent to warfarin and related agents, it does not require the frequent monitoring for dose adjustment (an ever-present problem with warfarin), and the clinicians' fear of drug–drug interactions does not exist.

One serious and unresolved issue with ximelagatran and all other direct thrombin inhibitors is the management of excessive bleeding during therapy. It is fortunate that the half-life of the prodrug and its active metabolite melagatran (which is the true thrombin inhibitor) is short so that cessation of therapy has been the accepted approach. Many clinicians believe that r-VIIa would be the agent of choice should serious bleeding occur. A recent trial of r-VIIa has been conducted in healthy volunteers given melagatran, with subsequent serial evaluation of the inhibition of thrombin generation and platelet activation [118]. Volunteers were given a 5-hour infusion to achieve a steady-state melagatran plasma concentration (0.5 μmol/L). They were then given a single bolus of r-VIIa (90 μg/kg) or placebo. The melagatran appropriately produced decreased evidence of thrombin generation and platelet activation, but the attempt at reversal with r-VIIa failed to completely reverse the effects of a high constant concentration of melagatran [118]. Albeit disappointing, the parameters of the study examined the potential repair by r-VIIa under the most severe circumstances.

Summary

It is clear that major clinical advantages are achieved when direct thrombin inhibitors are used in venous thromboembolism. These advantages include the inhibition of fibrin-bound thrombin and the inhibition of activation of platelet factor 4. These agents provide more reliable anticoagulant response patterns because they are not significantly bound to plasma proteins and few, if any, drug–drug interactions are seen.

The studies to date confirm that not all direct thrombin inhibitors are the same. The new reversible, short-acting catalytic site–specific drugs provide an excellent safety profile and high degree of efficacy for the prophylaxis and treatment of venous thromboembolism and pulmonary embolic states. The availability of the oral prodrug ximelagatran allows reproducible, effective, and safe direct thrombin inhibition without the requirement for coagulation laboratory monitoring; it appears destined to be the oral anticoagulant of the future.

References

[1] Howell WH. Heparin as an anticoagulant. Am J Physiol 1923;63:434–48.
[2] Murray DWG. Heparin in thrombosis and embolism. Br J Surg 1939;27:567.
[3] Campbell HA, Link KP. Studies on the hemorrhagic sweet clover disease. IV. The isolation and crystallization of the hemorrhagic agent. J Biol Chem 1941;138:21.
[4] Bingham JB, Meyer OO, Pohle FJ. A preparation from spoiled sweet clover (3,3′-methylene-bis (4-hycroxycoumarin). 1. Its effect on the prothrombin and coagulation time of the blood of dogs and humans. Am J Med Sci 1941;202:563.
[5] Furie B. Oral anticoagulant therapy. In: Hoffman R, editor. Hematology: basic principles and practice. 2nd edition. New York: Churchill Livingstone; 1995. p. 1795–801.
[6] Perkins WD. DVT prophylaxis for the nonsurgical patient. University of Texas Southwestern Medical School. Internal Medicine Grand Rounds. April 18, 2002.
[7] Jandl JH. Blood: textbook of hematology. Boston/Toronto: Little, Brown & Co.; 1987.
[8] Jenny NS, Mann KG. Thrombin. In: Colman RW, Hersh J, Marder VJ, Clowes AW, George JN, editors. Hemostasis and thrombosis: basic principles and clinical practice. 4th edition. Philadelphia: Lippencott Williams & Wilkins; 2001. p. 172–89.
[9] Greenberg CS, Orthner CL. Blood coagulation and fibrinolysis. In: Lee GR, Foerster J, Lukens J, Paraskevas F, Greer J, Rogers G, editors. Wintrobe's clinical hematology. 10th edition. Philadelphia: Lippencott Williams & Wilkins; 1999. p. 684–764.
[10] Furie B, Furie BC. Molecular basis of blood coagulation. In: Hoffman R, editor. Hematology: basic principles and practice. 2nd edition. New York: Churchill Livingstone; 1995. p. 1566–87.
[11] Mann KG, Jenny RJ, Krishnaswamy S. Cofactor proteins in the assembly and expression of blood clotting enzyme complexes. Annu Rev Biochem 1988;57:915–56.
[12] Krishnaswamy S, Mann KG, Nesheim ME. The prothrombinase-catalyzed activation of prothrombin proceeds through the intermediate meizothrombin in an ordered, sequential reaction. J Biol Chem 1986;261:8977–84.
[13] Doyle MF, Mann KG. Multiple forms of thrombin. IV. Relative activities of meizothrombins. J Biol Chem 1992;265:10693–701.
[14] Krishnaswamy S, Field KA, Edgington TS, et al. Role of membrane surface in the activation of human coagulation factor X. J Biol Chem 1992;267:26110–20.
[15] Mann KG. Normal hemostasis. In: Kelly WN, editor. Textbook of internal medicine. Philadelphia: Lippencott; 1992. p. 1240–5.
[16] Lawson JH, Krishnaswamy S, Butenas S, et al. Extrensic pathway proteolytic activity methods. Enzymology 1993;222:177–95.
[17] Rand MD, Lock JB, van Veer C, et al. Blood clotting in minimally altered whole blood. Blood 1996;88:3432–45.
[18] Cawthern KM, Veer C, Lock JB, et al. Blood coagulation in hemophilia A and hemophilia C. Blood 1998;91:4581–92.
[19] Brummel KE, Butenas S, Mann KG. An integrated study of fibrinogen during blood coagulation. J Biol Chem 1999;274:22862–70.
[20] Brummel K, Paradis SG, Butenas S, Mann KG. Thrombin functions during tissue factor-induced blood coagulation. Blood 2002;100:148–52.
[21] Bahou W, Coller B, Potter C, et al. The thrombin receptor extracellular domain contains sites crucial for peptide ligand-induced activation. J Clin Invest 1993;91:1405.
[22] Schmidt VA, Vitale E, Bahou WF. Genomic cloning and characterization of the human thrombin receptor gene. J Biol Chem 1996;271:9307.
[23] Van Obberghen-Schilling E, Pouyssegur J. Signaling pathways of the thrombin receptor. Thromb Haemost 1993;70:163–7.
[24] Stubbs MT, Bode W. A player of many parts: the spotlight on thrombin's structure. Thromb Res 1993;69:1–58.
[25] Tulinsky A. Molecular interactions of thrombin. Semin Thromb Hemost 1996;22:117–24.
[26] Weitz J, Hirsh J. New antithrombotic drugs. In: Colman RW, et al, editors. Hemostasis and

thrombosis: basic principles and clinical practice. 4th edition. Philadelphia: Lippencott Williams & Wilkins; 2002. p. 1529–68.

[27] Kumar R, Beguin S, Hemker HC. The effect of fibrin clots and clot-bound thrombin on the development of platelet procoagulant activity. Thromb Haemost 1995;74:962–8.

[28] Kumar R, Beguin S, Hemker HC. The influence of fibrinogen and fibrin on thrombin generation-evidence for feedback activation of the clotting system by clot bound thrombin. Thromb Haemost 1994;72:713–21.

[29] Broze Jr GJ. Tissue factor pathway inhibitor and the current concept of blood coagulation. Blood Coagul Fibrinolysis 1995;1:7–13.

[30] Hanson SR, Harker LA. Interruption of acute platelet-dependent thrombosis by the synthetic antithrombin D-phenylalanyl-L-prolyl-L-arginyl chloromethyl ketone. Proc Natl Acad Sci USA 1988;85:3184–8.

[31] Krupski WC, Bass A, Kelly AD, et al. Heparin resistant thrombus formation by endovascular stints in baboons: interruption by a synthetic antithrombin. Circulation 1990;82:570–2.

[32] Bittl JA, Strony J, Brinker JA, et al. Treatment with bivaliruden (Hirulog) as compared with heparin during coronary angioplasty for unstable or postinfarction angina. N Engl J Med 1995; 333:764–9.

[33] Bittl JA, Feit A. A randomized comparison of bivalirudin and heparin in patients undergoing coronary angioplasty for postinfarction angina. Am J Cardiol 1998;82:43–9.

[34] Warkentin TE. Limitations of conventional treatment options for heparin-induced thrombocytopenia. Semin Hematol 1998;35:17.

[35] Walenga JM, Jeske WP, Samama MM. Fondaparinux: a synthetic heparin pentasaccharide as a new antithrombotic agent. Expert Opin Investig Drugs 2002;11:397–407.

[36] Eriksson BI, Bauer KA, Lassen MR, et al. Fondaparinux compared with enoxaparin for the prevention of venous thromboembolism after hip-fracture surgery. N Engl J Med 2001;345: 1298–304.

[37] Walenga Jr JM, Hoppensteadt DA, Mayuga M, et al. Functionality of pentasaccharide depends upon endogenous antithrombin levels. Blood 2000;96:817a.

[38] Bick RL, Frenkel EP. Clinical aspects of heparin-induced thrombocytopenia and thrombosis and other side effects of heparin therapy. Clin Appl Thromb Hemost 1999;5(Suppl):S7–15.

[39] Frenkel EP. Thrombycytopenia and thrombocytosis. In: Bick RL, editor. Disorders of thrombosis and hemostasis: clinical and laboratory produce. 3rd edition. Philadelphia: Lippencott Williams & Wilkins; 2002. p. 91–115.

[40] Van Aken H, Bode C, Darius H, et al. Anticoagulation: the present and future. Clin Appl Thromb Hemost 2001;7:195.

[41] Hirsh J. Oral anticoagulant drugs. N Engl J Med 1991;324:1865.

[42] Beest FJAP, Meegen E, Rosendaal FR, et al. Characteristics of anticoagulant therapy and comorbidity related to overcoagulation. Thromb Haemost 2001;86:569.

[43] Markwardt F. Development of direct thrombin inhibitors in comparison with glycosaminoglycans. Semin Thromb Hemost 2001;27:523–30.

[44] Markwardt F. Coagulation inhibitors of blood sucking animals—a new line of developing antithrombotic drugs. Pharmazie 1993;49:313–6.

[45] Markwardt F. The development of hirudin as an antithrombotic drug. Thromb Res 1994;74: 1–23.

[46] Wallis RB. Hirudins: from leeches to man. Semin Thromb Hemost 1996;22:185–96.

[47] Markwardt F. Antithrombotimc agents from hematophagous animals. Clin Appl Thromb Hemost 1996;2:75–82.

[48] Dodt J, Otte M, Strube KH, et al. Thrombin inhibitors of bloodsucking animals. Semin Thromb Hemost 1996;22:203.

[49] Engelmann F, Stode C. Uber die bedeutung des blulegelextraktes fur die therapy der eklampsie. Munchner Medizinische Wochenschrift 1909;43:2203.

[50] Hass G. Uber versuche der blutauswaschung am lebenden met hilfe der dialyse. Arch Pharmacol 1926;16:158.

[51] Greinacher A, Volpel H, Janssens U, et al. Lepirudin (recombinant hirudin) for parenteral anticoagulation in patients with heparin-induced thrombocytopenia. Circulation 1999;100: 587–93.
[52] Greinacher A, Eichler P, Lubenow N, et al. Heparin-induced thrombocytopenia with thromboembolic complications: meta-analysis of 2 prospective trials to assess the value of parenteral treatment with lepirudin and its therapeutic a PTT range. Blood 2000;96:846–51.
[53] Greinacher A. Recombinant hirudin for the treatment of heparin-induced thrombocytopenia. In: Warkentin TE, Greinacher A, editors. Heparin induced thrombocytopenia. 2nd edition. New York: Marcel Dekker; 2001. p. 349–79.
[54] Greinacher A, Lubenow N. Recombinant hirudin in clinical practice. Circulation 2001; 103:1479.
[55] Reiner AP, Siscovick DS, Rosendaal FR. Hemostatic risk factors and arterial thrombotic disease. Thromb Haemost 2001;85:584–95.
[56] Hall SW, Gibbs CS, Leung LLK. Identification of critical residues on thrombin mediating its interaction with fibrin. Thromb Haemost 2001;86:1466–75.
[57] Ananyeva NM, Kouiavskaia DV, Shima M, et al. Intrinsic pathway of blood coagulation contributes to thrombogenicity. Blood 2002;99:4475–85.
[58] Song X, Huhle G, Wang L, et al. Generation of anti-hirudin antibodies in heparin-induced thrombocytopenia patients treated with r-hirudin. Circulation 1999;100:1528–32.
[59] Eichler P, Friesen HJ, Lubenow N. Antihirudin antibodies in patients with heparin-induced thrombocytopenia treated with lepirudin: incidence, effects on a PTT, and clinical relevance. Blood 2000;96:2373–8.
[60] Potzsch B, Hund S, Madlener K, et al. Monitoring of r-hirudin: anticoagulatioin during cardiopulmonary bypass: assessment of the whole blood ecarin clotting time. Thromb Haemost 1997;77:920.
[61] Potzsch B, Hund S, Madlener K, et al. Monitoring of recombinant hirudin: assessment of a plasma-based ecarin clotting time. Thromb Res 1997;86:373.
[62] Nowak G. Clinical monitoring of hirudin and direct thrombin inhibitors. Semin Thromb Hemost 2001;27:537.
[63] GUSTO IIa Investigators. Randomized trial of intravenous heparin versus recombinant hirudin for acute coronary syndromes. Circulation 1994;90:1631–7.
[64] Hirsh J. New anticoagulants. Am Heart J 2001;142:253.
[65] Prisco D, Falcian M, Antonucci E, et al. Hirudins for prophylaxis and treatment of venous thromboembolism. Semin Thromb Hemost 2001;27:543.
[66] Eriksson BI, Wille-Jorgensen P, Kalebo P, et al. Comparison of recombinant hirudin with a low-molecular-weight heparin to prevent thromboembolic complications after hip replacement. N Engl J Med 1997;337:1329–35.
[67] Wille-Jorgensen P. The potential role of new therapies in deep-vein thrombosis prophylaxis. Semin Hematol 2001;38(Suppl 5):20.
[68] Fox I, Dawson A, Loynds P. Anticoagulant activity of hirulog, a direct thrombin inhibitor, in humans. Thromb Haemost 1993;69:157.
[69] Diuquid D. Choosing a parenteral anticoagulant agent. N Engl J Med 2001;345:1340.
[70] Matsuo T, Koide M, Kario K. Development of argatraban, a direct thrombin inhibitor, and its clinical application. Semin Thromb Hemost 1997;23:517–22.
[71] Schwartz RP, Becker JP, Brooks RL, Hurstin MJ, Joffrion JL, Krappenberger GD. The preclinical and clinical pharmacology of Novaston (argatroban): a small-molecule, direct thrombin inhibitor. Clin Appl Thromb Hemost 1997;3:1–15.
[72] Jeske R, et al. Pharmacology of argatroban. Expert Opin Investig Drugs 1999;8:625.
[73] Hurstin ML, Alford KL, Becker JP, et al. Novastan™ (brand of Argatroban): a small-molecule, direct thrombin inhibitor. Semin Thromb Hemost 1997;23:503–16.
[74] Fareed J, Callas D, Hoppensteadt DA, Lewis BE, Bick RL, Waleng JM. Antithrombin agents as anticoagulants and antithrombotics: implications in drug development. Semin Hematol 1999; 36:42–56.

[75] Kondo LM, Wittkowsky AK, Wiggens BS. Argatroban for the prevention and treatment of thromboembolism in heparin-induced thrombocytopenia. Ann Pharmacother 2001;35:440–51.
[76] Swan SK, Hurstin MJ. The pharmacokinetics and pharmacodynamics of argatroban: effects of age, gendor or hepatic or renal dysfunction. Pharmacotherapy 2000;20:318–29.
[77] Sheth SB, DiCicco RA, Hurstin MJ, Montague T, Jorkasky DK. Interpreting the international normalized ratio (INR) in individuals receiving argatroban and warfarin. Thromb Haemost 2001;85:435–40.
[78] Lewis BE, Wallis DE, Berkowitz S, et al. Argatroban anticoagulant therapy in patients with heparin-induced thrombocytopenia. Circulation 2001;103:1838–43.
[79] Lewis BE, Matthai W, Grassman ED, Leya FS, Fareed J, Walenga JM. Results of a phase 2/3 trial of argatroban anticoagulation during PTCA of patients with heparin-induced thrombocytopenia. Circulation 1997;96:210–7.
[80] Jang IK, Brown DM, Giugliano RP. A multicenter, randomized study of argatroban versus heparin as adjunct to tissue plasminogen activator (TPA) in acute myocardial infarction with Novastan and tPA (MINT) study. J Am Coll Cardiol 1999;33:1879–85.
[81] Lewis BE, Wallis DE, Zehnder JL. Argatroban re-exposure in patients with heparin-induced thrombocytopenia (HIT). Blood 2000;96:52A.
[82] Van Aken H, Bode C, Darius H, et al. Anticoagulants: the present and future. Clin Appl Thromb Hemost 2001;7:195–203.
[83] Maraganore JM, Bourdon P, Jablonski J, et al. Design and characterization of hirulogs: a novel class of bivalent peptide inhibitors of thrombin. Biochemistry 1990;29:7095.
[84] Nutescu EA, Wittkowsky AK. Direct thrombin inhibitors for anticoagulation. Ann Pharmacother 2004;38:99–109.
[85] Witting JI, Bourdon P, Brezniak DV, et al. Thrombin-specific inhibition by and slow cleavage of hirulog-1. Biochem J 1992;283:737.
[86] Gustafsson D, Elg M. The pharmacodynamics and pharmacokinetics of the oral direct thrombin inhibitor ximelagatran and its active metabolite melagatran: a mini-review. Thromb Res 2003;109(Suppl 1):S9–19.
[87] Fenyvesi T, Joerg I, Glese C, Traeger I, Harenberg J. APTT-reagent and phenprocoumom effects on analysing direct thrombin inhibitor effects with APTT in molar comparison. Pathophysiol Haemost Thromb 2002;32(Suppl 2):85.
[88] Mattson C, Menschik-Lundion A. Prothrombin time assays are unsuitable for monitoring the effects of melagatran, the active form of the oral, direct thrombin inhibitor H376/95. Blood 2000;96(Part 2):98b.
[89] Fox I, Dawson A, Loynds P. Anticoagulant activity of hirulog, a direct thrombin inhibitor, in humans. Thromb Haemost 1993;69:157.
[90] Sarich TC, Eriksson UG, Mattson C, Wolzt M, Frison L, Fager G, et al. Inhibition of thrombin generation by the oral direct thrombin inhibitor ximelagatran in shed blood from healthy male subjects. Thromb Haemost 2002;87:300–5.
[91] Sarich TC, Wolzt M, Eriksson UG, Mattson C, Schmidt A, Elg S, et al. Effects of ximelagatran, an oral direct thrombin-inhibitor, r-hirudin and exoxaparin on thrombin generation and platelet activation in healthy male subjects. J Am Coll Cardiol 2003;41:557–64.
[92] Eriksson UG, Bredberg U, Hoffmann K-J, et al. Absorption, distribution, metabolism and excretion of ximelagatran, an oral direct thrombin inhibitor, in rats, dogs and humans. Drug Metab Dispos 2003;31:294–305.
[93] Ericksson UG, Bredberg U, Gislen K, et al. Pharmacokinetics and pharmacodynamics of ximelagatran, a novel oral direct thrombin inhibitor, in young healthy male subjects. Eur J Clin Pharmacol 2003;59:35–43.
[94] Gustafsson D, Antonsain T, Bylund R, et al. Effects of melagatran, a new low molecular weight inhibitor, in thrombin and fibrinolytic enzymes. Thromb Haemost 1998;79:110–8.
[95] Gustaffson D, Nystrom J, Carlsson S, et al. The direct thrombin inhibitor melagatran and its oral pro-drug H376/95: intestinal absorption, properties, biochemical and pharmacodynamics effects. Thromb Res 2001;101:171–81.

[96] Schutzer K-M, Wall U, Lonnerstedt C, Ohlsson L, Teng R, Sarich T, et al. Bioequivalence of ximelagatran, an oral direct thrombin inhibitor, as whole or crushed tablets or dissolved formulation. Curr Med Res Opin 2004;20:325–31.
[97] Johansson S, Eriksson UG, Samuelsson O, Attmon P, Mulec H, Frison L, et al. The influence of severe renal impairment on the pharmacokinetics of oral ximelagatran and subcutaneous melagatran. Clin Pharm Therapeutics 2002;71:96.
[98] Erikkson UG, Johansson S, Attmon PO, Mulec H, Frison L, Fager G, et al. Influence of severe renal impairment on the pharmacokinetics and pharmacodynamics of oral ximelagatran and subcutaneous melagatran. Clin Pharmacokinet 2003;42:743–53.
[99] Sarich TC, Teng R, Peters GR, Wollbratt M, Homolka R, Svensson M, et al. No influence of obesity in the pharmacokinetics and pharmacodynamics of melagatran, the active form of the oral direct thrombin inhibitor ximelagatran. Clin Pharmacokinet 2003;42:485–92.
[100] Johansson LC, Frison L, Logren U, Fager G, Gustafsson D, Eriksson UG. Influence of age on the pharmacokinetics and pharmacodynamics of ximelagatran, an oral direct thrombin inhibitor. Clin Pharmacokinet 2003;42:381–92.
[101] Johansson LC, Frison L, Nakanishi T, Fager G, Eriksson UG. No influence of ethnic origin on the PK and PD properties of ximelagatran in young healthy males. Clin Pharm Therapeutics 2003;73(Suppl S):22.
[102] Dorani H, Schutzer K, Wollbratt M, Sarich TC, Eriksson UG, Teng R, et al. No clinically significant interactions between the oral direct thrombin inhibitor ximelagatran and amiodarone, atorvastin, or digoxin. Clin Pharm Therapeutics 2004;75:78.
[103] Fager G, Cullberg M, Eriksson-Lepkowska M, Frison L, Eriksson UG. Pharmacokinetics and pharmacodynamics of melagatran, the active form of the oral direct thrombin inhibitor ximelagatran, are not influenced by acetylsalicylic acid. Europ J Clin Pharmac 2003;59:283–9.
[104] Johansson S, Schutzer K, Kessler M-E, Sarich T, Eriksson UG. No influence of alcohol intake on the pharmacokinetics or pharmacodynamics of the oral direct thrombin inhibitor, ximelagatran, in healthy volunteers. J Thromb Haemost 2003;1(Suppl 1):1991.
[105] Bredberg E, Andersson TB, Frison L, Thuressen A, Johansson S, Eriksson-Lepkowska M, et al. Ximelagatran, an oral direct thrombin inhibitor has a low potential for cytochrome P450-mediated drug-drug interactions. Clin Pharmacokinet 2003;42:765–77.
[106] Wahlander K, Eriksson-Lepkowska M, Frison L, Fager G, Eriksson UG. No influence of mild-to-moderate hepatic impairment in the pharmacokinetics and pharmacodynamics of ximelagatran an oral direct thrombin inhibitor. Clin Pharmacokinet 2003;42:755–65.
[107] Heit JA, Colwell CW, Francis CW, Ginsberg JS, Berkowitz SD, Whipple J, et al. Comparison of the oral direct thrombin inhibitor ximelagatran with enoxaparin as prophylaxis against venous thromboembolism after total knee replacement. Arch Intern Med 2001;161:2215–21.
[108] Clagett GP, Anderson Jr FA, Geerts W, Heit JA, Knudson M, Lieberman JR. Prevention of venous thromboembolism. Chest 1998;114:531S–60S.
[109] Geets WH, Heit JA, Clagett GP, et al. Prevention of venous thromboembolism. Chest 2001; 119(Suppl):132S–75S.
[110] Heit JA, Berkowitz SD, Bono R, et al. Efficacy and safety of low molecular weight heparin (ardeparin sodium) compared to warfarin for prevention of venous thromboembolism following total knee replacement: a double-blind, dose-ranging study. Thromb Haemost 1997;77:32–8.
[111] Eriksson BI, Lindbratt S, Kalebo P, et al. METHRO II: dose-response study of the novel oral, direct thrombin inhibitor, H376/95, and its subcutaneous formulation melagatran, compared to dalteparin as thromboembolic prophylaxis after total hip or knee replacement. Haemostases 2000;30(Suppl):20–1.
[112] Heit JA, Colwell CW, Francis CW, Ginsberg JS, Berkowitz SD, Whipple J, et al. Comparison of the oral direct thrombin inhibitor ximelagatran with enoxaparin as prophylaxis against venous thromboembolism after total knee replacement. Arch Intern Med 2001;161:2215–21.
[113] Francis CW, Davidson BL, Berkowitz SD, Lotke PA, Ginsberg JS, Lieberman JR, et al. Ximelagatran versus warfarin for the prevention of venous thromboembolism after total knee arthroplasty. Ann Intern Med 2002;137:648–55.

[114] Schulman S, Wahlander K, Lundstrom T, Clason SB, Eriksson H. Secondary prevention of venous thromboembolism with the oral direct thrombin inhibitor ximelagatran. N Engl J Med 2003;349:1713–21.

[115] Francis CW, Berkowitz SD, Comp PC, Lieberman JR, Ginsberg JS, Paiemont G, et al. Comparison of ximelagatran with warfarin for the prevention of venous thromboembolism after total knee replacement. N Engl J Med 2003;349:1703–12.

[116] Peterson P, Grind M, Adler J. Ximelagatran versus warfarin for stroke prevention in patients with non-valvular atrial fibrillation. SPORTIF II: a dose-guiding, tolerability and safety study. J Am Coll Cardiol 2003;41:1445–51.

[117] Executive Steering Committee of SPORTIF III Investigators. Stroke prevention with the oral direct thrombin inhibitor ximelagatran compared with warfarin in patients with non-valvular atrial fibrillation (SPORTIF III): a randomized controlled trial. Lancet 2003;362:1691–8.

[118] Wolzt M, Levi M, Sarich TC, Bostrom SL, Eriksson UG, Eriksson-Lepkowska M, et al. Effect of recombinant factor VIIa in melagatran-induced inhibition of thrombin generation and platelet activation in healthy volunteers. Thromb Haemost 2004;91:1090–6.

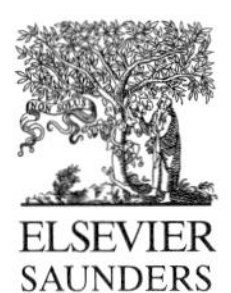
ELSEVIER
SAUNDERS

Hematol Oncol Clin N Am
19 (2005) 147–181

HEMATOLOGY/
ONCOLOGY
CLINICS OF
NORTH AMERICA

Thrombolytic Therapy: Current Clinical Practice

William F. Baker, Jr, MD, FACP[a,b,c,*]

[a]*Center for Health Sciences, University of California–Los Angeles, Los Angeles, CA, USA*
[b]*Thrombosis, Hemostasis, and Special Hematology Clinic, Kern Medical Center, 1830 Flower Street, Bakersfield, CA 93305, USA*
[c]*California Clinical Thrombosis Center, 9330 Stockdale Highway #300, Bakersfield, CA 93311, USA*

Thrombolytic therapy is an essential tool in the array of therapies designed to reopen arteries and veins occluded with thrombus. As the use of thrombolytic agents has entered mainstream practice, their application has expanded to include a wide variety of indications and settings. Thrombolysis is practiced in hospitals and emergency departments of all sizes and has been expanded to selected outpatient settings. It has been clear from the time the first trial was published in 1959 [1], that thrombolysis would become an important therapeutic option for patients with arterial and venous thrombosis. There remain a number of unresolved controversies, however, regarding the indications for thrombolysis, the agent of choice, and the appropriate adjunctive therapies to maintain vascular patency. Thrombolytic agents are used in patients with thrombosis of coronary arteries, precerebral and cerebral arteries, the aorta, iliac and mesenteric arteries, and peripheral arteries. The use of thrombolysis in venous thrombosis has included deep venous thrombosis (DVT) of the upper and lower extremities and vena cava, mesenteric veins, cerebral veins, and central access catheters. Thrombolytic agents also are effective therapy for intracardiac and mechanical valve thrombosis. Well-defined clinical practice guidelines are available from the American College of Cardiology/American Heart Association (ACC/AHA) [2] regarding the use of thrombolytic therapy in patients who have acute ST-segment elevation myocardial infarction (STEMI) and from the American Stroke Association (ASA) [3] regarding patients with acute ischemic stroke. Recommendations for practice also are available from the American College of Chest Physicians (ACCP) Sixth Consensus Conference on Antithrombotic Therapy

* California Clinical Thrombosis Center, 9330 Stockdale Highway #300, Bakersfield, CA 93311.
E-mail address: wbaker@thrombosiscenter.com

doi:10.1016/j.hoc.2004.09.008 ***hemonc.theclinics.com***

[4,5]. This article focuses on the current use of thrombolytic agents in general clinical practice, including the current clinical practice guidelines when available. The important structural and functional differences between thrombolytic agents and their physiologic effects are briefly summarized. The clinical trial data, which provide the basis for current recommendations, are summarized.

Overview

The clinical consequences of arterial or venous thrombosis may be associated with a high risk of significant morbidity or mortality. The achievement of rapid recanalization of the thrombosed artery or vein is the primary goal of thrombolysis. All thrombolytic agents activate plasminogen to plasmin, which then acts to degrade fibrin clots, fibrinogen, and other plasma proteins including factors V, VIII, IX, XI, and XII, components of complement, growth hormone, adrenocorticotropic hormone, and insulin [6,7]. Plasmin is inactivated by a number of plasmin inhibitors, including the rapidly acting and potent α_2-antiplasmin and the slow-acting α_2-macroglobulin [8,9]. The action of fibrinolytic agents in relationship to the intrinsic pathways of thrombosis and fibrinolysis is depicted in Fig. 1. The commercially available thrombolytic agents include urokinase (UK), streptokinase (SK), alteplase (recombinant tissue plasminogen activator [rt-PA]), tenecteplase [10–12], and reteplase (recombinant plasminogen activator [r-PA]) [156]. Agents that are not commercially available in the United States include anistreplase (anisoylated streptokinase activator complex), saruplase, lanoteplase, monteplase, pamiteplase, recombinant UK, recombinant prourokinase (rpro-UK), alfimerase [13], and staphylokinase [14]. Only those agents in general clinical use are discussed in this review.

Structure, function, and procoagulant effect of thrombolytic agents

Plasminogen activators are structurally similar in that they all possess an active site and a fibrin-binding site (kringle regions). Structural characteristics are compared with other functional proteins including fibronectin (finger domain), epidermal growth factor, plasminogen kringle regions (K1 through K5), serine protease trypsin, and the catalytically active center of the serine protease domain. A schematic representation of tissue plasminogen activator (t-PA) is shown in Fig. 2. The structural differences in thrombolytic agents are summarized in Table 1. SK is an antigenic bacterial enzyme, and is anisoylated to become anistreplase. UK is an endogenous plasminogen activator derived from tissue, kidney, and vascular cells and urine (UK-type plasminogen activators). The commercially available t-PA (rt-PA) is a recombinant product with a variety of derivatives produced by various alterations in the basic protein (r-PA, tenecteplase, and so forth) [14,156,198].

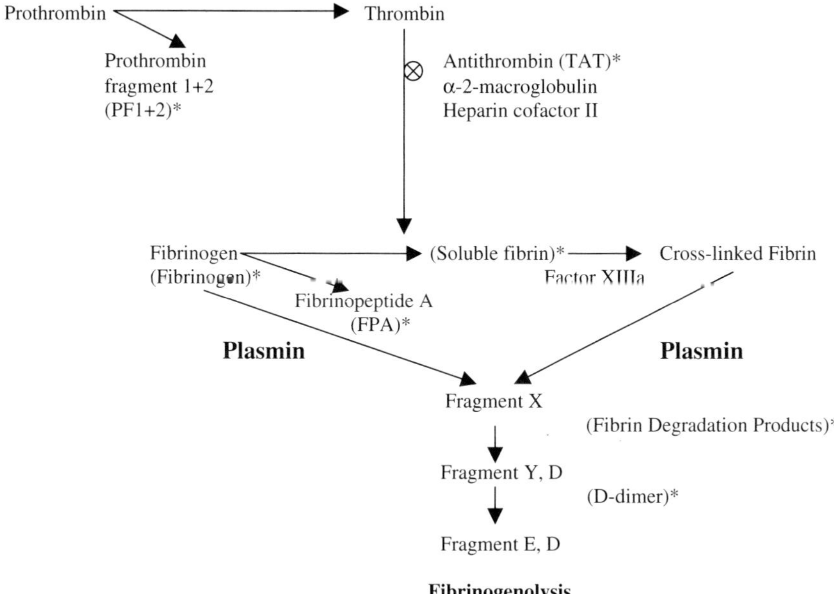

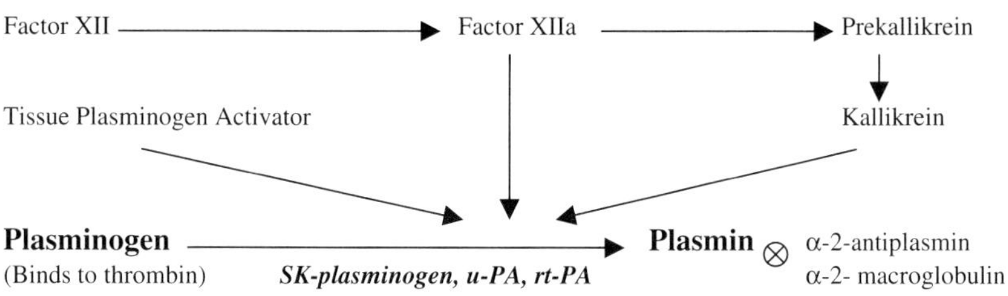

⊗ Inhibitors
Therapeutic thrombolytic agents SK, u-Pa, rt-PA
*Laboratory markers

Bick, RL. Disorders of Thrombosis and Hemostasis. Chicago: ASCP Press, 1992.

Fig. 1. Pathways of thrombosis and fibrinolysis. rt-PA, alteplase; SK, streptokinase; u-PA, urokinase-type plasminogen activators. (*From* Bick RL, editor. Disorders of hemostasis and thrombosis: clinical and laboratory practice. Chicago: ASCP Press; 1992. p. 398; with permission.)

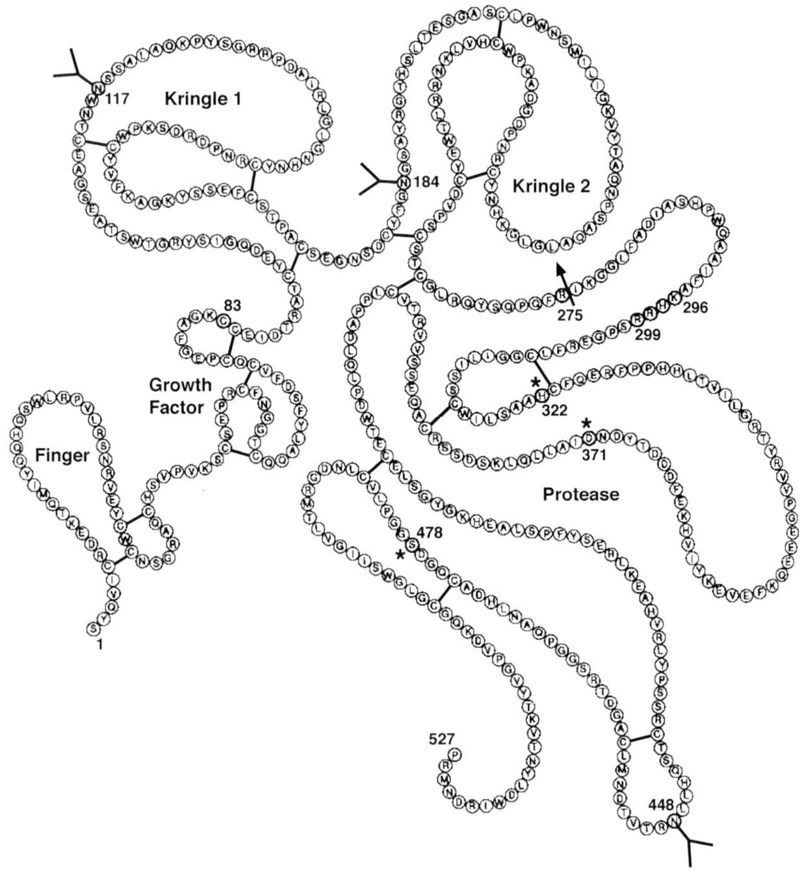

Fig. 2. Tissue-type plasminogen activator.

Therapeutic thrombolysis stimulates intrinsic fibrinolysis to control pathologic thrombosis. The "ideal" thrombolytic agent would induce local pathologic clot dissolution without producing systemic fibrinogenolysis or disrupting physiologic thrombi necessary for normal hemostatic balance. The attempt to more specifically target cross-linked fibrin is closely linked to the additional objective of minimizing the risk of bleeding. The properties of the ideal agent are outlined in Table 2. Because there is no ideal agent, a variety of adjunctive agents are required to achieve all of the goals of an ideal thrombolytic. Adjunctive therapies to sustain patency despite incomplete thrombolysis or post-thrombolytic hypercoagulability are summarized in Table 3 [15].

In addition to activating the intrinsic fibrinolytic system, thrombolytic agents induce a hypercoagulable state [16–20]. Patients with acute myocardial infarction, stroke, and other manifestations of acute arterial thrombosis are characterized by a significant risk of reocclusion due to underlying vascular pathology.

Table 1
Structural characteristics of thrombolytic agents

Agent	Molecular weight (kd)	Structure	Mutation
SK	47–50.2	414 amino acids 4 folded domains	Native
UK	54	411 amino acids 3 domains: EGF, K, P	Native
rt-PA	68	527 amino acids 5 domains: F,EGF, K1+K2, P, C	Native
r-PA	39.6	355 amino acids Absent: F, EGF, K1 K2, P preserved	Single-chain deletion
TNK t-PA	65	527 amino acids T103N, N117Q, KHRR 296–99AAAA	Point substitutions

Abbreviations: C, catalytic center; EGF, epidermal growth-factor domain; F, finger domain; K, kringle domain; P, serine protease domain; PGN, plasminogen; TNK t-PA, tenecteplase.
Data from Leopold J, Keaney J, Loscalzo J, Pharmacology of thrombolytic agents. In: Loscalzo J, Schafer A, editors. Thrombosis and hemorrhage. Baltimore: Williams and Wilkins; 1998. p. 1215–58; and Investigators of the International Joint Efficacy Comparison of Thrombolytics (INJECT). Randomized, double-blind comparison reteplase double-bolus administration with streptokinase in acute myocordial infarction (INJECT): trial to investigate equivalence. Lancet 1995;346:329–36.

To this risk is added the secondary procoagulant and proinflammatory effects of thrombolysis. By stimulating the intrinsic fibrinolytic system, the complement and kinin systems are activated and more thrombin is generated [18–21]. The procoagulant effect is greater with SK than with rt-PA [16,22].

In acute coronary thrombosis, the contact phase of coagulation, the intrinsic coagulation pathways, the intrinsic fibrinolytic system, and the platelets are activated [22–27]. Coronary thrombi are platelet rich, and platelet activation and aggregation are accentuated post therapeutic thrombolysis [28–30]. Some differences may exist between thrombolytic agents in the time course and degree of enhancement of platelet activity, but all stimulate measurable increases in platelet aggregation [31–33]. In addition to activation of coagulation, thrombolytic

Table 2
The "ideal" thrombolytic agent

Characteristics	Clinical advantages
Rapid thrombolysis	Prompt restoration of arterial or venous blood flow
Fibrin specificity	Targets areas of acute thrombus with reduced systemic fibrinolysis
Sustained duration of action	Maintains patency, no early reocclusion
Thrombus specific	Avoids effects on fibrinogen and other coagulation proteins yet does not impair primary hemostasis
Low risk of hemorrhage	Reduced risk of cerebral and other sites of occult hemorrhage; compatible with acute interventional procedures
Absence of systemic side effects	Nonantigenic; avoids systemic fibrinolysis
Low cost	Availability across a wide economic spectrum

Table 3
Adjunctive therapies to thrombolytic agents

Agent	Mechanism of action
Indirect antithrombin agents	
Heparin	Antithrombin activation to inhibit anti-Xa and factor II
Low molecular weight heparin	Antithrombin activation to inhibit anti-Xa
Direct thrombin inhibitors	
Hirudin(log)	Direct antithrombin inhibition
Argatroban	Direct antithrombin inhibition
Antiplatelet agents	
Aspirin	Cyclooxygenase inhibitor
Dipyridamole	Phosphodiesterase inhibition
Ticlopidine	Blocks exposure of platelet GpIIb/IIIa
Clopidogrel	Inhibits ADP-mediated activation of platelet GpIIb/IIIa
Abciximab	Antagonist to platelet GpIIb/IIIa
Tirofiban	Antagonist to platelet GpIIb/IIIa
Eptifibatide	Antagonist to platelet GpIIb/IIIa

Abbreviation: Gp, glycoprotein.

therapy for acute myocardial infarction is associated with activation of the inflammatory system. Patients receiving t-PA exhibit a significant early rise in markers of inflammation (interleukin-6, C-reactive protein) coincident with a rise in markers of coagulation (prothrombin fragment 1+2, high molecular weight kininogen, factor XII), not observed in the patients receiving heparin alone [21].

Clinical practice

Myocardial infarction

Since Herrick's [34] description of acute myocardial infarction in 1912, it has become well-accepted that nearly 90% of patients with acute myocardial infarction have acute coronary thrombosis [35]. The three critical factors that determine post–myocardial infarction outcome are (1) early diagnosis, (2) prompt treatment with aspirin, and (3) rapid restoration of blood flow through the infarct-related artery [36]. In addition to the demonstrated efficacy of thrombolytic therapy, randomized clinical trials also have demonstrated the utility of primary percutaneous coronary intervention (PCI) in restoring myocardial perfusion. Primary PCI refers to PCI performed without pretreatment with thrombolytic agents [37]. The specific clinical indications and settings in which primary PCI or thrombolysis are prescribed for acute STEMI has been the subject of numerous trials [38,39]. Key issues for both approaches remain the time from diagnosis to treatment and the time from initiation of treatment to restoration of grade 3 flow as designated by the Thrombolysis in Myocardial Infarction (TIMI) trial [36,40].

Numerous studies demonstrate the efficacy of thrombolytic agents in opening the thrombosed coronary artery (Table 4) [41–50]. Reperfusion success primarily is measured against the standard set by the TIMI trial, which designated occlusion

Table 4
Comparison of thrombolytic agents in acute myocardial infarction

Agent	Clot lysis[a] (%)	Fibrin specific	Half-life[b]	IC Bleed[b] (%)	Cost
Streptokinase	44–85	No	≈ 23 min	0.5	Low
Alteplase	60–88	> Urokinase	≈ 4 min	0.9	High
Reteplase	63–85	= Alteplase	≈ 58 min	0.8	High
Tenecteplase	54–88	> Alteplase	≈ 20 min	0.9	High

Abbreviation: IC, intracranial.

[a] Clot lysis reflects TIMI grade 2 or 3 flow.

[b] Values are approximations from a number of studies.

Data from Refs. [5,11,12,48,196,200–203].

as TIMI grade 0 to grade 1 flow and patency as TIMI grade 2 to grade 3 flow (grade 3 is designated as normal antegrade flow) [42]. Although mortality is reduced, failure to restore normal antegrade flow occurs in 45%, and the mortality rate with thrombolytic therapy remains at 7% to 10% [33].

The earlier the therapy is instituted after symptoms onset, the greater the potential for a reduction in time-dependent myocardial injury [40,51–56]. Early intervention also correlates with greater electrical stability and an increase in survival benefit [57].

The major factors that distinguish the various thrombolytic agents have been the early (90-minute) and late success at achieving reperfusion, the rate of re-occlusion, mortality, and the risk of hemorrhage. Studies have varied primarily in the choice of thrombolytic agent, the dose regimen, and the use of adjunctive agents. Randomized clinical trials that provide the foundation for current clinical practice and have important conclusions are summarized in Table 5. Because adjunctive agents have been demonstrated to play an essential role in achieving and maintaining coronary artery patency, clinical trials of adjunctive therapies are presented in Table 6. The benefit of each agent and combination of agents is balanced against the risk of bleeding (especially intracranial hemorrhage).

Current clinical practice in myocardial infarction

Thrombolysis versus primary percutaneous coronary intervention. The management of acute STEMI continues to include an important role for thrombolytic therapy. With the primary objective of treatment being the rapid opening of the infarct-related artery, providers of emergency cardiac care must have a plan in place to address acute coronary artery occlusion without delay. The current guidelines of the ACC/AHA recommend that all patients younger than 75 years who have cardiogenic shock resulting from acute STEMI undergo coronary revascularization within 36 hours [2,58]. Primary PCI is effective in promptly re-establishing coronary perfusion, and multiple clinical trials demonstrate superiority over thrombolytic therapy in short- and long-term outcome including morbidity [36]. In institutions that meet the ACC/AHA guidelines of performing 200 or more PCIs per year with available physicians who perform at least 75 such procedures per year, and if the “door-to-balloon” time is less than 120 minutes,

Table 5
Clinical trials of thrombolytic agents in acute myocardial infarction

Agent	Trial	Reference	Conclusions
SK	GISSI-1	[47]	Lysis achieved, mortality reduced (Aspirin only used in 14% and heparin only used in 62%)
SK	ISAM	[204]	Lysis achieved, mortality reduced
SK	ISIS-2	[48]	Lysis achieved, mortality reduced Reduced mortality with aspirin alone Aspirin with SK the most effective (aspirin "essential")
rt-PA	TIMI-1	[204]	Patency rate superior to SK
rt-PA	GISSI-2	[205]	Poor correlation between patency and mortality (Slow-infusion rt-PA or duteplase and delayed subcutaneous heparin)
rt-PA	ISIS-3	[206]	Poor correlation between patency and mortality (Slow infusion rt-PA or duteplase and delayed subcutaneous heparin)
rt-PA	GUSTO-1	[41,207]	Mortality reduction greatest with "accelerated" dosing Slight (1%) benefit over SK (Early intravenous heparin)
rt-PA	TIMI-4	[201]	Patency and mortality better compared with SK and APSAC (Accelerated dosing and early intravenous heparin)
r-PA	RAPID-1	[202]	Patency superior to rt-PA (TIMI-3 at 90 min)
r-PA	RAPID-2	[208]	Patency and mortality with r-PA superior to rt-PA
r-PA	INJECT	[199]	At least as effective as SK in reducing mortality
r-PA	GUSTO-3	[209]	Improved patency but not mortality over rt-PA (An absolute increase in TIMI-3 flow of 20% is required to improve mortality in acute myocardial infraction)
TNK t-PA	TIMI-10A	[203]	Patency similar to rt-PA (TIMI-3 at 90 min)
TNK t-PA	ASSENT-1	[10]	Higher doses ($\geq$ 0.5 mg/kg) superior to lower doses Reduced risk of ICH compared to alteplase
TNK t-PA	TIMI-10B	[12]	Patency similar to alteplase with reduced ICH risk Better outcomes compared with rt-PA if thrombolysis >4 h after symptoms onset Heparin dosing of 4000-U bolus then 800 U/h for $\leq$ 67-kg and 5000-U bolus and 1000 U/h for $\geq$ 67-kg patients results in less bleeding

Abbreviations: APSAC, anisoylated streptokinase activator complex; ICH, intracranial hemorrhage; TNK t-PA, tenecteplase.

primary PCI is recommended as the treatment of choice. It appears that although the performance of primary PCI within 2 hours of presentation is preferred, both short- and long-term mortality after 2 hours are improved. It appears that compared with thrombolysis, primary PCI success is not as dependent on the time to treatment [59,60]. Emergency transfer of the STEMI patient to a facility prepared to perform immediate PCI (without thrombolysis) leads to improved clinical outcomes [2,61].

Table 6
Clinical trials of adjunctive agents in thrombolytic therapy for acute myocardial infarction

Agent	Trial	Reference	Conclusions
Aspirin	ISIS-2	[48]	Aspirin alone reduces mortality and is synergistic with SK
Abciximab	TAMI-8	[210]	Improved patency compared to rt-PA alone
Abciximab	TIMI-14		Improved patency and mortality
Abciximab	SPEED	[211]	Improved patency and outcomes
Abciximab	GUSTO-V	[156]	Improved patency and outcomes
Abciximab	ASSENT-3	[212]	Improved patency and outcomes but increased ICH risk in patients over 75 years of age (Enoxaparin and abciximab are both superior to unfractionated heparin)
Eptifibatide	Ohman et al	[25]	Improved patency and faster resolution of EKG changes
Eptifibatide	INTRO-AMI	[213]	No improvement in survival or 20% improvement in TIMI grade 3 flow
Eptifibatide	INTEGRITI	[214]	No improvement in survival or 20% improvement in TIMI grade 3 flow
Heparin	GUSTO-1	[41]	IV heparin essential to improved outcomes
Heparin	TIMI-4		IV heparin improves late infarct-related artery patency
Heparin	TIMI-9	[215]	Lower doses of IV heparin are efficacious and reduce bleeding risk
Heparin	InTIME-2	[216]	Lower doses of IV heparin are efficacious and reduce bleeding risk
Dalteparin	FRAMI		Reduced risk of LV mural thrombus and reduced risk of recurrent myocardial infarction at 30 d
Dalteparin	ASSENT-Plus	[217]	Reduced in-hospital reinfarction rates with comparable outcomes at 30 d to 1 y
Enoxaparin	AMI-SK	[218]	Early resolution of ST-segment elevation and improved 5- to 7-d patency
Enoxaparin	HART-2	[219]	Improved efficacy and reduced ICH
Enoxaparin	ASSENT-3	[212]	Improved efficacy but with increased ICH in patients over 75 years of age (Enoxaparin and abciximab are both superior to unfractionated heparin)
Desirudin	TIMI-6	[220]	Reduced risk of reinfarction with increased bleeding risk
Desirudin	TIMI-9b	[221]	Reduced risk of reinfarction with increased bleeding risk
Lepirudin	HIT-3	[222]	Reduced risk of reinfarction with increased bleeding risk
Lepirudin	HIT-4	[223]	Reduced risk of reinfarction with increased bleeding risk
Bivalrudin	HERO-2	[223]	Reduced risk of reinfarction with increased bleeding risk

Abbreviations: ICH, intracranial hemorrhage; IV, intravenous; LV, left ventricle.

According to recent ACC/AHH guidelines, thrombolysis generally is preferred if presentation is 3 hours or less from symptoms onset and primary PCI is not immediately available. Primary PCI is preferred when (1) medical or door-to-balloon time is less than 90 minutes; (2) there is a high risk of myocardial infarction (cardiogenic shock, Killip class ≥ 3); (3) there is a contraindication to thrombolysis such as increased risk for bleeding and intracranial hemorrhage; (4) there is late presentation (symptoms onset more than 3 hours earlier); and (5) the

Box 1. Indications for thrombolytic therapy in acute ischemic stroke

Diagnosed ischemic stroke with a measurable neurologic deficit
Neurologic signs are not clearing spontaneously
Neurologic signs should not be minor and isolated
Onset of symptoms <3 hours before symptom onset
Blood pressure not elevated (systolic <185 mm Hg and diastolic <110 mm Hg)
CT brain scan does not reveal multilobar infarction (hypodensity greater than one third of cerebral hemisphere)
Patient and/or family understand the potential risks and benefits for thrombolytic therapy, particularly the risk for intracranial hemorrhage and clinical worsening

(*From* Adams HP, Adams RJ, Brott T, et al. Guidelines for the early management of patients with ischemic stroke: a scientific statement from the stroke council of the American Stroke Association. Stroke 2003;34:1067; with permission.)

diagnosis of STEMI is in doubt [2]. Contraindications to thrombolytic therapy are listed in Box 1.

Facilitated percutaneous coronary intervention. Facilitated PCI refers to treatment with low-dose thrombolytic agents alone or combined with platelet glycoprotein IIb/IIIa inhibitors before PCI. The objective is rapid reperfusion with pharmacologic therapy before definitive treatment. Randomized clinical trials of this facilitated approach to primary PCI have demonstrated no benefit and a significant increased rate of hemorrhage [62–65]. Several additional trials are proceeding to refine this technique to improve outcomes without the previously observed increase in bleeding [36].

Current guidelines and delivery of reperfusion therapy. The current ACC/AHA guidelines advise the administration of thrombolytic therapy to all patients who have symptoms suggesting acute myocardial infarction, regardless of age, sex, or race who present within 12 hours of symptoms onset; who demonstrate EKG changes of acute myocardial infarction (ST elevation or bundle branch block); and who have no contraindications to therapy. Acute management considers the time from symptoms onset to presentation and the availability of PCI. Recently published guidelines clearly indicate the preference of primary PCI over primary thrombolytic therapy (Fig. 3). It is abundantly clear, however, that although some approaches (eg, primary PCI versus primary thrombolysis) are preferred over

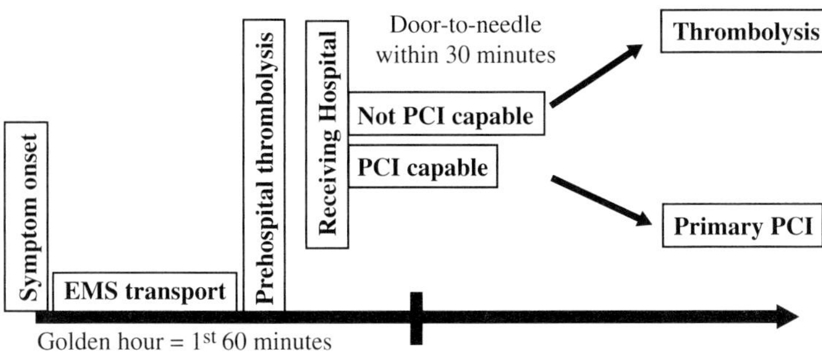

Fig. 3. Guidelines for management of acute myocardial infarction. EMS, emergency medical services. (*From* ACC/AHA guidelines for the management of patients with ST-elevation myocardial infarction: executive summary. A report of the American College of Cardiology/American Health Association Task Force on Practice Guidelines. J Am Coll Cardiol 2004;44:676; with permission.)

others, some form of reperfusion therapy should be prescribed for all patients with suspected STEMI [2].

Primary percutaneous coronary intervention. A major issue in the management of patients with acute myocardial infarction is the delay in initiation of therapy [40,54,55,66]. There appears to be a "golden hour"—starting from the onset of symptoms of acute myocardial infarction—during which acute intervention is most likely to be effective in limiting the extent of myocardial injury, with an associated reduction in morbidity and mortality. The goal for primary thrombolysis to achieve the optimal outcomes has been recognized as 120 minutes. This same 120 minutes also has been the standard for primary PCI. Optimal "door-to-needle" time has been established as 30 minutes. The 2004 ACC/AHA Guidelines in conjunction with the Task Force on the Management of Acute Myocardial Infarction of the European Society of Cardiology have lowered the medical contact-to-balloon or door-to-balloon time goal from within 120 minutes to 90 minutes [2,67]. This change reflects the recognition that the superiority of primary PCI over thrombolysis is best observed if therapy is delayed no more than 60 minutes from the stated 30-minute medical door-to-needle goal for thrombolytic therapy [68,69].

Not only are delays associated with the failure of the patient to access care but organizational and institutional delays also compound the problem. Efforts to improve public education, recognition, and elimination of sex bias [54] and movement of thrombolytic therapy to the emergency department [40] and into the field by way of first responders demonstrate a reduction in time before reperfusion therapy is initiated [53]. Thrombolysis in the setting of acute nontraumatic cardiopulmonary resuscitation has been demonstrated to reduce morbidity and mortality [52]. Out-of-hospital thrombolysis by trained paramedics with an available 12-lead EKG for accurate diagnosis also may reduce the total ischemic time and is recommended as a goal in well-developed and supported emergency medical services systems [2,56].

Cerebrovascular thrombosis

The administration of thrombolytic agents to patients with acute ischemic stroke is based on the understanding that most of these events (~80%) result from intravascular thrombosis [70,71]. The progression from acute cerebral ischemia to irreversible infarction is time dependent [72]. Early studies were limited by the lack of availability of CT imaging and were abandoned as the result of concern regarding intracranial hemorrhage [73,74]. Meta-analysis of the available trials, however, indicated the potential benefit of thrombolysis [75].

In 1995, the National Institute of Neurologic Disorders and Stroke Study Group (NINDS) published the first major clinical trial clearly demonstrating the benefit of thrombolytic therapy (rt-PA) in acute ischemic stroke [76]. Clinical outcome measures were standardized using the National Institutes of Health Stroke Scale in part I of the trial and, in part II, the Barthel index, the modified Rankin scale, and the Glasgow Outcome Scale were added. The study protocol included only patients within 3 hours of symptoms onset and without evidence of intracerebral hemorrhage on the pretreatment CT brain scan. Initial results indicated efficacy and safety in patients who presented within 3 hours of symptoms onset and without evidence of major acute abnormalities on CT brain scan. In view of the recognized association between uncontrolled hypertension and intracerebral hemorrhage, the blood pressure of all patients was carefully controlled within the range of < 185 mm Hg systolic and < 110 mm Hg diastolic. The dose of rt-PA was 0.9 mg/kg administered 10% as a bolus and the remainder as an infusion over 1 hour. Part I results demonstrated no significant difference at 24 hours between patients receiving rt-PA and those receiving placebo. Subsequent analysis and 3-month follow-up data, however, indicated benefit from rt-PA in all measurements of outcome. Part II patients treated with rt-PA were 30% less likely to be disabled than the placebo-treated patients. The 3-month mortality rate was 17% in the rt-PA group and 21% in the placebo group. All stroke subtypes faired similarly, and the risk of symptomatic cerebral hemorrhage was 6.4% for rt-PA patients and 0.6% for placebo patients. Although the risk of hemorrhage was greatest among the patients with cerebral edema, mass effect, and the greatest degree of clinical deficit, the potential for benefit also was greatest. At the 12-month follow-up mark, benefit again was demonstrated in the treated patients, with a 30% reduction in disability compared with placebo patients.

The European and Australasian trials (European Cooperative Acute Stroke Study I and II) [77,78] were of significantly different design and yielded different results. Lack of efficacy and an increased risk of intracranial hemorrhage emphasized importance of the 3-hour window between symptoms onset and intervention with thrombolysis.

The Alteplase Thrombolysis for Acute Noninterventional Therapy in Ischemic Stroke trial [79,80] was eventually terminated in 1998 due to lack of demonstrable benefit of rt-PA compared with placebo and to an excess of intracerebral hemorrhage. All three SK trials [81–83] also were terminated early because of an increase in early mortality and intracranial hemorrhage.

Intra-arterial administration of rpro-UK was evaluated in the Prourokinase for Acute Cerebral Thrombosis (PROACT) [84] and PROACT-II [85] trials. The original PROACT trial used rpro-UK infusion directly into the thrombosed artery by way of a supraselective catheter. Intravenous heparin infusion was administered concomitantly in all patients. Outcomes and mortality at 90 days favored the rpro-UK–treated patients but did not reach statistical significance. Hemorrhagic transformation occurred in 15.4% of rpro-UK–treated patients and in 7.1% of placebo-treated patients [84]. The PROACT-II trial compared intra-arterial rpro-UK (9 mg) plus heparin with heparin alone (heparin, 2000-U bolus and 500 U/h for 4 hours in each trial arm). Favorable outcomes were demonstrated to a modified Rankin scale score ≤ 2 in 40% of rpro-UK patients and in 25% of controls. Mortality was 25% and 27% in the rpro-UK and placebo arms, respectively, and the rate of symptomatic intracerebral hemorrhage was 10% for rpro-UK and 2% for controls. TIMI grade 3 flow was achieved in 66% of rpro-UK patients and in 10% of controls [85,86].

Following the guidelines of the NINDS and PROACT trials, a number of trials and case reports have appeared, continuing the practice of intravenous and cerebral intra-arterial thrombolysis. Therapy has included the use of UK and rt-PA. A variety of occluded cerebral arteries have been perfused, including the basilar artery [87]. In addition, trials have included the use of combined intravenous and intra-arterial therapy. Combined intravenous with intra-arterial thrombolysis trials have included the Emergency Management of Stroke Bridging Trial [88], the Interventional Management of Stroke Trial [89], and others [90,91]. Recanalization success varied in these combined trials from 55% to 75%, and there were improved clinical outcomes but an increased risk of intracranial hemorrhage [92]. Following tight guidelines to initiate intra-arterial t-PA or UK therapy within 3 hours of symptoms onset, recanalization is achieved in 75% of stroke patients, with a symptomatic intracranial hemorrhage rate of 11% and a mortality rate of 22% [93]. Fifty percent of patients exhibited a modified Rankin scale score of 0 to 1 at 1 to 3 months compared with 39% in the NINDS trial [93]. This finding confirms that further study is required to determine the safety and comparative efficacy of intra-arterial thrombolytic therapy for acute stroke.

Meta-analysis of thrombolytic therapy in acute ischemic stroke currently indicates that significant benefit may result from the administration of intravenous rt-PA in patients who present within 6 hours of symptom onset. The greatest benefit and lowest risk of hemorrhagic transformation, however, is measured in patients treated within 3 hours of symptoms onset [94,95]. Adherence to the NINDS [76] protocol offers the greatest potential for successful outcome at the lowest risk [4]. A meta-analysis of 15 published open-label studies was presented to assess the safety of rt-PA in acute stroke. The combined 2639 patients demonstrated a symptomatic cerebral hemorrhage rate of 5.2% (slightly lower than the rate of 6.4% in the NINDS trial). The total death rate was 13.4% and the percentage achieving a very favorable outcome was 37.1%, which were comparable to the NINDS results. Protocol deviations were noted at a rate of 19.8% and directly correlated with mortality, again supporting the need for strict adherence to NINDS criteria [96]. Thrombolysis is effective when administered within 3 hours of symptoms onset intravenously or within 3 to 6 hours intra-arterially. Greater success is predicted using MRI and other predictors of hemorrhagic transformation [97]. MRI assessment before and after rt-PA also allows for the prediction of long-term prognosis [98]. The recent report of combining reduced-dose rt-PA intravenously (single 20-mg bolus in 15 cases and a 10-mg bolus followed by a 40-mg infusion over 1 hour in 4 cases) combined with the platelet glycoprotein IIb/IIIa inhibitor tirofiban (body weight–adjusted dose according to the Platelet Receptor Inhibition in ischemic Syndrome Management in Patients Limited by Unstable Signs & symptoms [PRISM PLUS] protocol [224]) indicate improved recanalization of the middle cerebral artery and significant neurologic improvement in those successfully reperfused [99]. Additional study is required, however, before this combination of reduced-dose t-PA is combined with platelet glycoprotein IIb/IIIa agents in ischemic stroke.

Current clinical practice in acute ischemic stroke

Guidelines for the management of acute ischemic stroke have been published by a number of organizations, including the American Heart Association Emergency Cardiovascular Care Committee [100], the Canadian Stoke Consortium [101], the Pan European Consensus Meeting on Stroke Management [102], and the ACCP [4]. The ASA has provided the most recent comprehensive guidelines: Guidelines for the Early Management of Patients with Ischemic Stroke [3]. The ASA guidelines provide that immediate evaluation of patients with suspected acute ischemic stroke should include noncontrast enhanced CT brain scan. Because the major concern is determination of risk for hemorrhagic transformation, definition of the CT criteria that suggest increased (or potential benefit) of thrombolysis has been sought. A hyperdense middle cerebral artery sign indicative of thrombus or embolus in the first portion of the middle cerebral artery is an indicator of potential successful thrombolysis. The findings of loss of gray-white matter delineation in the cortical ribbon and sulcal effacement are associated with ischemia and poor outcomes [77,103–105]. The finding of generalized signs of cerebral infarction also increases the risk of hemorrhage with thrombolysis. The NINDS trial of rt-PA delivered within 3 hours of symptoms onset indicated an eightfold increased risk of symptomatic hemorrhage when the initial CT scan revealed evidence of early edema [76]. Other CT signs of infarction have been defined by additional study and remain an essential aspect of prethrombolysis assessment [3]. For potential rt-PA candidates, the ASA guidelines establish the time goal of 25 minutes for door-to–completed CT scan and an additional 20 minutes for time to completed interpretation (total 45 minutes) [3]. The results of history and physical examination and the CT scan findings determine the potential for successful thrombolysis. Box 1 lists indications and Box 2 lists contraindications to thrombolytic therapy for acute ischemic stroke. If the patient is determined to be a candidate and can be treated within 3 hours of symptoms onset, then rt-PA is recommended (with adjunctive administration of unfractionated heparin) in a dose of 0.9 mg/kg, with a maximum dose of 90 mg. The ASA protocol for thrombolytic therapy in acute ischemic stroke is presented in Box 3 [3]. Table 7 summarizes the regimens for hypertension management [3]. It is unfortunate that there remain many barriers to providing thrombolytic therapy for the large number of patients with acute ischemic stroke who might truly benefit. As with acute myocardial infarction, impediments to prompt intervention include public lack of awareness, delayed recognition of the significance of early symptoms, nonemergent care for stroke,

Box 2. Contraindications and relative contraindications to thrombolytic therapy in acute ischemic stroke

Absolute contraindications

- Presenting symptoms and signs should not suggest acute subarachnoid hemorrhage
- Head trauma or prior stroke within the previous 3 months
- Myocardial infarction within the previous 3 months
- Gastrointestinal or urinary tract hemorrhage within the previous 21 days
- Major surgery within the previous 14 days
- Arterial puncture at a noncompressible site within the previous 7 days
- History of previous intracranial hemorrhage
- Active bleeding or acute trauma (fracture) on examination
- Platelet count $< 100,000\ mm^3$
- Blood glucose < 50 mg/dL
- Seizure or postictal neurologic impairments

Relative contraindications

- Oral anticoagulation (international normalized ratio must be ≤ 1.5)
- Heparin within the previous 48 hours (activated partial thromboplastin time must be in the normal range)

(*Data from* Adams HP, et al. Guidelines for the early management of patients with ischemic stroke: a scientific statement from the stroke council of the American Stroke Association. Stroke 2003; 34:1056–83.)

Box 3. Protocol for thrombolytic therapy in patients with of acute ischemic stroke

1. Determine if the patient is a candidate for thrombolytic therapy.
2. Infuse alteplase (rt-PA) 0.9 mg/kg (maximum of 90 mg) over 60 minutes with 10% of the dose given as a bolus over 1 minute.
3. Admit the patient to an intensive care unit or stroke unit for monitoring.
4. Neurologic assessment to be performed every 15 minutes during the infusion of rt-PA and every 30 minutes for the first 2 hours for the next 6 hours, then every hour for 24 hours from the time of initial treatment.
5. If the patient develops a severe headache, acute hypertension, nausea, or vomiting, discontinue the infusion and perform and emergency CT brain scan.
6. Measure blood pressure every 15 minutes for the first 2 hours, every 30 minutes for the next 6 hours, and then every hour until 24 hours from the time of initial treatment.
7. Increase the frequency of blood pressure measurements if a systolic blood pressure ≥180 mm Hg systolic or ≥105 mm Hg diastolic is recorded. Administer antihypertensive medications to maintain the blood pressure at or below these levels (see Box 5).

(*From* Adams HP, Adams RJ, Brott T, et al. Guidelines for the early management of patients with ischemic stroke: a scientific statement from the stroke council of the American Stroke Association. Stroke 2003;34:1067; with permission.)

delays in diagnostic testing, inefficient emergency department and hospital systems, delayed consent for therapy and physicians' uncertainty related to difficulties in administering therapy within 3 hours of symptoms onset, and inconclusive diagnosis [106].

Venous thromboembolism

The indications for thrombolytic therapy in venous thromboembolism are less clear than in other clinical settings. Although acute pulmonary embolism (PE) may cause hemodynamic instability and sudden death, the presentation of DVT usually is less acute, and time-dependent tissue injury does not occur in the same manner as acute arterial occlusion. Complete clot lysis is not critical or likely in

Table 7
Protocol for the management of hypertension in patients with acute ischemic stroke treated with thrombolytic therapy

Blood pressure level (mmHg)	Treatment
Pretreatment with alteplase	
Systolic >185 mm Hg or	Labetalol 10–20 mg IV over 1–2 min
Diastolic >110 mm Hg	May repeat × 1 or apply nitropaste 1–2 in If blood pressure is not reduced and maintained at the target levels (≤185 mm Hg systolic and ≤110 mm Hg diastolic), do not administer rt-PA
During and after thrombolysis	
Monitor BP	Check BP every 15 min for 2 h, then every 30 min for 6 h, then every h for 16 h
Diastolic >140 mm Hg	Sodium nitroprusside 0.5 μg/kg/min IV infusion as an initial bolus and titrate to desired BP
Systolic >230 mm Hg or	Labetalol 10 mg IV over 1-2 min
Diastolic 121–140 mm Hg	May repeat or double the labetalol every 10 in to a maximum dose of 300 mg or give the initial labetalol bolus and then start a labetalol drip at 2–8 mg/min or Nicardipine 5 mg/h IV infusion as initial dose then titrate to the desired BP level by increasing the dose 2.5 mg/h every 5 min to a maximum of 15 mg/h. If the BP is still not controlled by labetalol, consider sodium nitroprusside
Systolic 180–230 mm Hg or	Labetalol 10 mg IV over 1–2 min
Diastolic 105–120 mm Hg	May repeat or double labetalol every 10–20 min to a maximum dose of 300 mg or give the initial labetalol bolus and then start a labetalol drip at 2–8 mg/min

Abbreviations: BP, blood pressure; IV, intravenous.
From Adams HP, et al. Guidelines for the early management of patients with ischemic stroke: a scientific statement from the stroke council of the American Stroke Association. Stroke 2003; 34:1056–83; with permission.

the low-flow venous circulation [107–111]. Compared with arterial thrombi, venous thrombi usually are present for a much longer period of time and in a greater state of cross-linked maturation when clinically diagnosed. The objective of thrombolysis is to acutely relieve hemodynamic instability due to massive PE to (1) restore venous flow more quickly in hopes of acutely reducing the pain and swelling of iliofemoral DVT and (2) reduce the risk of postphlebitic syndrome (~25%–40% among patients with proximal DVT [112–119] and 95% of patients with iliofemoral thrombosis treated with anticoagulation alone) [120]. The major question has been whether acute intervention with thrombolytic agents is superior to standard anticoagulation therapy with unfractionated heparin or low molecular weight heparin.

Deep venous thrombosis

Thrombolytic therapy for DVT has produced evidence of early benefit with relatively low risk. Although the incidence of symptomatic postphlebitic syndrome may be reduced from 40% in heparin patients to 10% in patients treated with thrombolysis [121], there is controversy regarding the long-term clinical impact of early thrombolytic therapy [113,114,116,117]. Recommendations are to consider thrombolysis (preferably catheter directed) in young patients with acute iliofemoral thrombosis at high risk for postphlebitic syndrome and at low risk for hemorrhage [120]. Food and Drug Administration approval is for 48 hours of UK and for 72 hours of SK [122]. Dosing for DVT is the same as PE; however, the infusion of SK or UK may be required for a longer time interval to achieve satisfactory clinical improvement. Catheter-directed therapy has emerged as an option for the delivery of thrombolytic agents. Recanalization rates as high as 90% are achieved, and the procedure may be combined with the placement of an intravascular stent [123–126]. Clots as old as 4 weeks may be amenable to treatment. It is unfortunate that the rate of intracerebral hemorrhage has been reported as high as 11% [127], that death may still result from PE, and that the long-term clinical benefit of early clot lysis remains unclear [122].

Pulmonary embolism

In the treatment of acute PE, SK, UK, and rt-PA have been well studied [128]. Large clinical trials performed in the 1970s demonstrated that infusion of SK for 24 hours and UK for 12 hours were similarly efficacious and superior to heparin in the rate of early recanalization [107–109]. rt-PA has demonstrated similar efficacy [110,111,129–131]. At 24 hours, reduction in pulmonary vascular resistance by 25% was demonstrated with thrombolysis compared with 4% with intravenous unfractionated heparin alone. Ventilation/perfusion lung scans were improved at 24 and 72 hours with thrombolysis but comparable to heparin later [107,108,132]. The risk of intracranial hemorrhage in patients treated with thrombolytic agents for venous thromboembolism consistently has been in the range of 1% to 2% [133]. Double-bolus r-PA also has been compared with rt-PA, with similar efficacy and safety [134].

Thrombolytic regimens for venous thromboembolism are different than for arterial disease. SK is used as a 250,000-U loading dose followed by infusion of 100,000 U/hour for 24 hours. UK is dosed as a 4400-IU/kg loading dose followed by infusion of 2200 IU/kg/hour for 12 hours [122]. Laboratory monitoring with SK and UK primarily is directed to document systemic fibrinogenolysis. Prolongation of the activated partial thromboplastin time or thrombin time allows documentation of fibrinogenolysis. Heparin may be initiated when the activated partial thromboplastin time or thrombin time return to less than two times normal. rt-PA is administered as a 100-mg infusion over 2 hours. Catheter-directed rt-PA therapy has been used as a 10-mg bolus followed by a 1- to 2-mg/hour infusion for 8 to 12 hours or as a 2- to 4-mg/hour infusion [135]. r-PA currently is not approved for use in PE but has been studied at a dose of two intravenous boluses of 10 U, 30 minutes apart [134]. Heparin should not be infused concurrently with SK or UK but is optional with rt-PA and r-PA. Although frequently employed [136], there is no clear evidence that catheter-directed therapy is superior to systemic therapy with rt-PA [137].

Following any thrombolytic agent, full-dose anticoagulation with intravenous unfractionated heparin or low molecular weight heparin is required to prevent rethrombosis. Current clinical use of thrombolytic agents in patients who have PE most often is confined to those with hemodynamic instability [138] or echocardiographic evidence of right ventricular dysfunction [122,139–141]. The recommendation of the AHA has been to consider rt-PA therapy in patients with the potential for greatest benefit, such as those with syncope, hypotension, or submassive PE in the presence of premorbid cardiac or pulmonary disease [142]. The ACCP guidelines indicate the potential usefulness of thrombolysis in patients with acute massive embolism who are hemodynamically unstable. The ACCP recommendations indicate the complexities involved in choosing thrombolytic therapy by advising that the use of thrombolysis in acute PE should be individualized by patient and should provide for considerable physician latitude in selecting therapy [122]. As a life-saving measure, rt-PA also has been used in patients for whom thrombolytic therapy ordinarily is considered contraindicated, including patients who have had recent general surgery [143] or neurosurgery [144], who are pregnant [145], and who have cardiac arrest requiring cardiopulmonary resuscitation [146,147]. In patients with massive PE, thrombolysis has been combined with embolus fragmentation by a rotating pigtail catheter [148,149].

Current clinical practice in venous thromboembolism

The use of thrombolytic therapy for DVT and PE varies greatly based on the unique clinical presentation and the experience of the treating physicians and institutions. Randomized clinical trial data are lacking to clearly define the role of thrombolysis in DVT. The well-described and accepted practice is to offer thrombolysis to young, active, and otherwise healthy patients who have iliofemoral thrombosis (at highest risk for postphlebitic syndrome and associated lifetime morbidity). Generally, it is recommended that patients who present with massive PE accompanied by hemodynamic instability be treated with thrombolysis unless there is a contraindication. No clear advantage of catheter-directed therapy versus systemic intravenous therapy has been shown.

Substantial controversy exists regarding the indications for thrombolytic therapy in patients who have submassive PE (echocardiographic evidence of right ventricular enlargement or hypokinesis without hemodynamic instability) or who are at risk for progression to shock and long-term pulmonary disability [150,151]. There is considerable uncertainty regarding this subset. The argument in favor of thrombolysis is that on the basis of the Management Strategies and Prognosis of Pulmonary Embolism (MAPPET) registry [152,153] and the MAPPET-3 study [152], thrombolysis should be considered strongly when there is echocardiographic evidence of right ventricular dysfunction, particularly with an elevated cardiac troponin I or T level, even if the blood pressure is normal at the time [154]. It also is clear that if thrombolysis is withheld initially, then management should include critical care monitoring and prompt thrombolysis if clinical deterioration is observed [150,155]. The opposing viewpoint is largely based on the Urokinase Pulmonary Embolism Trial (UPET) [107] that demonstrated no significant difference in recurrent PE between thrombolysis patients and those treated with heparin alone. In addition, it is noted that although a significant early benefit of thrombolysis is seen in measures of pulmonary obstruction and right ventricular function, this benefit is not sustained at 2 weeks and 1 year. Although more rapid resolution of pulmonary obstruction occurs at 24 hours, it is not sustained after 24 hours and there is no reduction in mortality [107]. In addition, concerns are raised regarding the safety of thrombolysis because the rate of intracranial hemorrhage appears to be substantially higher in thrombolysis patients (2.1%) [157] compared with heparin patients (0.2%) [138,151]. The call is made for randomized clinical trials to determine whether thrombolysis or heparin anticoagulation alone is the optimal strategy for patients with or without shock or who have right ventricular dysfunction without shock [151]. Current clinical practice varies based on the bias of the treating physicians and institutions. The indications for thrombolysis in venous thromboembolism are presented in Box 4. Box 5 summarizes the controversy concerning thrombolysis in submassive PE. There are no clear guidelines regarding the use of thrombolytic therapy in patients with massive or submassive PE.

Peripheral arterial thrombosis

Acute thrombosis of peripheral arteries presents a problem similar to acute coronary thrombosis; that is, acute, time-dependent tissue ischemia proceeding to infarction. The application of thrombolytic therapy to acute peripheral arterial thrombosis has been met with considerable success in opening the occluded artery [158–165]. The clinical outcome with thrombolysis is contrasted with the recognized benefit of early surgical intervention. The benefit of thrombolysis is balanced against the risk of intracranial hemorrhage.

Most patients with peripheral arterial occlusion have atherosclerosis and other risk factors associated with an increased risk of hemorrhage. Thrombolysis may be especially efficacious for small peripheral artery occlusion that is not amenable to surgical therapy. In addition to thrombolysis for acute thrombosis, angioplasty with the placement of an intra-arterial stent or surgery may still be required for definitive treatment to sustain vascular patency [158–165].

Box 4. Indications for thrombolytic therapy in venous thromboembolism

Severe iliofemoral thrombosis in a young patient at risk for severe postphlebitic syndrome
Massive PE with hemodynamic instability
Submassive PE but hemodynamically stable (controversial)

Box 5. Thrombolytic therapy for submassive pulmonary embolism

Definition

Echocardiographic evidence of right ventricular enlargement or hypokinesis without hemodynamic instability (persistent hypotension or shock) at presentation in a patient with confirmed acute PE

Comparison between anticoagulation with heparin alone versus thrombolysis with heparin anticoagulation

Pros

1. The MAPPET-3 randomized clinical trial confirms the benefit of primary thrombolysis.
2. rt-PA reduced the incidence of the primary endpoint (in-hospital death or the need for escalation in treatment) from 25% to 11%.
3. Although the reduction in hospital death was not statistically significant, rt-PA improved the "clinical course."
4. The need for emergency thrombolysis was reduced.
5. No fatal bleeding or intracranial hemorrhage was observed.

Cons

1. The hemodynamic benefits of thrombolytic therapy are short lasting.
2. Thrombolysis is a potentially life-threatening treatment due to the risk of bleeding (especially intracranial hemorrhage).
3. With the exception of massive PE resulting in cardiogenic shock, thrombolytic therapy does not reduce the in-hospital or long-term mortality compared with heparin alone.
4. The incidence of recurrent PE in the UPET trial was not reduced.

Current clinical practice in peripheral arterial occlusion

Thrombolytic therapy is applied widely for the treatment of thrombosis of the iliac and peripheral arteries and arterial grafts. Treatment with thrombolysis frequently is followed by percutaneous transluminal angioplasty, with stent placement. A 4-year hiatus of UK from the United States market resulted in the use of alternative thrombolytic agents. Evolution of interventional radiology techniques also has led to general use of catheter-directed therapy as the preferred mode of delivery, when available. The Surgery versus Thrombolysis for Ischemia of the Lower Extremities [176] and Thrombolysis or Peripheral Arterial Surgery

[166] trials demonstrated the utility and effectiveness of catheter-directed therapy for thrombolysis with rt-PA or UK [167]. A lower survival rate has been demonstrated with catheter-directed therapy compared with surgery [167]. Although a graded infusion protocol involving decreasing doses is administered after an initial high-dose rate has been employed with UK [168,169], the continuous-infusion protocol is the most widely practiced approach [13]. The role of anticoagulation with heparin and the potential value of other adjunctive therapies such as platelet glycoprotein IIb/IIIa agents has not been well established [13].

The primary unresolved issue remains the choice of thrombolytic agent [13]. Analysis of many studies indicates that increased doses are effective at more rapid reperfusion, without ultimately improving the degree of clot lysis [13]. Particularly with UK [170], rt-PA [171,172], and r-PA [173,174], more prompt lysis is accomplished at the expense of higher risk of hemorrhage [13]. rt-PA appears superior to UK in clot lysis and tibial artery perfusion if an end-hole perfusion technique is used. There is no apparent advantage between the two agents with intraclot perfusion [175]. Reported bleeding rates are similar

Table 8
Clinical applications of thrombolytic agents

Agent	Clinical use	Dose
Streptokinase	AMI	1.5 mU IV over 1 h or 20 kU intracoronary then 2 kU/min for 60 min
	PE	2.5 kU IV over 0.5 h then 100 kU/h for 24 h (72 h if concurrent DVT)
	DVT	2.5 kU IV over 0.5 hour then 100 kU/h for 72 h
	PAO	2.5 kU IV over 0.5 hour then 100 kU/h for 24–72 h
	AV	2.5 kU intracannula then clamp for 2 h
Urokinase	AMI	6 kU/kg/min for up to 2 h IC
	PE	4.4 kU/kg bolus then 4.4 kU/h for 12 h IV
	PAO	4 kU/min for 4 h then 4 kU/min for up to 48 h
	CC	5 kU intracatheter
Alteplase	AMI	15 mg bolus IV then 50 mg infusion over 30 min then 35 mg over next 60 min (>67 kg); if $\leq$ 67 kg use weight-based (maximum dose of 100 mg)
	PE	100 mg by IV infusion over 2 h
	AIS	0.9 mg/kg IV over 60 min with 10% of dose as initial bolus (maximum 90 mg total dose)
	DVT	10 mg intracatheter then 1 mg to 2 mg/h for 12 h (not FDA approved)
Reteplase	AMI	10 U IV over 2 min, wait 28 min then repeat
	PE	10 U IV over 2 min, wait 28 min then repeat (not FDA approved)
Tenecteplase	AMI	30–50 mg IV bolus (weight-based)

Abbreviations: AIS, acute ischemic stroke; AMI, acute myocardial infarction; AV, arteriovenous cannulae occlusion; CC, catheter clearance; DVT, deep vein thrombosis; FDA, Food and Drug Administration; IV, intravenous; kU, thousand units; mU, million units; PAO, peripheral arterial occlusion; PE, pulmonary embolus.

[175,176]. Catheter-directed thrombolysis with r-PA is effective at clot lysis (venous and arterial), but the risk of hemorrhage has varied from 6% to 19.2% [173,174,177,178]. Tenecteplase has been studied in two small trials and found to be efficacious at clot lysis, with a low bleeding rate [179,180].

Currently, thrombolysis for lower-extremity arterial thrombosis employs catheter-directed therapy. The choice of thrombolytic agent is a matter of experience, individual preference, and cost [13]. Randomized clinical trials involving large numbers of patients applying the standard of the Society of Interventional Radiology Acute Limb Ischemia Reporting Standards [181] are needed.

Box 6. Contraindications to thrombolytic therapy[a]

- Recent (within 10 days) major surgery
- Recent (within 10 days) puncture of noncompressible organ or vessel
- Recent (within 10 days) gastrointestinal or genitourinary bleeding
- Recent (within 10 days) trauma
- Recent (within 3 months) intracranial or intraspinal surgery, serious head trauma, or stroke
- Uncontrolled hypertension, with blood pressure $\geq$180 mm Hg systolic or $\geq$110 mm Hg diastolic
- Intracranial neoplasm, arteriovenous malformation, or aneurysm
- Strong probability of intracardiac thrombus
- Subacute bacterial endocarditis
- Acute pericarditis
- Hemorrhagic diathesis
- Major hepatic dysfunction (r-PA may be safer due to renal metabolism)
- Pregnancy
- Hemorrhagic opthalmopathy (eg, diabetic retinopathy)
- Current use of anticoagulants (especially warfarin)
- Septic thrombophlebitis or thrombosed and infected arteriovenous fistula
- Demonstrated allergy to thrombolytic agent (especially SK, anistreplase)
- Administration of SK or anistreplase within the preceding 2 years or more (antibodies may persist as long as 54 months)
- Age >75 years (relative contraindication)

[a] Contraindications are relative and not absolute. Benefit versus risk should be weighed on a patient-by-patient basis.

Miscellaneous disorders

Broad experience with thrombolysis in the treatment of arterial and venous thrombosis has led to a wide array of clinical applications. Cerebral venous sinus thrombosis [182] and intraventricular hemorrhage [183,184] have been treated effectively with thrombolysis. Unusual foci of thrombosis amenable to treatment with catheter-directed thrombolysis include the axillary/subclavian vein [185,186], the mesenteric artery and venous system, the superior and inferior vena cava (particularly when compressed by tumor), portal vein thrombosis [187–189], and peripheral arterial occlusion due to heparin-induced thrombocytopenia with thrombosis. Thrombolytic therapy has been recommended as first-line strategy in patients with mechanical valves who experience valve thrombosis, with evidence that many may not subsequently require surgery [190,191]. More recent studies indicate, however, that thrombolysis should be reserved for patients with tricuspid valve thrombosis, for patients who are not candidates for surgery, or as an emergency measure before transfer to a center capable of performing heart valve replacement [192,193]. Thrombosis of other devices for which thrombolytic agents are used include vena caval filters, peripheral and central access catheters [194], arteriovenous cannulae, and dialysis catheters. In all instances, the potential benefit must be weighed against the potential for life-threatening hemorrhage [195].

Complications of thrombolytic therapy

The primary risk of thrombolytic therapy is hemorrhage. Of greatest concern is life-threatening major hemorrhage and intracranial hemorrhage. Clinical trials clearly indicate that the risk of hemorrhage is greater with thrombolytic therapy than with placebo or with anticoagulation alone in all clinical settings [196,197]. Careful case selection and strict adherence to established protocols will help to mitigate the risk of hemorrhage. Clinical applications of the available thrombolytic agents are summarized in Table 8 and contraindications are summarized in Box 6. Table 9 summarizes the management of complications.

Table 9
Complications of thrombolytic therapy

Complication	Etiology	Management
Hemorrhage	Fibrinogenolysis (fibrinogen low)	ε-aminocaproic acid or aprotonin (particularly during thrombolysis), FFP, cryoprecipitate (may be required up to 36 h)
	Platelet dysfunction (TBT prolonged)	Platelet transfusion (requirement determined by TBT)
Embolization	Partial thrombolysis	Continue thrombolytic infusion, add adjunctive agents
Hypotension rash, fever	Anaphylaxis	Intravenous fluids, vasopressors, glucocorticoids, antihistamines

Abbreviations: FFP, fresh frozen plasma; TBT, template bleeding time.

Summary

The therapeutic use of thrombolytic agents is the natural result of the increasing understanding of the pathophysiologic mechanisms underlying normal and deranged thrombosis and fibrinolysis. Plasminogen activators capable of increasing the production of plasmin exhibit considerable efficacy in the treatment of a variety of arterial and venous thrombotic disorders. The ideal thrombolytic agent has yet to be developed, but the desired clinical result—rapid opening of the thrombosed vessel without reocclusion, without activation of systemic fibrinogenolysis, and without risk of hemorrhage—is well defined. Clinical studies clearly demonstrate that the addition of a variety of adjunctive agents to the available thrombolytics enhances benefit without inordinate risk. The use of intravascular angioplasty with or without stenting as primary therapy and in addition to thrombolysis increases the potential short- and long-term success at resolving arterial thrombosis. Despite well-established indications, there still are many barriers to effective delivery of thrombolysis. Many controversies regarding the clinical application of thrombolytic therapy remain to be resolved by ongoing and future randomized clinical trials. Current clinical practice will change as new trial data become available.

References

[1] Fletcher A, et al. The maintenance of a sustained thrombolytic state in man: II. Clinical observations on patients with myocardial infarction and other thromboembolic disorders. J Clin Invest 1959;38:11–9.

[2] Antman EM, et al. ACC/AHA guidelines for the management of patients with ST-elevation acute myocardial infarction: executive summary. A report of the American College of Cardiology/American Heart Association Task Force on Practice Guidelines (Writing Committee to Revise the 1999 Guidelines for the Management of Patients with Acute Myocardial Infarction). J Am Coll Cardiol 2004;44:671–719.

[3] Adams HP, et al. Guidelines for the early management of patients with ischemic stroke: a scientific statement from the stroke council of the American Stroke Association. Stroke 2003; 34:1056–83.

[4] Albers GW, et al. Antithrombotic and thrombolytic therapy for ischemic stroke. Chest 2001; 119(Suppl 1):300S–30S.

[5] Ohman EM, et al. Intravenous thrombolysis in acute myocardial infarction. Chest 2001; 119(Suppl 1):253S–77S.

[6] McNicol G. The fibrinolytic system. Postgrad Med J 1973;49(Suppl):10–7.

[7] Bick R. Physiology of hemostasis. In: Bick R, editor. Disorders of hemostasis and thrombosis: clinical and laboratory practice. Chicago: ASCP Press; 1992. p. 1–27.

[8] Bick R. Physiology of hemostasis and thrombosis. In: Weinberg RW, Wilke BP, Geffner J, editors. Disorders of hemostasis and thrombosis: principles of clinical practice. New York: Thieme; 1985. p. 1–30.

[9] Aoki N, Moroi M, Matsuda M. The behavior of alpha-2-plasmin inhibitor in fibrinolytic states. J Clin Invest 1977;60:361.

[10] Van de Werf F, Cannon CP, Luyten A, et al. Safety assessment of a single bolus administration of TNK tissue-plasminogen activator in acute myocardial infarction: the ASSENT-1 trial. Am Heart J 1999;137:786–91.

[11] Assessment of the Safety and Efficacy of a new Thrombolytic Regimen Investigators. Single bolus tenecteplase compared with front-loaded alteplase in acute myocardial infarction: the ASSENT-2 double-blind randomized trial. Lancet 1999;354:716.
[12] Cannon CP, Gibson CM, McCabe CH, et al. TNK-tissue plasminogen activator compared with front-loaded alteplase in acute myocardial infarction. Results of the TIMI 10B trial. Circulation 1998;98:2805–14.
[13] Razavi MK, Lee DS, Hofmann LV. Catheter-directed thrombolytic therapy for limb ischemia: current status and controversies. J Vasc Interv Radiol 2004;15(1 Pt 1):13–23.
[14] Deitcher SR, Jaff MR. Pharmacologic and clinical characteristics of thrombolytic agents. Rev Cardiovasc Med 2002;3(Suppl 2):S25–33.
[15] Brouwer MA, Clappers N, Verheugt FW. Adjunctive treatment in patients treated with thrombolytic therapy. Heart 2004;90(5):581–8.
[16] Hoffmeister HM, et al. Thrombolytic therapy in acute myocardial infarction: comparison of procoagulant effects of streptokinase and alteplase regimens with focus on kallikrein system and plasmin. Circulation 1998;98:2527–33.
[17] Rapold H. Promotion of thrombin activity by thrombolytic therapy without simultaneous anticoagulation. Lancet 1990;1:481–2.
[18] Eisenberg P, Sherman LA, Jaffe AD. Paradoxic elevation of fibrinopeptide A after streptokinase: evidence for continued thrombosis despite fibinolysis. J Am Coll Cardiol 1987; 10:527–9.
[19] Ewald GS, Eisenberg P. Plasmin-mediated activation of the contact system in response to pharmacological thrombolysis. Circulation 1995;91:28–36.
[20] Eisenberg P, et al. Factors responsible for the differential procoagulant effects of diverse plasminogen activators in plasma. Fibrinolysis 1991;5:217–24.
[21] Merlini PA, et al. Activation of the contact system and inflammation after thrombolytic therapy in patients with acute myocardial infarction. Am J Cardiol 2004;93(7):822–5.
[22] Davies M, Thomas A, Knapman P. Intra-myocardial platelet aggregation in patients with unstable angina suffering sudden ischemic cardiac death. Circulation 1986;73:418–27.
[23] Nicolini FA, et al. Combination of platelet fibrinogen receptor antagonist and direct thrombin inhibitor at low doses markedly improves thrombolysis. Circulation 1994;89:1802–9.
[24] Roux S, et al. Effects of heparin, aspirin, and synthetic glycoprotein IIb/IIIa receptor antagonist on coronary reperfusion and reocclusion after thrombolysis with tissue-type plasminogen activator in the dog. J Pharmacol Exp Ther 1993;264:501–8.
[25] Ohman EM, et al. Combined accelerated tissue-plasminogen activator and glycoprotein IIb/IIIa integrin receptor blockade with Integrilin in acute myocardial infarction: results of a randomized, placebo-controlled dose-ranging trial. Circulation 1997;95:846–54.
[26] Moliterno DJ, et al. More complete and stable reperfusion with platelet IIb/IIIa antagonism plus thrombolysis for AMI: the PARADIGM trial [abstract]. Circulation 1996; 94(Suppl I):I553.
[27] Rote W, et al. Prevention of rethrombosis after coronary thrombolysis in chronic canine model: adjunctive therapy with monoclonal antibody 7E3 F(ab′) 2 fragment. J Cardiovasc Pharmacol 1994;23:194–202.
[28] Cronberg S. Effect of fibrinolysis on adhesion and aggregation of human platelets. Thromb Diathesis Haemorrhage 1968;19:474–82.
[29] Terres W, et al. Effects of streptokinase, urokinase, and recombinant tissue plasminogen activator on platelet aggregability and stability of platelet aggregates. Cardiovasc Res 1990; 24(6):471–7.
[30] Fitzgerald D, et al. Marked platelet activation in vivo after intravenous streptokinase in patients with acute myocardial infarction. Circulation 1988;77:142–50.
[31] Nordt TK, et al. Augmented platelet aggregation as predictor of reocclusion after thrombolysis in acute myocardial infarction. Thromb Haemost 1998;80:881–6.
[32] Gurbel PA, et al. Effects of reteplase and alteplase on platelet aggregation and major receptor expression during the first 24 hours of acute myocardial infarction treatment. J Am Coll Cardiol 1997;31:1466–73.

[33] Coulter S, et al. High levels of platelet inhibition with abciximab despite heightened platelet activation and aggregation during thrombolysis for acute myocardial infarction: results from TIMI (Thrombolysis in Myocardial Infarction) 14. Circulation 2000;101:2690–5.
[34] Herrick J. Clinical features of sudden obstruction of the coronary arteries. JAMA 1912;59: 2015–20.
[35] DeWood M, et al. Prevalence of total coronary occlusion during the early hours of transmural myocardial infarction. N Engl J Med 1980;303:897–902.
[36] Keeley EC, Grines CL. Primary coronary intervention for acute myocardial infarction. JAMA 2004;291(6):736–9.
[37] The Global Use of Strategies to Open Occluded Coronary Arteries in Acute Coronary Syndromes. (GUSTO IIb) Angioplasty Substudy Investigators. A clinical trial comparing primary coronary angioplasty with tissue plasminogen activator for acute myocardial infarction. N Engl J Med 1997;336:1621–8.
[38] Gibson CM, et al. Early and long-term clinical outcomes associated with reinfarction following fibrinolytic administration in the thrombolysis in myocardial infarction trials. J Am Coll Cardiol 2003;42:7–16.
[39] Keeley EC, Boura JA, Grines CL. Primary angioplasty versus intravenous thrombolytic therapy for acute myocardial infarction. Lancet 2003;361:13–20.
[40] McLean S, et al. Improving door-to-drug time and ST segment resolution in AMI by moving thrombolysis administration to the emergency department. Accid Emerg Nurs 2004;12(1):2–9.
[41] The GUSTO Investigators. An international randomized trial comparing four thrombolytic strategies for acute myocardial infarction. N Engl J Med 1993;329:673.
[42] Chesebro JH, et al. Thrombolysis in Acute Myocardial Infarction (TIMI) trial, phase 1: a comparison between intravenous plasminogen activator and intravenous streptokinase. Circulation 1987;76:142–54.
[43] Verstraete M, et al. Randomized trial of intravenous recombinant tissue-type plasminogen activator versus intravenous streptokinase in acute myocardial infarction. Lancet 1985; 1:842–7.
[44] Verstraete M, et al. Double blind randomized trial of intravenous tissue-type plasminogen activator versus placebo in acute myocardial infarction. Lancet 1985;2:956–69.
[45] Sheehan FH, et al. The effect of intravenous thrombolytic therapy on left ventricular function: a report on tissue-type plasminogen activator and streprokinase from the thrombolysis in myocardial infarction (TIMI phase I) trial. Circulation 1987;75:817–29.
[46] PRIMI Trial Study Group. Randomized double-blind trial of recombinant prourokinase against streptokinase in acute myocardial infarction. Lancet 1989;1:863.
[47] Gruppo Italiano per lo Studio della Straptochinasi nell'Infarto Miocardico (GISSI)-1. Effectiveness of intravenous thrombolytic treatment in acute myocardial infarction. Lancet 1986;1:397–402.
[48] Second International Study of Infarct Survival (ISIS-2) Collaborative Group. Randomized trial of intravenous streptokinase, oral aspirin, both or neither among 17,187 cases of suspected acute myocardial infarction. J Am Coll Cardiol 1988;12(6 Suppl A):3A–13A.
[49] AIMS Trial Study Group. Effect of intravenous APSAC on mortality after acute myocardial infarction: preliminary report of placebo-controlled clinical trial. Lancet 1988;1:545.
[50] Wilcox R, et al. Trial of tissue plasminogen activator for mortality reduction in acute myocardial infarction: Anglo-Scandinavia study of early thrombolysis (ASSET). Lancet 1988; 2(8610):525–30.
[51] Morrison LJ, et al. Mortality and prehospital thrombolysis for acute myocardial infarction: a meta analysis. JAMA 2000;283(20):2686–92.
[52] Lederer W, et al. Long-term survival and neurological outcome of patients who received recombinant tissue plasminogen activator during out-of-hospital cardiac arrest. Resuscitation 2004;61(2):123–9.
[53] Smallwood A. Nurse-initiated thrombolysis: a systematic review of the literature. Nurs Crit Care 2004;9(1):4–12.

[54] Grace SL, et al. Presentation, delay, and contraindication to thrombolytic treatment in females and males with myocardial infarction. Womens Health Issues 2003;13(6):214–21.
[55] Zed PJ, et al. Fibrinolytic administration for acute myocardial infarction in a tertiary ED: factors associated with an increased door-to-needle time. Am J Emerg Med 2004;22(3):192–6.
[56] Steg PG, et al. Impact of time to treatment on mortality after prehospital fibrinolysis or primary angioplasty: data from the CAPTIM randomized clinical trial. Circulation 2003;108(23): 2851–6.
[57] Carnendran L, Steinberg JS. Does an open infarct-related artery after myocardial infarction improve electrical stability? Prog Cardiovasc Dis 2000;42(6):439–54.
[58] Ryan T, et al. Update: ACC/AHA guidelines for the management of patients with acute myocardial infarction: a report of the American College of Cardiology/American Heart Association Task Force on Practice Guidelines (Committee on Management of Acute Myocardial Infarction). J Am Coll Cardiol 1999;34:890–911.
[59] Brodie BR, et al. Importance of time to reperfusion for 30-day and late survival and recovery of left ventricular function after primary angioplasty. J Am Coll Cardiol 1998;32:1312–9.
[60] Brodie BR, et al. Importance of tome to reperfusion on outcomes with primary coronary angioplasty for acute myocardial infarction. Am J Cardiol 2001;88:1085–90.
[61] Dalby M, et al. Transfer for primary angioplasty versus immediate thrombolysis in acute myocardial infarction. Circulation 2003;108:1809–14.
[62] O'Neill WW, et al. A prospective, placebo-controlled, randomized trial of intravenous streptokinase and angioplasty versus lone angioplasty therapy of acute myocardial infarction. Circulation 1992;86:1710–7.
[63] Widimsky P, et al. Multicenter randomized trial comparing transport to primary angioplasty vs immediate thrombolysis vs combined strategy for patients with acute myocardial infarction presenting to a community hospital without a catheterization laboratory. Eur Heart J 2000; 21:823–31.
[64] Vermeer F, et al. Prospective randomised comparison between thrombolysis, rescue PTCA, and primary PTCA in patients with extensive myocardial infarction admitted to a hospital without PTCA facilities. Heart 1999;82:426–31.
[65] Ross AM, et al. A randomized trial comparing primary angioplasty with a strategy of short-acting thrombolysis and immediate planned rescue angioplasty in acute myocardial infarction. J Am Coll Cardiol 1999;34:1954–62.
[66] Cohen M, Arjomand H, Pollack Jr CV. The evolution of thrombolytic therapy and adjunctive antithrombotic regimens in acute ST-segment elevation myocardial infarction. Am J Emerg Med 2004;22(1):14–23.
[67] The Task Force on the Management of Acute Myocardial Infarction of the European Society of Cardiology. Management of acute myocardial infarction in patients presenting with ST-segment elevation. Eur Heart J 2003;24:28–66.
[68] Juliard JM, et al. Relation of mortality of primary angioplasty during acute myocardial infarction to door-to-Thrombolysis in Myocardial Infarction (TIMI) time. Am J Cardiol 2003; 91:1401–5.
[69] Williams DO. Treatment delayed is treatment denied. Circulation 2004;109:1806–8.
[70] Fieschi C, et al. Clinical and instrumental evaluation of patients with ischemic stroke within the first six hours. J Neurol Sci 1989;91(3):311–21.
[71] del Zoppo GJ, et al. Recombinant tissue plasminogen activator in acute thrombotic and embolic stroke. Ann Neurol 1992;32(1):78–86.
[72] Siesjo BK. Pathophysiology and treatment of focal cerebral ischemia. Part II: mechanisms of damage and treatment. J Neurosurg 1992;77(3):337–54.
[73] Levine SR, Brott TG. Thrombolytic therapy in cerebrovascular disorders. Prog Cardiovasc Dis 1992;34(4):235–62.
[74] Brott T, Broderick J, Kothari R. Thrombolytic therapy for stroke. Curr Opin Neurol 1994; 7(1):25–35.
[75] Wardlaw JM, Warlow CP. Thrombolysis in acute ischemic stroke: does it work? Stroke 1992; 23(12):1826–39.

[76] The National Institute of Neurological Disorders and Stroke rtPA Study Group. Tissue plasminogen activator for acute ischemic stroke. N Engl J Med 1995;333:1581.
[77] Hacke W, Kaste M, Fieschi C, et al. Intravenous thrombolysis with recombinant tissue plasminogen activator for acute hemisperic stroke: the European Cooperative Stroke Study. JAMA 1995;274:1017.
[78] Hacke W, et al. Randomised double-blind placebo-controlled trial of thrombolytic therapy with intravenous alteplase in acute ischaemic stroke (ECASS II). Second European–Australasian Acute Stroke Study Investigators. Lancet 1998;352(9136):1245–51.
[79] Clark WM, et al. Recombinant tissue-type plasminogen activator (alteplase) for ischemic stroke 3 to 5 hours after symptom onset. The ATLANTIS Study: a randomized controlled trial Alteplase Thrombolysis for Acute Noninterventional Therapy in Ischemic Stroke. JAMA 1999; 282(21):2019–26.
[80] Clark WM, et al. The rtPA (alteplase) 0- to 6-hour acute stroke trial, part A (A0276g): results of a double-blind, placebo-controlled, multicenter study. Thrombolytic therapy in acute ischemic stroke study investigators. Stroke 2000;31(4):811–6.
[81] Multicenter Acute Stroke Trial–Italy (MAST-I) Group. Randomized controlled trial of streptokinase, aspirin and combination of both in treatment of acute ischemic stroke. Lancet 1995; 346:1509.
[82] The Australian Streptokinase (ASK) Trial Study Group. Streptokinase for acute ischemic stroke with relationship to time of admission. JAMA 1996;276:961.
[83] The Multicenter Stroke Trial–Europe Study Group. Thrombolytic therapy with streptokinase in acute ischemic stroke. N Engl J Med 1996;335:145.
[84] del Zoppo G, Higashida RT, Furlan R, et al. PROACT: a phase II randomized trial of recombinant prourokinase by direct delivery in acute middle cerebral artery stroke. Stroke 1998;29:4.
[85] Furlan A, Higashida R, Wechsler L, et al. A randomized trial of intra-arterial prourokinase for acute ishemic stroke due to middle cerebral artery occlusion. JAMA 1999;282:2003.
[86] Furlan A. Intra-arterial thrombolysis for acute stroke. Cleve Clin J Med 2004;71(Suppl 1):S31–8.
[87] Arnold M, et al. Clinical and radiological predictors of recanalisation and outcome of 40 patients with acute basilar artery occlusion treated with intra-arterial thrombolysis. J Neurol Neurosurg Psychiatry 2004;75(6):857–62.
[88] Lewandowski CA, et al. Combined intravenous and intra-arterial r-TPA versus intra-arterial therapy iof acute ischemic stroke: Emergency Management of Stroke (EMS) Bridging Trial. Stroke 1999;30:2598–605.
[89] Tomsick TS, et al. Combined IV–IA rtPA treatment in major ischemic stroke [abstract]. Stroke 2002;33:359.
[90] Keris V, et al. Combined intraarterial/intravenous thrombolysis fro acute ischemic stroke. Am J Neuroradiol 2001;22:352–8.
[91] Lee DH, et al. Local intraarterial urokinase thrombolysis of acute ischemic stroke with or without intravenous abciximab: a pilot study. J Vasc Interv Radiol 2002;13:769–74.
[92] Ng PP, et al. Intraarterial thrombolysis trials in acute ischemic stroke. J Vasc Interv Radiol 2004;15(1 Pt 2):S77–85.
[93] Bourekas EC, et al. Intraarterial thrombolytic therapy within 3 hours of the onset of stroke. Neurosurgery 2004;54(1):39–44 [discussion: 44–6].
[94] Wardlaw JM, Warlow CP, Counsell C. Systematic review of evidence on thrombolytic therapy for acute ischaemic stroke. Lancet 1997;350(9078):607–14.
[95] Hacke W, et al. Thrombolysis in acute ischemic stroke: controlled trials and clinical experience. Neurology 1999;53(7 Suppl 4):S3–14.
[96] Graham GD. Tissue plasminogen activator for acute ischemic stroke in clinical practice: a meta-analysis of safety data. Stroke 2003;34(12):2847–50.
[97] Schellinger PD, Kaste M, Hacke W. An update on thrombolytic therapy for acute stroke. Curr Opin Neurol 2004;17(1):69–77.
[98] Chalela JA, et al. Early magnetic resonance imaging findings in patients receiving tissue plasminogen activator predict outcome: insights into the pathophysiology of acute stroke in the thrombolysis era. Ann Neurol 2004;55(1):105–12.

[99] Straub S, et al. Systemic thrombolysis with recombinant tissue plasminogen activator and tirofiban in acute middle cerebral artery occlusion. Stroke 2004;35(3):705–9.
[100] Alberts MJ, et al. Recommendations for the establishment of primary stroke centers: Brain Attack Coalition. JAMA 2001;283:3102–9.
[101] Norris JW, et al. Canadian guidelines for intravenous thrombolytic treatment in acute stroke: a consensus statement of the Canadian Stroke Consortium. Can J Neurol Sci 1998;25:257–9.
[102] Aboderin I, Venables G. Stroke management in Europe: Pan European Consensus Meeting on Stroke Management. J Intern Med 1996;240:173–80.
[103] Moulin T, et al. Early CT signs in acute middle cerebral artery infarction: predictive value for subsequent infarct locations and outcome. Neurology 1996;47:366–75.
[104] von Kummer R, et al. Detectability of cerebral hemisphere ischaemic infarcts by CT within 6 h of stroke. Neuroradiology 1996;38:31–3.
[105] von Kummer R, et al. Acute stroke: usefulness of early CT findings before thrombolytic therapy. Radiology 1997;205:327–33.
[106] Kwan J, Hand P, Sandercock P. A systematic review of barriers to delivery of thrombolysis for acute stroke. Age Ageing 2004;33(2):116–21.
[107] Bell W, Black E, DeMets D. Urokinase pulmonary embolism trial. JAMA 1970;214:2163.
[108] Bell W, et al. Urokinase-streptokinase embolism trial, phase 2 results. JAMA 1974;229: 1606–13.
[109] Marder VJ. The use of thrombolytic agents: choice of patient, drug administration, laboratory monitoring. Ann Intern Med 1979;90(5):802–8.
[110] Goldhaber SZ, et al. Randomized controlled trial of recombinant tissue plasminogen activator versus urokinase in th treatment of acute pulmonary embolism. Lancet 1988;2:293.
[111] Goldhaber SZ, et al. Randomized controlled trial of tissue plasminogen activator in proximal deep venous thrombosis. Am J Med 1990;88(3):235–40.
[112] Immelman E, Jeffrey P. The post-phlebitic syndrome. Pathophysiology prevention and management. Clin Chest Med 1984;5:537.
[113] Arnesen H, Hoiseth A, Ly B. Streptokinase of heparin in the treatment of deep vein thrombosis. Follow-up results of a prospective study. Acta Med Scand 1982;211(1–2):65–8.
[114] Elliot MS, et al. A comparative randomized trial of heparin versus streptokinase in the treatment of acute proximal venous thrombosis: an interim report of a prospective trial. Br J Surg 1979;66(12):838–43.
[115] Watz R, Savidge GF. Rapid thrombolysis and preservation of valvular venous function in high deep vein thrombosis. A comparative study between streptokinase and heparin therapy. Acta Med Scand 1979;205(4):293–8.
[116] Common HH, et al. Deep vein thrombosis treated with streptokinase or heparin. Follow-up of a randomized study. Angiology 1976;27(11):645–54.
[117] Johansson L, et al. Comparison of streptokinase with heparin: late results in the treatment of deep venous thrombosis. Acta Med Scand 1979;206(1–2):93–8.
[118] Kakkar VV, Lawrence D. Hemodynamic and clinical assessment after therapy for acute deep vein thrombosis. A prospective study. Am J Surg 1985;150(4A):54–63.
[119] Prandoni P, et al. The long-term clinical course of acute deep venous thrombosis. Ann Intern Med 1996;125:1–7.
[120] Navarro F, Dean S. Young patients with iliofemoral deep venous thrombosis should receive thrombolytic therapy. Med Clin North Am 2003;87(6):1165–77.
[121] Turpie AG, et al. Tissue plasminogen activator (rt-PA) vs heparin in deep vein thrombosis. Results of a randomized trial. Chest 1990;97(Suppl 4):172S–5S.
[122] Hyers TM, et al. Antithrombotic therapy for venous thromboembolic disease. Chest 2001; 119(Suppl 1):176S–93S.
[123] Comerota AJ, et al. A strategy of aggressive regional therapy for acute iliofemoral venous thrombosis with contemporary venous thrombectomy or catheter-directed thrombolysis. J Vasc Surg 1994;20(2):244–54.
[124] Semba CP, Dake MD. Iliofemoral deep venous thrombosis: aggressive therapy with catheter-directed thrombolysis. Radiology 1994;191(2):487–94.

[125] Verhaeghe R, Maleux G. Endovascular local thrombolytic therapy of ileofemoral and inferior caval vein thrombosis. Semin Vasc Med 2001;1(1):123–8.
[126] Bjarnason H, et al. Iliofemoral deep venous thrombosis: safety and efficacy outcome during 5 years of catheter-directed thrombolytic therapy. J Vasc Interv Radiol 1997;8(3):405–18.
[127] Mewissen MW, et al. Catheter-directed thrombolysis for lower extremity deep venous thrombosis: report of a national multicenter registry. Radiology 1999;211(1):39–49.
[128] Marder VJ, Sherry S. Thrombolytic therapy: current status. N Engl J Med 1988;318(23): 1512–20.
[129] Goldhaber SZ, et al. Alteplase versus heparin in acute pulmonary embolism: randomised trial assessing right-ventricular function and pulmonary perfusion. Lancet 1993;341(8844):507–11.
[130] Goldhaber SZ, Agnelli G, Levine MN. Reduced dose bolus alteplase vs conventional alteplase infusion for pulmonary embolism thrombolysis. An international multicenter randomized trial. The Bolus Alteplase Pulmonary Embolism Group. Chest 1994;106(3):718–24.
[131] Meneveau N, et al. Comparative efficacy of a two-hour regimen of streptokinase versus alteplase in acute massive pulmonary embolism: immediate clinical and hemodynamic outcome and one-year follow-up. J Am Coll Cardiol 1998;31(5):1057–63.
[132] Konstantinides S, et al. Comparison of alteplase versus heparin for resolution of major pulmonary embolism. Am J Cardiol 1998;82(8):966–70.
[133] Sharma GV, Burleson VA, Sasahara AA. Effect of thrombolytic therapy on pulmonary-capillary blood volume in patients with pulmonary embolism. N Engl J Med 1980;303(15):842–5.
[134] Tebbe U, et al. Hemodynamic effects of double bolus reteplase versus alteplase infusion in massive pulmonary embolism. Am Heart J 1999;138(1 Pt 1):39–44.
[135] Goldhaber SZ. Management of deep vein thrombosis and pulmonary embolism. Clin Cornerstone 2000;2(4):47–55.
[136] Murphy JM, et al. Percutaneous catheter and guidewire fragmentation with local administration of recombinant tissue plasminogen activator as a treatment for massive pulmonary embolism. Eur Radiol 1999;9:959–64.
[137] Verstraete M, et al. Intravenous and intrapulmonary recombinant tissue-type plasminogen activator in the treatment of acute massive pulmonary embolism. Circulation 1988;77(2): 353–60.
[138] Dalen JE, Alpert JS, Hirsch J. Thrombolytic therapy for pulmonary embolism: is it effective? Is it safe? When is it indicated? Arch Intern Med 1997;157(22):2550–6.
[139] McConnell MV, et al. Regional right ventricular dysfunction detected by echocardiography in acute pulmonary embolism. Am J Cardiol 1996;78(4):469–73.
[140] Goldhaber SZ, Bounameaux H. Thrombolytic therapy in pulmonary embolism. Semin Vasc Med 2001;1(2):213–20.
[141] Goldhaber SZ. Thrombolysis for pulmonary embolism. N Engl J Med 2002;347:1131–2.
[142] Hirsh J, Hoak J. Management of deep vein thrombosis and pulmonary embolism: a statement for healthcare professionals. Circulation 1996;93:2212–45.
[143] Nasraway SA, Kabani N, Lawrence KR. Thrombolytic therapy for pulmonary embolism: reversal of shock in the early postoperative period. Pharmacotherapy 1994;14(5):616–9.
[144] Severi P, et al. Urokinase thrombolytic therapy of pulmonary embolism in neurosurgically treated patients. Surg Neurol 1994;42(6):469–70.
[145] Mazeka PK, Oakley CM. Massive pulmonary embolism in pregnancy treated with streptokinase and percutaneous catheter fragmentation. Eur Heart J 1994;15(9):1281–3.
[146] Kurkciyan I, et al. Pulmonary embolism as a cause of cardiac arrest: presentation and outcome. Arch Intern Med 2000;160(10):1529–35.
[147] Bottinger BW, et al. High-dose bolus injection of urokinase. Use during cardiopulmonary resuscitation for massive pulmonary embolism. Chest 1994;106(4):1281–3.
[148] Schmitz-Rode T, et al. Massive pulmonary embolism: percutaneous emergency treatment by pigtail rotation catheter. J Am Coll Cardiol 2000;36(2):375–80.
[149] Lapanum W, et al. Major pulmonary embolism and shock. Persistent hypotension after thrombolysis treated with improvised mechanical fragmentation of thrombus. Med J Aust 2003;179(9):495–6.

[150] Konstantinides S. Thrombolysis in submassive pulmonary embolism? Yes. J Thromb Haemost 2003;1:1127–9.
[151] Dalen JE. Thrombolysis in submassive pulmonary embolism? No. J Thromb Haemost 2003;1: 1130–2.
[152] Kasper W, et al. Management strategies and determinants of outcome in acute major pulmonary embolism: results of a multicenter registry. J Am Coll Cardiol 1997;30:1165–71.
[153] Konstantinides S, et al. Association between thrombolytic treatment and the prognosis of hemodynamically stable patients with major pulmonary embolism. Circulation 1997;96:882–8.
[154] Konstantinides S, et al. Heparin plus alteplase compared with heparin alone in patients with submassive pulmonary embolism. N Engl J Med 2002;347:1143–50.
[155] Konstantinides S. Should thrombolytic therapy be used in patients with pulmonary embolism? Am J Cardiovasc Drugs 2004;4(2):69–74.
[156] The Global Use of Strategies to Open Occluded Coronary Arteries (GUSTO) V Investigators. A comparison of heparin plus full, bolus dose reteplase with half-dose reteplase plus abciximab plus heparin in patients with acute myocardial infarction. Lancet 2001;357:1905.
[157] O'Meara JJ, et al. A decision analysis of streptokinase plus heparin as compared with heparin alone for deep-vein thrombosis. N Engl J Med 1994;330:1864–9.
[158] Verstraete M, Vermylen J, Donati MB. The effect of streptokinase infusion on chronic arterial occlusions and stenoses. Ann Intern Med 1971;74(3):377–82.
[159] Cotton LT, Flute PT, Tsapogas MJ. Popliteal artery thrombosis treated with streptokinase. Lancet 1962;2:1081–3.
[160] Amery A, et al. Outcome of recent thromboembolic occlusions of limb arteries treated with streptokinase. BMJ 1970;4(736):639–44.
[161] Sicard GA, et al. Thrombolytic therapy for acute arterial occlusion. J Vasc Surg 1985;2(1): 65–78.
[162] Hallett Jr JW, et al. Statistical determinants of success and complications of thrombolytic therapy for arterial occlusion of lower extremity. Surg Gynecol Obstet 1985;161(5):431–7.
[163] Chaise LS, et al. Selective intra-arterial streptokinase therapy in the immediate postoperative period. JAMA 1982;247(17):2397–400.
[164] Hess H, et al. Local low-dose thrombolytic therapy of peripheral arterial occlusions. N Engl J Med 1982;307(26):1627–30.
[165] Berni GA, et al. Streptokinase treatment of acute arterial occlusion. Ann Surg 1983;198(2): 185–91.
[166] Ouriel K, Veith F, Sasahara AA. Investigators for the Thrombolysis or Peripheral Artery Surgery (TOPAS). A comparison of recombinant urokinase with vascular surgery as initial treatment for acute arterial occlusion of the legs. N Engl J Med 1998;338:1105.
[167] Ouriel K, et al. A comparison of thrombolytic therapy with operative revascularization in the initial treatment of acute peripheral arterial ischemia. J Vasc Surg 1994;19(6):1021–30.
[168] Working Party on Thrombolysis in the Management of Limb Ischemia. Thrombolysis in the management of lower limb peripheral arterial occlusion: a consensus document. Am J Cardiol 1998;81:207–18.
[169] McNamara TO, Fischer JR. Thrombolysis of peripheral arterial and graft occlusions: improved results using high-dose urokinase. AJR Am J Roentgenol 1985;144(4):769–75.
[170] Ouriel K, Veith FJ, Sasahara AA. Thrombolysis or peripheral arterial surgery: phase I results. TOPAS Investigators. J Vasc Surg 1996;23:64–73.
[171] Ward AS, Andaz SK, Bygrave S. Peripheral thrombolysis with tissue plasminogen activator: results of two treatment regimens. Arch Surg 1994;129:861–5.
[172] Braithwaite BD, Buckenham TM, Galland RB, on behalf of the Thrombolysis Study Group. Prospective randomized trial of high-dose versus low-dose tissue plasminogen activator infusion in the management of acute limb ischemia. Br J Surg 1997;84:646–50.
[173] Ouriel K, et al. Reteplase in the treatment of peripheral arterial and venous occlusions: a pilot study. J Vasc Interv Radiol 2000;11:849–54.
[174] Castaneda F, et al. Declining-dose study of reteplase treatment for lower extremity arterial occlusions. J Vasc Interv Radiol 2002;13:1093–8.

[175] Mahler F, Schneider E, Hess H. Recombinant tissue plasminogen activator versus urokinase for local thrombolysis of femoropopliteal occlusions: a prospective, randomized multicenter trial. J Endovasc Ther 2001;8:638–47.
[176] The STILE Investigators. Results of a prospective randomized trial evaluating surgery versus thrombolysis for ischemia of the lower extremity. The STILE Trial. Ann Surg 1994;220:251.
[177] Davidian MM, et al. Initial results of reteplase in the treatment of acute lower extremity arterial occlusions. J Vasc Interv Radiol 2000;11:289–94.
[178] Castaneda F, et al. Catheter-directed thrombolysis in deep venous thrombosis with the use of reteplase: immediate results and complications from a pilot study. J Vasc Interv Radiol 2002; 13:577–80.
[179] Razavi MK, et al. Initial clinical results of tenecteplase (TNK) in catheter-directed thrombolytic therapy. J Endovasc Ther 2002;9:593–8.
[180] Burkart DJ, et al. Thrombolysis of occluded peripheral arteries and veins with tenecteplase: a pilot study. J Vasc Interv Radiol 2002;13:1099–102.
[181] Patel N, et al. SCVIR reporting standards for the treatment of acute limb ischemia with the use of transluminal removal of arterial thrombus. J Vasc Interv Radiol 2001;12:559–70.
[182] Weatherby SJ, et al. Good outcome in early pregnancy following direct thrombolysis for cerebral venous sinus thrombosis. J Neurol 2003;250(11):1372–3.
[183] Murry KR, Rhoney DH, Coplin WM. Urokinase in the treatment of intraventricular hemorrhage. Ann Pharmacother 1998;32(2):256–8.
[184] Amin-Hanjani S, Ogilvy CS, Barker Jr FG. Does intracisternal thrombolysis prevent vasospasm after aneurysmal subarachnoid hemorrhage? A meta-analysis. Neurosurgery 2004; 54(2):326–34 [discussion: 334–5].
[185] Lee WA, et al. Surgical intervention is not required for all patients with subclavian vein thrombosis. J Vasc Surg 2000;32(1):57–67.
[186] Urschel Jr HC, Razzuk MA. Paget-Schroetter syndrome: what is the best management? Ann Thorac Surg 2000;69(6):1663–8 [discussion: 1668–9].
[187] Leebeek FW, et al. Budd-Chiari syndrome, portal vein and mesenteric vein thrombosis in a patient homozygous for factor V Leiden mutation treated by TIPS and thrombolysis. Br J Haematol 1998;102(4):929–31.
[188] Bhattacharjya T, et al. Percutaneous portal vein thrombolysis and endovascular stent for management of post transplant portal venous conduit thrombosis. Transplantation 2000;69(10): 2195–8.
[189] Henao EA, Bohannon WT, Silva Jr MB. Treatment of portal venous thrombosis with selective superior mesenteric artery infusion of recombinant tissue plasminogen activator. J Vasc Surg 2003;38(6):1411–5.
[190] Silber H, et al. The St. Jude valve. Thrombolysis as the first line of therapy for cardiac valve thrombosis. Circulation 1993;87:30–7.
[191] Shapira Y, et al. Thrombolysis is an effective and safe therapy in stuck bileaflet mitral valves in the absence of high-risk thrombi. J Am Coll Cardiol 2000;35(7):1874–80.
[192] Roudaut R, et al. Fibrinolysis of mechanical prosthetic valve thrombosis: a single center study of 127 cases. J Am Coll Cardiol 2003;41:653–8.
[193] Durrleman N, et al. Prosthetic valve thrombosis: twenty-year experience at the Montreal Heart Institute. J Thorac Cardiovasc Surg 2004;127(5):1388–92.
[194] Agazzi A, et al. Local thrombolytic therapy in cancer patients with central venous catheter occlusion in urgent need of antiblastic treatment: a single institution experience. J Thromb Thrombolysis 2003;15(2):109–11.
[195] Marder VJ. Thrombolytic therapy: foundations and results. In: Colman R, Hirsh J, Marder VJ, et al, editors. Hemostasis and thrombosis: basic principles and clinical practice. 4th edition. Philadelphia: Lippincott; 2001. p. 1475.
[196] Gore J, Granger C, Simoons M, et al. Stroke after thrombolysis. Mortality and functional outcomes in the GUSTO-1 trial. Global Use of Strategies to Open Occluded Coronary Artery. Circulation 1995;92:2811.

[197] Kandzari DE, et al. Risk factors for intracranial hemorrhage and nonhemorrhagic stroke after fibrinolytic therapy (from the GUSTO-i trial). Am J Cardiol 2004;93(4):458–61.

[198] Leopold J, Keaney J, Loscalzo J. Pharmacology of thrombolytic agents. In: Loscalzo J, Schafer A, editors. Thrombosis and hemorrhage. Baltimore: Williams and Wilkins; 1998. p. 1215–58.

[199] Investigators of the International Joint Efficacy Comparison of Thrombolytics (INJECT). Randomized, double-blind comparison of reteplase double-bolus administration with streptokinase in acute myocardial infarction (INJECT): trial to investigate equivalence. Lancet 1995; 346:329.

[200] Gurwitz JH, et al. Risk for intracranial hemorrhage after tissue plasminogen activator treatment for acute myocardial infarction. Participants in the National Registry of Myocardial Infarction 2. Ann Intern Med 1998;129(8):597–604.

[201] Cannon CP, et al. Comparison of front-loaded recombinant tissue-type plasminogen activator, anistreplase and combination thrombolytic therapy for acute myocardial infarction: results of the Thrombolysis in Myocardial Infarction (TIMI) 4 trial. J Am Coll Cardiol 1994;24:1604–10.

[202] Smalling R, et al. More rapid, complete, and stable coronary thrombolysis with bolus administration of reteplase compared with alteplase infusion in acute myocardial infarction. Circulation 1995;91:2725–32.

[203] Cannon CP, et al. TNK-tissue plasminogen activator in acute myocardial infarction. Results of the Thrombloysis in Myocardial infarction (TIMI) 10. A dose-ranging trial. Circulation 1997; 95:351.

[204] The TIMI Study Group. Thrombolysis in Myocardial Infarction (TIMI) trial phase I findings. N Engl J Med 1985;312:932.

[205] Gruppo Italiano per lo Studio della Sopravvivenza nell'Infarto Miocardico. GISSI-2: a factorial randomized trial of alteplase versus streptokinase and heparin versus no heparin among 12,490 patients with acute myocardial infarction. Lancet 1990;336:65.

[206] Third International Study of Infarct Survival (ISIS-3) Collaborative Group. ISIS3: a randomized comparison of streptokinase versus tissue plasminogen activator versus anistreplase and of aspirin plus heparin versus aspirin alone among 14,299 cases of suspected acute myocardial infarction. Lancet 1992;339:753.

[207] The GUSTO Angiographic Investigators. The effects of tissue plasminogen activator, streptokinase, or both on coronary-artery patency, ventricular function, and survival after acute myocardial infarction. N Engl J Med 1993;329:1615.

[208] Bode C, et al. Randomized comparison of coronary thrombolysis achieved with double-bolus reteplase (recombinant plasminogen activator) and front-loaded alteplase (recombinant tissue plasminogen activator) in patients with acute myocardial infarction. Circulation 1995;94:891.

[209] The Global Use of Strategies to Open Occluded Coronary Arteries. (GUSTO-III) Investigators. A comparison of reteplase with alteplase for acute myocardial infarction. N Engl J Med 1997; 337:1118.

[210] Kleiman N, et al. Profound inhibition of platelet aggregation with monoclonal antibody 7E3 fab following thrombolytic therapy: results of the TAMI 8 pilot study. J Am Coll Cardiol 1993; 22:381–9.

[211] Strategies for Patency Enhancement in the Emergency Department (SPEED) Trial Group. Trial of abciximab with and without low-dose reteplase for acute myocardial infarction: Strategies for Patency Enhancement in the Emergency Department (SPEED). Circulation 2000;101:2788.

[212] The Assessment of the Safety and Efficacy of a New Thrombolytic Regimen Investigators. Efficacy and safety of tenecteplase in combination with enoxaparin, abcixmab, or unfractionated heparin: the ASSENT-3 randomized trial in acute myocardial infarction. Lancet 2001;358:605.

[213] Brener S, et al. Eptifibatide and low-dose tissue plasminogen activator in acute myocardial infarction. The Integrilin and Low-Dose Thrombolysis in Acute Myocardial Infraction (INTRO-AMI) trial. J Am Coll Cardiol 2003;39:377–86.

[214] Giugliano RP, et al. Combination reperfusion therapy with eptifibatide and reduced-dose tenecteplase for ST-elevation myocardial infarction. Results of the Integrilin and tenecteplase in

acute myocardial infarction (INTEGRITI) phase II angiographic trial. J Am Coll Cardiol 2003; 41:1251–60.

[215] Antman EM, et al. Abciximab facilitates the rate and extent of thrombolysis: results of the thrombolysis in myocardial infarction (TIMI) 14 trial. The TIMI 14 Investigators. Circulation 1999;99(21):2720–32.

[216] The InTIME-II Investigators. Intravenous NPA for the treatment of single-bolus lanoteplase vs accelerated alteplase for the treatment of patients with acute mycardial infarction. Eur Heart J 2000;21:2005.

[217] Wallentin L, et al. Low molecular weight heparin (dalteparin) compared to unfractionated heparin as an adjunct to rt-PA (alteplase) for improvement of coronary artery patency in acute myocardial infarction-the ASSENT Plus study. Eur Heart J 2003;24:897–908.

[218] Simoons ML, et al. Improved reperfusion and clinical outcome with enoxaparin as an adjunct to streptokinase thrombolysis in acute myocardial infarction. The AMI-SK study. Eur Heart J 2002;23:1282–90.

[219] Ross AM, et al. Randomized comparison of enoxaparin, a low- molecular-weight heparin, with unfractionated heparin adjunctive to recombinant tissue plasminogen activator thrombolysis and aspirin: second trial of Heparin and Aspirin Reperfusion Therapy (HART II). Circulation 2001;104:648–52.

[220] Lee L. Initial experience with hirudin and streptokinase in acute myocardial infarction: results of the Thrombolysis in Myocardial Infarction (TIMI) 6 trial. Am J Cardiol 1995;75:7–13.

[221] Antman EM. Hirudin in acute myocardial infarction: Thrombolysis and Thrombin in Myocardial Infarction (TIMI) 9b trial. Circulation 1996;94:911–21.

[222] Neuhaus K, et al. Safety observations from the pilot phase of the randomized r-Hirudin for Improvement of Thrombolysis (HITT-III) study: a study of the Arbeirsgemeinschaft Leitender Kardiologischer Krankenhausarzte (ALKK). Circulation 1994;90:1638–42.

[223] The Hirulog and Early Reperfusion or Occlusion (HERO) 2 Trial Investigators. Thrombin-specific anticoagulation with bivalrudin versus heparin in patients receiving fibrinolytic therapy for acute myocardial infarction: The HERO-2 randomized trial. Lancet 2001;358:1855.

[224] Zhao XQ, et al. Intracoronary thrombus and platelet glycoprotein IIb/IIIa receptor blockade with tirofiban in unstable angina or non-Q-wave myocardial infarction. Angiographic results from the PRISM-PLUS trial (Platelet receptor inhibition for ischemic syndrome management in patients limited by unstable signs and symptoms.) PRISM-PLUS Investigators. Circulation 1999;100(15):1609–15.

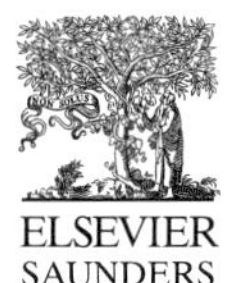

ELSEVIER
SAUNDERS

Hematol Oncol Clin N Am
19 (2005) 183–202

HEMATOLOGY/
ONCOLOGY
CLINICS OF
NORTH AMERICA

Catheter-Related Thrombosis in Cancer Patients: Pathophysiology, Diagnosis, and Management

Rachel P. Rosovsky, MD, David J. Kuter, MD, DPhil*

Hematology/Oncology Unit, Massachusetts General Hospital, Harvard Medical School, 100 Blossom Street, Boston, MA 02114, USA

Central venous catheters (CVCs) have become an integral part of treating patients in and out of the hospital and essential for the management of cancer patients. In the United States, more than 5 million CVCs are inserted every year [1], including over 200,000 ports implanted into cancer patients. These devices allow the administration of alimentation, chemotherapy, blood products, and antimicrobial therapy and allow the withdrawal of blood samples from the central circulation. Eliminating frequent venipunctures clearly increases a patient's level of comfort. Whether the use of CVCs translates into extending or improving the quality of life currently is being investigated in a number of different studies [2].

It was not until 1952 that Aubaniac [3–7] described cannulating the subclavian vein of a wounded soldier for the purpose of resuscitation. In the subsequent 50 years, a number of devices have been introduced for the semipermanent cannulation of the central venous system (Box 1). In 1973, Broviac et al [8] developed the first long-term CVC for parenteral nutrition. This was followed by the Hickman catheter in 1979, which was the first permanent venous access device used for cancer chemotherapy [9]. Totally implantable venous access devices (Fig. 1), ones that contain their own ports attached to a centrally placed catheter and are totally subcutaneous (SC), became available in the early 1980s

Funded, in part, by National Institutes of Health grant HL72299 to D.J. Kuter as part of the Transfusion Medicine and Hemostasis Network.

The authors do not have a relationship with any commercial company or direct or indirect financial interest in this subject matter.

* Corresponding author.

E-mail address: kuter.david@mgh.harvard.edu (D.J. Kuter).

doi:10.1016/j.hoc.2004.09.007

Box 1. Types of central venous catheters

Short-term devices (1–14 days)

Percutaneous internal jugular, subclavian, femoral lines
Peripherally implanted central catheters

Long-term devices (months–years)

Surgically tunneled catheters (Hickman, Broviac, Groshong, Quinton)
Totally implanted venous access devices (Mediport, Infus-a-Port, Port-a-Cath [Smith Medical MD, Inc, St. Paul, Minnesota])

[10]. The most recent advancement has been the peripherally implanted central catheters [11].

These devices are associated with a number of early and late complications (Box 2). Of these, thrombosis is a particularly frequent complication. Given the widespread use of CVCs in oncology, this review focuses on the thrombotic complications of CVCs in cancer patients. CVC-related thrombosis refers to all types of thrombi, including fibrin sheaths, intraluminal clots, and DVTs; whereas CVC-related DVT refers only to those mural thrombi that partially or completely block the blood vessel.

Types of thrombi associated with central venous catheters

Fibrin sheath formation

Soon after insertion, a fibrin sheath forms around almost all catheters. In an autopsy study of patients who had CVCs, 55 of 55 (100%) patients developed

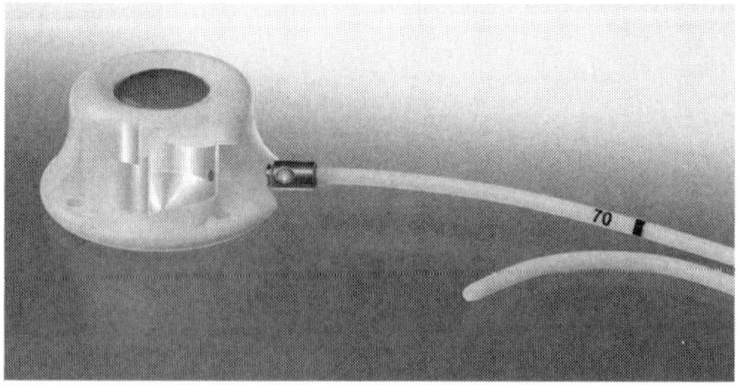

Fig. 1. Cutaway photo of Port-a-Cath implantable port showing the injection site, reservoir, and attached catheter. (Courtesy of Smith Medical MD, Inc, St. Paul, Minnesota.)

Box 2. Incidence of complications of central venous catheters

Early

Arrhythmia: 13%
Arterial puncture: 2.8% to 3.8%
Malposition of reservoir: 2%
Pneumothorax: 1% to 1.8%
Wound dehiscence: 1.5%
Hemorrhage: 1.1% to 1.2%
Failure of insertion: 1.2%

Late

Infection: 4% to 38%
Catheter fracture and embolization: 3%
Migration of catheter tip: 7.4%
Thrombosis: ~41% (range, 12%–74%)
  Asymptomatic: ~29% (range, 5%–62%)
  Symptomatic: ~12% (range, 5%–41%)

Sequelae of CVC-related thrombosis

Postphlebitic syndrome: 15% to 35%
Pulmonary embolization: ~11% (range, 7%–31%)
  Symptomatic: ~6% (range, 3%–14%)
  Asymptomatic: ~5% (range, 3%–15%)

this sheath, and in phlebographic studies, 45 of 57 (78%) had a fibrin sheath [12,13]. A venographic study by De Cicco et al [14] showed that 83 of 95 (87%) patients had these sheaths. Finally, these sheaths were present in 16 of 16 (100%) patients who were analyzed at the removal of their CVC after 3 to 34 (median 12.5) months of use [15].

Although the time of formation of the fibrin sheath has not been adequately studied, partial data from several studies show that the sheath develops within 24 hours of catheter insertion [12]. Furthermore, detailed studies by quantitative electron microscopy and by quantitative microbiologic testing of these fibrin sheaths over time show that they are always colonized by cocci [16–18].

The presence of these sheaths, however, does not predict subsequent deep venous thrombosis (DVT) of the vessel in which the catheter is placed. In one study, only 1 of 16 patients with a fibrin sheath developed thrombosis over a median of 12.5 months [15]. Furthermore, embolization of the fibrin sheath is uncommon and rarely is symptomatic, given the small volume of the embolus [14].

Intraluminal thrombosis of central venous catheters

A very common, and usually under-reported, event is the development of clotting within the lumen of the catheter [19–21]. This event usually is uncovered when the catheter fails to allow blood to be withdrawn or fails to allow infusion through a port. The frequency of this event varies widely among different studies. Anderson et al [21] reported 40 of 43 (93%) patients had this complication. In a large study by Schwarz et al [20], 122 of 923 (13.2%) patients had this problem, for a frequency of 0.81 events per 1000 catheter days, comparable with the 0.6 per 1000 catheter days reported by Ray [19]. It is fortunate that these intraluminal thrombi can be lysed in most situations (80%–95%) with fibrinolytic agents such as urokinase, streptokinase, and tissue plasminogen activator [22,23].

The inability to withdraw blood ("ball-valve effect") does not, however, predict the presence of intraluminal thrombosis. This phenomenon is of low specificity in predicting thrombosis of the catheter lumen or the blood vessel in which the catheter resides. In a study by Gould et al [24], 57% of thrombosed CVCs versus 27% of nonthrombosed CVCs failed to draw blood. When the CVCs that had problems with blood withdrawal were analyzed by venography, 58% had thrombosis and 42% did not have thrombosis [25], leading to the conclusion that nonthrombotic mechanical problems commonly prevented blood flow.

Central venous catheter–related blood vessel thrombosis (deep venous thrombosis)

The major thrombotic complication of CVCs is DVT. These mural thrombi may partially or completely block the blood vessel and, as described in greater detail later, involve 12% to 74% of all CVCs. Most CVCs (~71%) are asymptomatic. In those that are symptomatic, symptoms include arm/neck/head swelling or pain, headache, numbness of the extremity, erythema of the extremity, phlegmasia, venous distention, prominent vascular markings of the skin, or jaw pain.

Table 1 lists studies of patients with CVCs who developed symptoms and then clot in the affected blood vessel documented by venogram or ultrasound [21,24,26–38]. On average, 12% of all patients who had CVCs developed symptomatic thrombi, but there was a wide range (5%–41%) of all CVC insertions. The cause of this wide variability is due, in part, to the wide variation in catheter type, position, duration of insertion, and the underlying diseases. In addition, there is a lack of uniform standards in reporting this sort of information.

In a smaller group of studies, all patients underwent venographic studies at some time after their CVC placement, irrespective of symptoms [13,14,16,34, 39–48]. These venographic studies (Table 2) showed that approximately 41% (range, 12%–74%) of all patients who had CVCs developed thrombi. In those few studies in which symptoms also were assessed, 29% (range, 5%–62%) of all patients with CVCs had asymptomatic thrombi and 12% (range, 5%–54%) of all patients with CVCs had symptomatic thrombi. The latter value is identical to the

Table 1
Central venous catheter–related deep vein thrombosis—symptomatic

Author [reference no.]	N	Symptomatic DVT n (%)
Conlan et al [28]	46	19 (41)
Anderson et al [21]	168	22 (13)
Boraks et al [26]	115	15 (13)
Knofler et al [35]	77	11 (14)
Carr and Rabinowitz [27]	65	14 (21)
Craft et al [29]	153	12 (8)
de Gregorio et al [30]	188	13 (5)
Eastman et al [31]	160	26 (16)
Eastridge and Lefor [32]	209	21 (10)
Eastridge and Lefor [32]	113	7 (6)
Goey et al [33]	14	5 (36)
Gould et al [24]	255	35 (14)
Wermes et al [37]	137	10 (7)
Minassian et al [36]	209	24 (11)
Haire et al [63]	217	23 (11)
Heaton et al [38]	43	5 (12)
Total	2169	262 (12)

12% incidence seen in Table 1 for those individuals for whom only symptomatic thrombi were assessed [14,34,40,42,45,49]. Therefore, only about one in three mural thrombi results in symptoms. Indeed, in a study of 12 individuals who had totally occlusive clots of the upper extremity, only 4 (33%) had any symptoms [14].

The time of onset of these CVC-related clots has been studied longitudinally in only a small number of individuals. In the most extensive study by De Cicco

Table 2
Central venous catheter–related deep vein thrombosis—symptomatic and asymptomatic

Study	N	Total DVT n (%)	Symptomatic DVT n (%)	Asymptomatic DVT n (%)
Balestreri et al [13]	57	32 (56)		
De Cicco et al [14]	95	63 (66)	4 (4)	59 (62)
Horne et al [44]	35	14 (40)		
Monreal et al [45]	13	8 (62)	7 (54)	1 (8)
Bern et al [40]	40	15 (38)	13 (33)	2 (5)
Raad et al [47]	72	26 (36)		
Pucheu et al [46]	72	11 (15)		
Barzaghi et al [39]	38	28 (74)		
Glaser et al [42]	24	12 (50)	3 (13)	9 (38)
Horne et al [49]	50	20 (40)	5 (10)	15 (30)
Haire et al [34]	17	6 (35)	2 (12)	4 (24)
Reichardt et al [48]	94	11 (12)	5 (5)	6 (6)
Total	607	246 (41)	39 (12)	96 (29)

et al [14], serial venography was done, on average, 8, 30, and 105 days after insertion of CVCs. Of the CVCs that ultimately developed clots, 64% occurred by day 8 and 98% occurred by day 30 [14]. In other studies, 98% of all blood clots occurred in the first 8 days in one study [50] and 68% of all blood clots occurred within the first 30 days in another study [51]. Further analysis of the time course of thrombus formation is essential in helping to guide future studies addressing the timing and duration of anticoagulation prophylaxis to prevent CVC-related DVT (vide infra).

Sequelae of central venous catheter thrombosis

Autopsy studies

The pathologic effects of CVCs on blood vessels were studied in 74 consecutive autopsies of cancer patients who had CVCs in which the cannulated vessel was compared with the contralateral vessel that was not cannulated [47]. Venous pathology (hemorrhage, thrombosis, calcification, ulceration, and inflammation) was found in 49% of the cannulated blood vessels but in only 9% of those that were not cannulated. Furthermore, mural thrombosis was seen in 30% of the cannulated vessels and in only 1% of those not cannulated; in the latter case, the one patient with mural thrombosis and no recent catheter exposure had a cannula in this blood vessel several months earlier.

Infection of central venous catheters

Thrombosis is a major risk factor for infection of CVCs. This complication was first suggested by Press et al [52] in 1984 who found that bacteremia was much more common in patients with a documented CVC-related thrombosis. Subsequent studies have confirmed this finding. In the previously mentioned autopsy study of patients with CVCs, 7 of 31 (23%) CVCs with clots and 0 of 41 (0%) CVCs without clots documented at autopsy previously had experienced an associated bacteremia [16,17,47]. In a separate study, 5 of 28 (18%) CVCs with clot had clinical infection versus 0 of 10 (0%) CVCs without clot [39]. The odds ratio for infection related to thrombosis is 4.1 (confidence interval: 1.5–11.4) [31], and prophylactic heparin/vancomycin/ciprofloxacin or heparin/vancomycin flushes reduced blood infection threefold compared with heparin alone [53]. This finding is not surprising because almost all cannulated blood vessels contain a fibrin sheath that is seeded with adherent cocci [16–18,47].

Postphlebitic syndrome

After removal of CVCs from thrombosed vessels, the thrombi often persist. In a small study of 30 patients, venography was performed at variable times after the routine removal of a CVC. Nine (30%) patients had total occlusion of the blood vessel. Of these nine, only two had prior symptoms of thrombosis [49]. It is unfortunate that few other studies have looked at the long-term resolution and collateral blood vessel formation in patients with CVC-related thrombosis. Given the widespread use of CVCs in oncology, further studies in this area are warranted.

Fifteen percent to 35% of patients with CVC-related DVT develop the postphlebitic syndrome (see Box 2). Massoure et al [54] analyzed patients with upper-extremity DVT and found that 14 of 40 (35%) developed the postphlebitic syndrome. Prandoni et al [55] found that 4 of 27 (15%) patients with upper-extremity DVT developed a postphlebitic syndrome. The long-term complications of this syndrome are hard to assess in the cancer population, given the oftentimes short survival of those affected with CVC-related thrombosis.

Pulmonary emboli

DVT of the upper extremity has long been considered as being of trivial importance for embolization due to its location and modest size. Nonetheless, symptomatic pulmonary emboli (PE) have been reported in approximately 6% of all patients with upper-extremity DVT (see Box 2). Most of the patients in these studies [14,21,54] had CVCs and most had cancer, but these studies also included some patients who lacked CVCs and some noncancer patients. The subjects in the three studies, therefore, are heterogeneous but 2 of 40 (5%), 3 of 22 (14%), and 2 of 63 (3%) patients, respectively, who had upper-extremity DVT were found to have symptomatic PE [14,21,54].

In four separate studies [45,55–57] in which ventilation/perfusion (V/Q) scans were performed on all patients with upper-extremity DVT irrespective of pulmonary symptoms, the average total PE rate of 11% was twice that of the symptomatic PE rate (~5.5%). Although usually not fatal, in these four studies, 4 of 20 (20%), 13 of 86 (15%), 16 of 237 (7%), and 8 of 27 (30%) patients, respectively, were found to have a significant V/Q mismatch and a diagnosis of PE [45,55–57]. This rate is comparable to the rate of asymptomatic PE seen in patients with symptomatic lower-extremity DVT.

Risk factors for central venous catheter–related thrombosis

Patient

The patient risk factors related to CVC thrombosis are multiple. Most have not been studied in a comprehensive fashion but some can be substantiated by a number of studies, primarily in oncology patients.

The presence of malignancy seems to result in a higher rate of CVC-related thrombosis than the lack of malignancy. In oncology patients, there also is some suggestion that some types of malignancy may be associated with an increased rate of CVC-related thrombosis. Anderson et al [21] reported that 45% of patients with adenocarcinoma of the lung developed symptomatic CVC-related thrombosis, whereas only 9% of those with head and neck cancer developed CVC-related thrombosis. This may be related to the activation of the coagulation system in these different malignancies, tumor-related changes in blood flow, or levels of tissue factor or tissue factor pathway inhibitor. It is probably related to the general increased risk of thrombosis that occurs in oncology patients, as discussed elsewhere [58–61].

Most studies show that the inherited thrombophilia risk factors likely are not a major predictor of CVC-related thrombosis. One study, however, reported that low antithrombin III levels were associated with an increased risk of thrombosis [41]. Another study found that 32% of patients who had CVC-related thrombosis had a diagnosis of a hypercoagulable state; most had an elevated anticardiolipin antibody but no increase in prothrombin 20210A mutation, factor V Leiden, protein C deficiency, or protein S deficiency [62]. In children, however, it was found that 63% of those who had CVC-related thrombosis had an inherited risk factor, and most were compound heterozygotes [35]. In a related study, this increased risk for CVC-related thrombosis appeared to occur only in children with acute lymphoblastic leukemia [37].

Acquired thrombophilia risks may be more important causes of CVC-related thrombosis but are more difficult to document. One component of Virchow's triad is vessel damage. Numerous studies have documented local endothelial cell injury to blood vessels due to chemotherapy or to the CVC itself. Endothelial cell erosion in cannulated blood vessels has been reported [21]. Furthermore, there is a lower thrombomodulin level and a higher plasminogen activator inhibitor/tissue plasminogen activator level in blood from patients with CVC-related thrombosis than from those without thrombosis [43].

Other hematologic values such as the fibrinogen level and platelet count have been measured in patients with CVC-related thrombosis, but the data are conflicting [34,40,63]. It is, perhaps, clearer to say that most CVC-related thrombi are not related to elevations of fibrinogen or platelet count.

Finally, the type of chemotherapy does appear to be related to the rate of CVC-related thrombosis. Clotting occurred in 6 of 11 (55%) catheters through which sclerosing chemotherapy was infused but in only 9 of 29 (31%) infused with nonsclerosing chemotherapy [40].

Device

In the effort to develop catheters that minimize trauma to blood vessels and are less thrombogenic, major changes in catheter design and materials have been made. The substitution of Silastic or flexible plastic for polyethylene has been a major change, as has the use of different plasticizers.

The position of the catheter in the vascular system is a major determinate of CVC-related thrombosis. More thrombosis is seen when the catheter tip is placed high in the superior vena cava than when the catheter tip is placed low in the superior vena cava [20,29,32,64,65]. A possible explanation is the increased chance of damage to the blood vessel when the catheter tip is in the higher position rather than the lower. In addition, CVCs inserted from the left subclavian vein clotted more commonly than CVCs inserted from the right subclavian vein [14,24,27,66]. In a recent study, 14 of 16 (87%) left-side CVCs versus 49 of 79 (62%) right-side CVCs were reported to clot [14].

Finally, the number of catheter lumens is a major predictor of catheter thrombosis. Triple-lumen Hickman catheters failed at three times the rate of double-lumen catheters [32]. Presumably, the mechanism of action for this finding is that with a stiffer catheter, there is more occlusion of the blood vessel or more trauma to the blood vessel.

Overall, CVCs are a "stress test" of the coagulation system in cancer patients and can precipitate thrombosis due to multiple mechanisms related to the host or the device.

Diagnosis of central venous catheter–related deep venous thrombosis

Although contrast venography is considered the "gold standard" for diagnosing CVC-related DVT, it is expensive, invasive, and requires the need for contrast agents. Consequently, ultrasound with Doppler and color imaging currently is used. The criteria used to diagnose a clot by ultrasound include the absence of spontaneous flow or presence of turbulent flow, abnormal waveforms peripheral to an occluded segment that do not vary with respirations or cardiac pulsations, and visualization of a thrombi or inability to compress the veins.

Studies evaluating the efficacy of ultrasound in the diagnosis of suspected upper-extremity DVTs report sensitivities of 54% to 100% and specificities of 94% to 100% [67]. It is unfortunate that there are only a limited number of studies that directly address the accuracy of ultrasound in diagnosing suspected CVC-related DVT. Koksoy et al [68] studied 44 patients with CVC-related DVT and found that color Doppler ultrasound had a sensitivity and specificity of 94% and 96%, respectively. Of importance, the sensitivity of duplex ultrasound decreases significantly when used in the asymptomatic patient.

Two factors that influence the sensitivity of ultrasound are the location of the clot and the presence of the catheter. Clots located in the jugular, axillary, or subclavian veins are picked up more frequently than those located in the innominate or superior vena caval veins [69]. In addition, the presence of a catheter can alter not only the venous tone but also the venous flow, making it more difficult to interpret findings visualized on ultrasound.

Newer diagnostic tools currently are being investigated and include magnetic resonance venography and spiral CT. Preliminary studies show promising results with these newer modalities; however, randomized trials are necessary to compare them with the current standard of venography [70,71].

In practice, color Doppler ultrasound is the first tool used to diagnose suspected CVC-related DVT. If a negative result is obtained and the clinical suspicion is high, however, additional testing with serial ultrasounds or venography is warranted. Diagnosing asymptomatic clots remains a challenge.

Treatment of central venous catheter–related deep venous thrombosis

Due to the lack of prospective or comparative studies, there are currently no standard guidelines for the treatment of CVC-related DVT. Consequently, patients with this complication are treated in a manner similar to those who have lower-extremity DVT. Unfractionated heparin (UFH) or low molecular weight heparin (LMWH) is given for 5 to 7 days, and then patients are continued on warfarin sodium (Coumadin). Recent studies favor LMWH because it has been shown to be as effective as UFH and can be given as an outpatient treatment [72]. In addition, cancer patients may benefit more from LMWH than warfarin [73]. Pentasaccharides and oral direct thrombin inhibitors have not yet been studied in this situation. The optimal duration of anticoagulation is unknown. Most studies show that 6 months is effective; however, patients with active cancer may benefit from indefinite use.

The authors have routinely used the following approach:

1. If the CVC is nonfunctional, then it is removed and replaced as necessary in another vascular bed. If it is functional, then the CVC is kept in place if still needed.
2. All patients with adequate renal clearance receive dalteparin (150 IU/kg SC daily) or enoxaparin (1.5 mg/kg SC daily).
3. In the absence of active malignancy, all patients are then converted to warfarin (international normalized ratio [INR] 2–3) and treated for 3 to 6 months. In the presence of active malignancy, all are kept on the LMWH for at least 3 to 6 months.
4. Patients with heparin-induced thrombocytopenia are treated with fondaparinux (5 mg SC daily).
5. Patients with reduced renal function are treated initially with UFH, followed by warfarin.

Two other, more aggressive options—systemic thrombolysis and thrombectomy—have not been studied in a randomized fashion and, as a result, are not practiced routinely. In addition, the strategy to remove the catheter has not been extensively studied and remains controversial. Inserting another catheter is costly and associated with increased morbidity.

If a patient has a contraindication to anticoagulation therapy, then a superior caval vein filter can be placed. This filter has the potential to prevent subsequent complications with CVC-related DVT, such as PE or superior vena cava syndrome [74]. The long-term implications of filters, however, must be taken into account when considering their use. The authors believe that the use of such devices is rarely indicated.

If the thrombus is located at the tip or sleeve of the catheter, then local measures are effective. Low-dose thrombolytic therapy such as alteplase, urokinase, or streptokinase can be given locally and has been shown to restore patency in most patients [75]. Occasionally, patients will need repeated boluses to achieve flow.

The optimal way to treat CVC-related DVT is to try to prevent it from occurring in the first place. Much controversy exists as to the best way to accomplish this, and there are ongoing studies addressing this issue.

Costs of central venous catheter–related thrombosis

Loss of function of the CVC due to thrombosis often leads to the need to replace such ports at an average cost of approximately $5,000. Furthermore, partial obstruction or complete obstruction of the port lumen leads to efforts to clear the thrombosis with fibrinolytic drugs such as recombinant tissue plasminogen activator, urokinase, and streptokinase. A typical 1-mg tissue plasminogen activator flush costs $27.50, and the nursing time and frustration involved in trying to clear clogged catheters may dramatically increase the cost to open an occluded port. Finally, and difficult to quantify in monetary terms, is the associated patient anxiety, discomfort, and morbidity, and the need, at times, for prolonged systemic anticoagulation that comes from an occluded lumen or from an occluded blood vessel.

These costs have prompted major efforts to reduce CVC-related thrombosis. These efforts include the use of biomaterials, polymers, and plasticizers of low thrombogenicity. Impregnation of catheters with antithrombotic substances such as heparin/antithrombin III has been studied [76]. Early attempts to impregnate catheters with UFH resulted in rapid leaching from the catheter surface. Recent catheters, however, have a different bonding procedure that allows the heparin to remain attached longer. In addition, catheter designs have been developed to optimize blood flow around the catheter.

The most common procedure used to reduce CVC-related thrombosis is the routine flushing of catheter ports with UFH or other substances. Flushing occurs routinely, from once weekly to thrice weekly. Studies have shown that a 50-U UFH flush is as effective as a 1000-U UFH flush [66]. Surprisingly, recent studies show that a simple saline flush is as effective as a 100-U UFH flush in this regard [77].

The main effort to reduce CVC-related thrombosis, however, has been the use of low-dose systemic prophylactic anticoagulation with warfarin or heparin (UFH or LMWH).

The use of low-dose warfarin to prevent central venous catheter–related deep venous thrombosis

Most early studies suggest that low-dose warfarin is effective in preventing CVC-related DVT. In a 1990 randomized open, prospective study of oncology patients who had Port-a-Cath catheters, Bern et al [40] compared the administration of warfarin (1 mg/d) with no warfarin for 90 days. All patients underwent a venogram at the time of thrombotic symptoms or at 90 days. The total DVT rate determined by venographic methods decreased from 37.5% (15/40) in patients without warfarin to 9.5% (4/42) in patients taking warfarin. The symptomatic thrombi rate decreased from 32.5% (13/40) in patients without warfarin to 9.5% (4/42) in patients taking warfarin ($P = 0.001$).

Boraks et al [26] obtained similar results in a nonrandomized study in which patients prospectively received warfarin (1 mg/d) and were assessed for clinically symptomatic (but venographically verified) thrombi. In those patients prospectively treated with warfarin (1 mg/d), symptomatic thrombi occurred in 5 of 108 (5%) compared with 15 of 115 (13%) patients in a historical control group that did not receive warfarin ($P = 0.03$). Furthermore, the time to thrombosis was a median of 72 days in those who received warfarin (1 mg/d) but was only 16 days in those who did not receive warfarin.

Subsequently, a number of other studies were performed to assess the utility of low-dose warfarin prophylaxis. Three studies have shown a probable benefit of low-dose warfarin, which was of borderline statistical significance, given the small number of patients studied. In a prospective nonrandomized study, 1 mg/d of warfarin resulted in 0 of 52 (0%) CVC clots versus 4 of 65 (6%) CVC clots in patients not receiving warfarin ($P = 0.06$) [27]. In a retrospective nonrandomized study, symptomatic CVC thrombi developed in 4 of 96 (4%) patients treated with 1 mg/d of warfarin but in 24 of 209 (11%) patients who received no warfarin ($P = 0.04$) [36]. Of 949 Quinton-type catheters that received 1 mg/d of warfarin per day, the clinical DVT rate was 5.1% and clinical complications were not apparent [64].

Two recent studies, however, showed no benefit of low-dose warfarin. In a nonrandomized study of 160 patients with melanoma or renal cell cancer being treated with interleukin-2, warfarin (1 mg/d) did not reduce the CVC-related DVT rate [31]. In a nonblinded study of patients with hematologic malignancies, Heaton et al [38] randomized 88 patients with a double-lumen subclavian Hickman CVC to warfarin (1 mg/d) or no therapy. After 90 days, there was no difference in the rate of clinically significant thrombi for those treated with warfarin; 8 of 45 (18%) of patients treated with warfarin versus 5 of 43 (12%) of patients not treated had clinically evident thrombi.

The use of heparin to prevent central venous catheter–related deep venous thrombosis

In a randomized open-label, prospective study by Monreal et al [45], oncology patients who had Port-a-Cath catheters received dalteparin (2500 U/d) or no therapy and underwent a venogram at the time of symptoms or at 90 days. Of the 16 patients who received dalteparin, only 1 developed a DVT, which was symptomatic. Of the 13 patients who received no treatment, 8 (62%) developed a DVT, seven of which were symptomatic. Because of the highly statistically significant difference in outcome ($P = 0.002$), this study was closed early to accrual.

Similar studies done with larger numbers of patients, however, failed to show any difference in CVC-related DVT rates. Pucheu et al [46] prospectively compared 2500 anti-Xa units of dalteparin SC daily with untreated historical controls using ultrasonography at 1, 3, and 12 months to screen for thrombosis. Documented thrombi occurred in only 3 of 46 (6.5%) patients who received dalteparin, and all were without symptoms. In the historical control group, 11 of 72 (15%) patients developed documented clots, which was not a statistically significant difference. In the largest randomized, blinded placebo-controlled study ever performed to evaluate CVC prophylaxis in cancer patients, 194 patients received placebo injections and 294 received dalteparin (5000 U SC daily) for 16 weeks [48]. Clinical DVT occurred in 5.3% of the placebo group and in 5.8% of the dalteparin-treated patients, which was not a statistically significant difference. The low rate of DVT in the placebo group was nearly the lowest seen in any CVC prophylaxis study (see Table 1) and may reflect changes in catheter design, local care, or patient selection. There was no difference in infection rate.

The only other relevant data on the use of heparin to prevent CVC-related DVT comes from a meta-analysis of 14 studies by Randolph et al [78]. Only 2 of these studies were with oncology patients and the remainder was with patients who had a wide range of catheters placed for varying indications and procedures. What is striking about this meta-analysis is that various prophylactic heparin regimens, ranging from UFH to LMWH, decreased the relative rate of DVT to 0.43, the relative rate of bacterial colonization to 0.18, and the relative rate of bacteremia to 0.26. The decrease in infectious complications again confirms the association of thrombosis with infection.

Use of anticoagulation of central venous catheters in clinical practice

Older guidelines

The guidelines from the Sixth American College of Chest Physicians (ACCP) Conference on Antithrombotic Therapy were prepared before the recent studies with warfarin [31,38] and dalteparin [46,48] failed to show any benefit. These earlier guidelines state that warfarin 1 mg/d or LMWH administered once a day are valid prophylactic options for CVC [79–81]. Despite these recommendations, less than 10% of patients with CVCs receive systemic prophylaxis [27]. There are multiple reasons for this.

The chief reason is the conflicting data from the studies mentioned above. The studies with low-dose warfarin simply do not provide a clear-cut answer. These studies suffer from the small number of patients studied, the high dropout rate, the failure to use venographic endpoints in most studies, and the fact that most were not placebo-controlled.

A second reason for the lack of routine systemic prophylaxis for CVCs is a genuine concern about the bleeding risk of systemic anticoagulation in potentially thrombocytopenic or anorectic chemotherapy patients. Ten percent of the patients in the study by Bern et al [40] developed a prothrombin time greater than 15 seconds and required holding of their warfarin; 5% of the patients in the study by Boraks et al [26] developed a PT greater than 20 seconds and required holding of the warfarin. Ten of 45 patients in the study by Heaton et al [38] had an INR >1.5 and required small doses of vitamin K; there was no related bleeding. These findings suggest that there may be a need for monitoring patients who are on low-dose warfarin.

Considerable recent data has questioned the safety of low-dose warfarin in those patients receiving 5-flurouracil–based chemotherapy. Magagnoli and colleagues [82,83] have demonstrated an increased likelihood of an elevated INR and possible bleeding when low-dose warfarin is used in patients with 5-flurouracil–based chemotherapy regimens. 5-Flurouracil seems to interfere with the synthesis of hepatic cytochrome P4502C9 [84], inhibit the metabolism of the more active Senantiomer of warfarin, decrease its clearance, and thereby enhance the hypoprothrombinemic effect of warfarin [85]. Indeed, in patients on full-dose warfarin who then receive 5-flurouracil, the average warfarin dose to maintain a therapeutic INR declines by nearly half and requires careful weekly monitoring [86]. Similar effects have been noted with capecitabine, the prodrug of 5-flurouracil [87,88]. Therefore, 5-flurouracil or capecitabine chemotherapy regimens join marginal nutrition and impaired hepatic function as major risk factors for bleeding with low-dose warfarin prophylaxis.

The heparins also have some disadvantages: there is the major inconvenience of daily SC injection of UFH or LMWH, as well as the cost of the latter. In addition, in the asthenic or elderly cancer patient with reduced glomerular filtration rate, even low prophylactic doses of LMWH may accumulate and cause bleeding. This adverse effect of LMWH is amplified in patients with reduced renal function due to disease or chemotherapy.

Newer guidelines

The guidelines from the Seventh ACCP Conference on Antithrombotic Therapy recently were published and found that the routine use of low-dose warfarin or LMWH to try to prevent thrombosis related to long-term indwelling CVCs in cancer patients is not warranted [89]. These guidelines are based on the latest prophylactic anti-coagulation studies, many of which failed to find a benefit with either LMWH or low-dose warfarin and even raised concerns regarding safety of the latter medication [82,83].

Summary

CVC-related DVT is a common clinical problem that may affect nearly half of all cancer patients with CVCs. Although the DVT rate is high, only one-third of the thrombosed CVCs become symptomatic. Nonetheless, CVC-related DVT can result in clinical symptoms, the loss of catheter function, increased rate of infection, postphlebitic syndrome of the upper extremity, PE, and increased costs.

CVC-related DVT can best be diagnosed with ultrasound that has high sensitivity and specificity in symptomatic patients. Although clots associated with catheter tips may be lysed with thrombolytic agents, there is no standard of care for larger CVC-related DVT. Most clots are treated acutely with UFH or LMWH and the catheter is removed if it is nonfunctional. Patients are subsequently treated for at least 3 months, preferably with daily injections of LMWH if malignancy is still present.

Prophylactic flushes with UFH or saline are the standard of care to maintain CVC patency but they are inadequate to prevent blood vessel thrombosis. The benefit of systemic prophylaxis with LMWH or warfarin has not been established. Despite considerable evidence of effect for CVCs in nononcology patients, the lack of benefit seen in a recent large study of LMWH does not support the prophylactic use of LMWH in cancer patients with CVCs. Although many older studies support the use of low-dose warfarin, most recent studies do not. Current data has even questioned the safety of unmonitored low-dose warfarin in cancer patients receiving 5-flurouracil–based chemotherapy. The routine use of warfarin, therefore, cannot be justified. This is further supported by the newest ACCP guidelines, which recommends against the use of fixed-dose warfarin as prophylaxis to try to prevent thrombosis related to long-term indwelling CVCs in cancer patients and suggests that clinicians not use LMWH [89].

Larger, placebo-controlled studies of low-dose warfarin prophylaxis in CVCs could be considered, using both venographic and clinical endpoints. However, it may be more fruitful to consider instead the use of newer factor Xa inhibitors such as the pentasaccharides fondaparinux and idraparinux [90–95] or direct thrombin inhibitors such as ximelegatran [92,96–99]. The pentasaccharides appear to provide more effective prophylaxis of venous thromboembolism [90,93,100] and have less bleeding than LMWH; one of them, idraparinux has a prolonged half-life making weekly dosing possible [95]. The oral direct thrombin inhibitors may allow more stable oral anticoagulant than warfarin in that they are not affected by diet, antibiotics, or inhibitors of the CYP450 system, such as 5-flurouracil and capecitabine.

Given its common occurrence, further efforts to understand and prevent CVC-related thrombosis are of importance. These efforts should include not only studies of anticoagulant efficacy but also studies to determine the risk factors for CVC-related thrombosis, the timing of the onset and duration of therapy, as well as the natural history of CVC-related DVT.

References

[1] McGee DC, Gould MK. Preventing complications of central venous catheterization. N Engl J Med 2003;348:1123–33.

[2] Cadman A, Lawrance JA, Fitzsimmons L, et al. To clot or not to clot? That is the question in central venous catheters. Clin Radiol 2004;59:349–55.
[3] Polderman KH, Girbes AR. Central venous catheter use. Part 2: infectious complications. Intensive Care Med 2002;28:18–28.
[4] Aubaniac R. The subclavian vein puncture—advantages and technique. 1952. Nutrition 1990; 6:139–40 [discussion: 41].
[5] Aubaniac R. [A new route for venous injection or puncture: the subclavicular route, subclavian vein, brachiocephalic trunk.] Sem Hop 1952;28:3445–7.
[6] Aubaniac R. [Subclavian intravenous injection: advantages and technique.] Presse Med 1952;60:1456.
[7] Aubaniac R. [Subclavian intravenous transfusion: advantages and technique]. Afr Francaise Chir 1952;8:131–5.
[8] Broviac JW, Cole JJ, Scribner BH. A silicone rubber atrial catheter for prolonged parenteral alimentation. Surg Gynecol Obstet 1973;136:602–6.
[9] Hickman RO, Buckner CD, Clift RA, et al. A modified right atrial catheter for access to the venous system in marrow transplant recipients. Surg Gynecol Obstet 1979;148:871–5.
[10] Niederhuber JE, Ensminger W, Gyves JW, et al. Totally implanted venous and arterial access system to replace external catheters in cancer treatment. Surgery 1982;92:706–12.
[11] Bregenzer T, Conen D, Sakmann P, et al. Is routine replacement of peripheral intravenous catheters necessary? Arch Intern Med 1998;158:151–6.
[12] Hoshal Jr VL, Ause RG, Hoskins PA. Fibrin sleeve formation on indwelling subclavian central venous catheters. Arch Surg 1971;102:253–8.
[13] Balestreri L, De Cicco M, Matovic M, et al. Central venous catheter-related thrombosis in clinically asymptomatic oncologic patients: a phlebographic study. Eur J Radiol 1995;20: 108–11.
[14] De Cicco M, Matovic M, Balestreri L, et al. Central venous thrombosis: an early and frequent complication in cancer patients bearing long-term Silastic catheter. A prospective study. Thromb Res 1997;86:101–13.
[15] Starkhammar H, Bengtsson M, Morales O. Fibrin sleeve formation after long term brachial catheterisation with an implantable port device. A prospective venographic study. Eur J Surg 1992;158:481–4.
[16] Raad II, Hohn DC, Gilbreath BJ, et al. Prevention of central venous catheter-related infections by using maximal sterile barrier precautions during insertion. Infect Control Hosp Epidemiol 1994;15:231–8.
[17] Raad I, Costerton W, Sabharwal U, et al. Ultrastructural analysis of indwelling vascular catheters: a quantitative relationship between luminal colonization and duration of placement. J Infect Dis 1993;168:400–7.
[18] Tenney JH, Moody MR, Newman KA, et al. Adherent microorganisms on luminal surfaces of long-term intravenous catheters. Importance of *Staphylococcus epidermidis* in patients with cancer. Arch Intern Med 1986;146:1949–54.
[19] Ray S, Stacey R, Imrie M, et al. A review of 560 Hickman catheter insertions. Anaesthesia 1996;51:981–5.
[20] Schwarz RE, Coit DG, Groeger JS. Transcutaneously tunneled central venous lines in cancer patients: an analysis of device-related morbidity factors based on prospective data collection. Ann Surg Oncol 2000;7:441–9.
[21] Anderson AJ, Krasnow SH, Boyer MW, et al. Thrombosis: the major Hickman catheter complication in patients with solid tumor. Chest 1989;95:71–5.
[22] Hurtibise MR, Bottino JC, Lawson M. Restoring patency of occluded central venous catheters. Arch Surg 1980;115:212–3.
[23] Lawson M, Bottino JC, Hurtibise MR. The use of urokinase to restore patency of occluded central venous catheters. Am J Intraven Ther Clin Nutr 1982;9:29–32.
[24] Gould JR, Carloss HW, Skinner WL. Groshong catheter-associated subclavian venous thrombosis. Am J Med 1993;95:419–23.

[25] Stephens LC, Haire WD, Kotulak GD. Are clinical signs accurate indicators of the cause of central venous catheter occlusion? JPEN J Parenter Enteral Nutr 1995;19:75–9.
[26] Boraks P, Seale J, Price J, et al. Prevention of central venous catheter associated thrombosis using minidose warfarin in patients with haematological malignancies. Br J Haematol 1998;101: 483–6.
[27] Carr KM, Rabinowitz I. Physician compliance with warfarin prophylaxis for central venous catheters in patients with solid tumors. J Clin Oncol 2000;18:3665–7.
[28] Conlan MG, Haire WD, Lieberman RP, et al. Catheter-related thrombosis in patients with refractory lymphoma undergoing autologous stem cell transplantation. Bone Marrow Transplant 1991;7:235–40.
[29] Craft PS, May J, Dorigo A, et al. Hickman catheters: left-sided insertion, male gender, and obesity are associated with an increased risk of complications. Aust N Z J Med 1996;26: 33–9.
[30] de Gregorio MA, Miguelena JM, Fernandez JA, et al. Subcutaneous ports in the radiology suite: an effective and safe procedure for care in cancer patients. Eur Radiol 1996;6:748–52.
[31] Eastman ME, Khorsand M, Maki DG, et al. Central venous device-related infection and thrombosis in patients treated with moderate dose continuous-infusion interleukin-2. Cancer 2001;91:806–14.
[32] Eastridge BJ, Lefor AT. Complications of indwelling venous access devices in cancer patients. J Clin Oncol 1995;13:233–8.
[33] Goey SH, Verweij J, Bolhuis RL, et al. Tunnelled central venous catheters yield a low incidence of septicaemia in interleukin-2-treated patients. Cancer Immunol Immunother 1997;44:301–4.
[34] Haire WD, Edney JA, Landmark JD, et al. Thrombotic complications of subclavian apheresis catheters in cancer patients: prevention with heparin infusion. J Clin Apheresis 1990;5:188–91.
[35] Knofler R, Siegert E, Lauterbach I, et al. Clinical importance of prothrombotic risk factors in pediatric patients with malignancy—impact of central venous lines. Eur J Pediatr 1999; 158(Suppl 3):S147–50.
[36] Minassian VA, Sood AK, Lowe P, et al. Longterm central venous access in gynecologic cancer patients. J Am Coll Surg 2000;191:403–9.
[37] Wermes C, von Depka Prondzinski M, Lichtinghagen R, et al. Clinical relevance of genetic risk factors for thrombosis in paediatric oncology patients with central venous catheters. Eur J Pediatr 1999;158(Suppl 3):S143–6.
[38] Heaton DC, Han DY, Inder A. Minidose (1 mg) warfarin as prophylaxis for central vein catheter thrombosis. Intern Med J 2002;32:84–8.
[39] Barzaghi A, Dell'Orto M, Rovelli A, et al. Central venous catheter clots: incidence, clinical significance and catheter care in patients with hematologic malignancies. Pediatr Hematol Oncol 1995;12:243–50.
[40] Bern MM, Lokich JJ, Wallach SR, et al. Very low doses of warfarin can prevent thrombosis in central venous catheters. A randomized prospective trial. Ann Intern Med 1990;112:423–8.
[41] De Cicco M, Matovic M, Balestreri L, et al. Antithrombin III deficiency as a risk factor for catheter-related central vein thrombosis in cancer patients. Thromb Res 1995;78:127–37.
[42] Glaser DW, Medeiros D, Rollins N, et al. Catheter-related thrombosis in children with cancer. J Pediatr 2001;138:255–9.
[43] Horne III MK, Merryman PK, Mayo DJ, et al. Reductions in tissue plasminogen activator and thrombomodulin in blood draining veins damaged by venous access devices. Thromb Res 1995;79:369–76.
[44] Horne III MK, Mayo DJ, Alexander HR, et al. Upper extremity impedance plethysmography in patients with venous access devices. Thromb Haemost 1994;72:540–2.
[45] Monreal M, Alastrue A, Rull M, et al. Upper extremity deep venous thrombosis in cancer patients with venous access devices—prophylaxis with a low molecular weight heparin (Fragmin). Thromb Haemost 1996;75:251–3.
[46] Pucheu A, Leduc B, Sillet-Bach I, et al. Experimental prevention of deep venous thrombosis with low-molecular-weight heparin using implantable infusion devices. Ann Cardiol Angeiol (Paris) 1996;45:59–63.

[47] Raad II, Luna M, Khalil SA, et al. The relationship between the thrombotic and infectious complications of central venous catheters. JAMA 1994;271:1014–6.
[48] Reichardt P, Kretzschmar A, Biakhov M, et al. A phase III randomized, double-blind, placebo-controlled study evaluating the efficacy and safety of daily low-molecular-weight heparin (dalteparin sodium, Fragmin) in preventing catheter-related complications (CRCs) in cancer patients with central venous catheter (CVCs). Proc Am Soc Clin Oncol 2002;21:369a.
[49] Horne III MK, May DJ, Alexander HR, et al. Venographic surveillance of tunneled venous access devices in adult oncology patients. Ann Surg Oncol 1995;2:174–8.
[50] Curelaru I, Bylock A, Gustavsson B, et al. Dynamics of thrombophlebitis in central venous catheterization via basilic and cephalic veins. Acta Chir Scand 1984;150:285–93.
[51] Lokich JJ, Becker B. Subclavian vein thrombosis in patients treated with infusion chemotherapy for advanced malignancy. Cancer 1983;52:1586–9.
[52] Press OW, Ramsey PG, Larson EB, et al. Hickman catheter infections in patients with malignancies. Medicine (Baltimore) 1984;63:189–200.
[53] Henrickson KJ, Axtell RA, Hoover SM, et al. Prevention of central venous catheter-related infections and thrombotic events in immunocompromised children by the use of vancomycin/ciprofloxacin/heparin flush solution: a randomized, multicenter, double-blind trial. J Clin Oncol 2000;18:1269–78.
[54] Massoure PL, Constans J, Caudry M, et al. Upper extremity deep venous thrombosis: 40 hospitalized patients. J Mal Vasc 2000;25:250–5.
[55] Prandoni P, Polistena P, Bernardi E, et al. Upper-extremity deep vein thrombosis. Risk factors, diagnosis, and complications. Arch Intern Med 1997;157:57–62.
[56] Monreal M, Lafoz E, Ruiz J, et al. Upper-extremity deep venous thrombosis and pulmonary embolism. A prospective study. Chest 1991;99:280–3.
[57] Monreal M, Davant E. Thrombotic complications of central venous catheters in cancer patients. Acta Haematol 2001;106:69–72.
[58] Durica SS. Venous thromboembolism in the cancer patient. Curr Opin Hematol 1997;4:306–11.
[59] Letai A, Kuter DJ. Cancer, coagulation, and anticoagulation. Oncologist 1999;4:443–9.
[60] Prandoni P, Piccioli A, Girolami A. Cancer and venous thromboembolism: an overview. Haematologica 1999;84:437–45.
[61] Valente M, Ponte E. Thrombosis and cancer. Minerva Cardioangiol 2000;48:117–27.
[62] Leebeek FW, Stadhouders NA, van Stein D, et al. Hypercoagulability states in upper-extremity deep venous thrombosis. Am J Hematol 2001;67:15–9.
[63] Haire WD, Lieberman RP, Edney J, et al. Hickman catheter-induced thoracic vein thrombosis. Frequency and long-term sequelae in patients receiving high-dose chemotherapy and marrow transplantation. Cancer 1990;66:900–8.
[64] Nightingale CE, Norman A, Cunningham D, et al. A prospective analysis of 949 long-term central venous access catheters for ambulatory chemotherapy in patients with gastrointestinal malignancy. Eur J Cancer 1997;33:398–403.
[65] Stanislav GV, Fitzgibbons Jr RJ, Bailey Jr RT, et al. Reliability of implantable central venous access devices in patients with cancer. Arch Surg 1987;122:1280–3.
[66] Brown-Smith JK, Stoner MH, Barley ZA. Tunneled catheter thrombosis: factors related to incidence. Oncol Nurs Forum 1990;17:543–9.
[67] Mustafa BO, Rathbun SW, Whitsett TL, et al. Sensitivity and specificity of ultrasonography in the diagnosis of upper extremity deep vein thrombosis: a systematic review. Arch Intern Med 2002;162:401–4.
[68] Koksoy C, Kuzu A, Kutlay J, et al. The diagnostic value of colour Doppler ultrasound in central venous catheter related thrombosis. Clin Radiol 1995;50:687–9.
[69] Chait P, Dinyari M, Massicote P. The sensitivity and specificity of linegrams and ultrasound compared with venography for the diagnosis of central venous line related thrombosis in symptomatic children: The LUV Study. Thromb Haemost 2001;P697.
[70] Haire WD, Lynch TG, Lund GB, et al. Limitations of magnetic resonance imaging and ultrasound-directed (duplex) scanning in the diagnosis of subclavian vein thrombosis. J Vasc Surg 1991;13:391–7.

[71] Forneris G, Quarello F, Pozzato M, et al. [Spiral x-ray computed tomography in the diagnosis of central venous catheterization complications.] Nephrologie 2001;22:495–9.
[72] Savage KJ, Wells PS, Schulz V, et al. Outpatient use of low molecular weight heparin (dalteparin) for the treatment of deep vein thrombosis of the upper extremity. Thromb Haemost 1999;82:1008–10.
[73] Lee AY, Levine MN, Baker RI, et al. Low-molecular-weight heparin versus a coumarin for the prevention of recurrent venous thromboembolism in patients with cancer. N Engl J Med 2003;349:146–53.
[74] Spence LD, Gironta MG, Malde HM, et al. Acute upper extremity deep venous thrombosis: safety and effectiveness of superior vena caval filters. Radiology 1999;210:53–8.
[75] Ponec D, Irwin D, Haire WD, et al. Recombinant tissue plasminogen activator (alteplase) for restoration of flow in occluded central venous access devices: a double-blind placebo-controlled trial—the Cardiovascular Thrombolytic to Open Occluded Lines (COOL) efficacy trial. J Vasc Interv Radiol 2001;12:951–5.
[76] Chan AKC, Du YJ, Berry LR, et al. Covalent antithrombin-heparin complex coated catheter prevents thrombosis in a rabbit central venous catheter model. Thromb Haemost 2001; 86(Suppl 1):310S.
[77] Stephens LC, Haire WD, Tarantolo S, et al. Normal saline versus heparin flush for maintaining central venous catheter patency during apheresis collection of peripheral blood stem cells (PBSC). Transfus Sci 1997;18:187–93.
[78] Randolph AG, Cook DJ, Gonzales CA, et al. Benefit of heparin in central venous and pulmonary artery catheters: a meta-analysis of randomized controlled trials. Chest 1998;113:165–71.
[79] Geerts WH, Heit JA, Clagett GP, et al. Prevention of venous thromboembolism. Chest 2001; 119:132S–75S.
[80] Guyatt G, Schunemann H, Cook D, et al. Grades of recommendation for antithrombotic agents. Chest 2001;119:3S–7S.
[81] Hirsh J, Dalen J, Guyatt G. The sixth (2000) ACCP guidelines for antithrombotic therapy for prevention and treatment of thrombosis. American College of Chest Physicians. Chest 2001;119:1S–2S.
[82] Magagnoli M, Masci G, Carnaghi C, et al. Minidose warfarin is associated with a high incidence of international normalized ratio elevation during chemotherapy with FOLFOX regimen. Ann Oncol 2003;14:959–60.
[83] Masci G, Magagnoli M, Zucali PA, et al. Minidose warfarin prophylaxis for catheter-associated thrombosis in cancer patients: can it be safely associated with fluorouracil-based chemotherapy? J Clin Oncol 2003;21:736–9.
[84] Brown MC. An adverse interaction between warfarin and 5-fluorouracil: a case report and review of the literature. Chemotherapy 1999;45:392–5.
[85] Zhou Q, Chan E. Effect of 5-fluorouracil on the anticoagulant activity and the pharmacokinetics of warfarin enantiomers in rats. Eur J Pharm Sci 2002;17:73–80.
[86] Kolesar JM, Johnson CL, Freeberg BL, et al. Warfarin-5-FU interaction—a consecutive case series. Pharmacotherapy 1999;19:1445–9.
[87] Copur MS, Ledakis P, Bolton M, et al. An adverse interaction between warfarin and capecitabine: a case report and review of the literature. Clin Colorectal Cancer 2001;1:182–4.
[88] Reigner B, Blesch K, Weidekamm E. Clinical pharmacokinetics of capecitabine. Clin Pharmacokinet 2001;40:85–104.
[89] Geerts WH, Pineo GF, Heit JA, et al. Prevention of venous thromboembolism. Chest 2004;126: 338S–400S.
[90] Turpie AG, Bauer KA, Eriksson BI, et al. Fondaparinux vs enoxaparin for the prevention of venous thromboembolism in major orthopedic surgery: a meta-analysis of 4 randomized double-blind studies. Arch Intern Med 2002;162:1833–40.
[91] Eriksson BI, Bauer KA, Lassen MR, et al. Fondaparinux compared with enoxaparin for the prevention of venous thromboembolism after hip-fracture surgery. N Engl J Med 2001; 345:1298–304.

[92] Eriksson H, Wahlander K, Gustafsson D, et al. A randomized, controlled, dose-guiding study of the oral direct thrombin inhibitor ximelagatran compared with standard therapy for the treatment of acute deep vein thrombosis. THRIVE I. J Thromb Haemost 2003;1:41–7.

[93] Bauer KA, Eriksson BI, Lassen MR, et al. Fondaparinux compared with enoxaparin for the prevention of venous thromboembolism after elective major knee surgery. N Engl J Med 2001;345:1305–10.

[94] Bauer KA. Fondaparinux sodium: a selective inhibitor of factor Xa. Am J Health Syst Pharm 2001;58(Suppl 2):S14–7.

[95] Idraparinux Sodium. SANORG 34006, SR 34006. Drugs R D 2004;5:164–5.

[96] Colwell CW, Berkowitz SD, Davidson BL, et al. Comparison of ximelagatran, an oral direct thrombin inhibitor, with enoxaparin for the prevention of venous thromboembolism following total hip replacement. A randomized, double-blind study. J Thromb Haemost 2003;1:2119–30.

[97] Gustafsson D. Oral direct thrombin inhibitors in clinical development. J Intern Med 2003; 254:322–34.

[98] Halperin JL. Ximelagatran compared with warfarin for prevention of thromboembolism in patients with nonvalvular atrial fibrillation: rationale, objectives, and design of a pair of clinical studies and baseline patient characteristics (SPORTIF III and V). Am Heart J 2003; 146:431–8.

[99] de Moerloose P, Boehlen F. Two new antithrombotic agents (fondaparinux and ximelagatran) and their implications in anesthesia. Can J Anaesth 2002;49:S5–10.

[100] Eriksson BI, Lassen MR. Duration of prophylaxis against venous thromboembolism with fondaparinux after hip fracture surgery: a multicenter, randomized, placebo-controlled, double-blind study. Arch Intern Med 2003;163:1337–42.

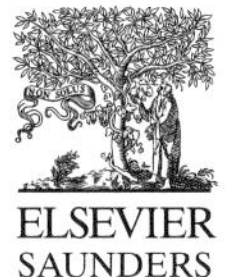

ELSEVIER
SAUNDERS

Hematol Oncol Clin N Am
19 (2005) 203–208

HEMATOLOGY/
ONCOLOGY
CLINICS OF
NORTH AMERICA

Index

Note: Page numbers of article titles are in **boldface** type.

doi:10.1016/S0889-8588(04)00167-4

B

C

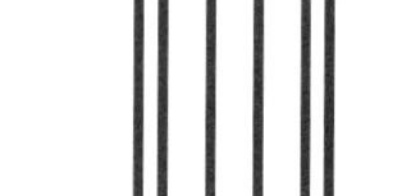

BUSINESS REPLY MAIL

FIRST-CLASS MAIL   PERMIT NO 7135   ORLANDO FL

POSTAGE WILL BE PAID BY ADDRESSEE

PERIODICALS ORDER FULFILLMENT DEPT
ELSEVIER
6277 SEA HARBOR DR
ORLANDO FL 32821-9816